FIRST AID FOR THE®

USMLE STEP 3

Second Edition

TAO LE, MD, MHS
Assistant Clinical Professor
Chief, Section of Allergy and Clinical Immunology
Department of Medicine
University of Louisville

VIKAS BHUSHAN, MD
Diagnostic Radiologist

ROBERT W. GROW, MD, MS
Resident Physician
Department of Emergency Medicine
Mayo Clinic

VÉRONIQUE TACHÉ, MD
Fellow, Maternal-Fetal Medicine
Department of Reproductive Medicine
University of California, San Diego

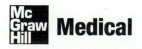

Medical

New York / Chicago / San Francisco / Lisbon / London / Madrid / Mexico City
Milan / New Delhi / San Juan / Seoul / Singapore / Sydney / Toronto

First Aid for the® USMLE Step 3, Second Edition

1 2 3 4 5 6 7 8 9 0   QPD/QPD   0 9 8 7

ISBN 978-0-07-148796-2
MHID 0-07-148796-4
ISSN 1554-1363

NOTICE

Medicine is an ever-changing science. As new research and clinical experience broaden our knowledge, changes in treatment and drug therapy are required. The authors and the publisher of this work have checked with sources believed to be reliable in their efforts to provide information that is complete and generally in accord with the standards accepted at the time of publication. However, in view of the possibility of human error or changes in medical sciences, neither the authors nor the publisher nor any other party who has been involved in the preparation or publication of this work warrants that the information contained herein is in every respect accurate or complete, and they disclaim all responsibility for any errors or omissions or for the results obtained from use of the information contained in this work. Readers are encouraged to confirm the information contained herein with other sources. For example and in particular, readers are advised to check the product information sheet included in the package of each drug they plan to administer to be certain that the information contained in this work is accurate and that changes have not been made in the recommended dose or in the contraindications for administration. This recommendation is of particular importance in connection with new or infrequently used drugs.

This book was set in Electra LH by Rainbow Graphics.
The editors were Catherine A. Johnson and Penny Linskey.
The production supervisors were Phil Galea and Tom Kowalczyk.
Project management was provided by Rainbow Graphics.
Quebecor World Dubuque was printer and binder.

This book is printed on acid-free paper.

To the contributors to this and future editions, who took time to share their experience, advice, and humor for the benefit of students.

and

To our families, friends, and loved ones, who endured and assisted in the task of assembling this guide.

CONTENTS

AUTHORS

Aditya Bardia, MBBS, MPH

Resident Physician
Department of Internal Medicine
Mayo Clinic

Jonas Green, MD, MPH

Resident Physician
Department of General Internal Medicine
University of California, Los Angeles

Aline Hansen-Guzmán, MD

Resident Physician
Department of Family and Community Medicine and
Department of Obstetrics and Gynecology
University of California Davis Health System

Martha Karakelides, MD

Resident Physician
Department of Internal Medicine
Mayo Clinic

Esther H. Krych, MD

Resident Physician
Department of Pediatric and Adolescent Medicine
Mayo Clinic

Gautam Kumar MBBS, MRCP(UK)

Fellow
Division of Cardiovascular Diseases
Department of Medicine
Mayo Clinic

Christopher Moreland, MD

Resident Physician
Department of Internal Medicine
University of California, Davis Medical Center

Jason H. Szostek, MD

Resident Physician
Department of Internal Medicine
Mayo Clinic

Julie Suzumi Young, MD, MS

Resident, Psychiatry
Department of Psychiatry and Behavioral Health
University of California, Davis

Amy Mikail Wolf, MD, MPH

Resident Physician
Department of Internal Medicine
University of California, Davis

FACULTY REVIEWERS

Jeremy Cooke, MD

Assistant Professor
Department of Emergency Medicine
The University of California, Davis Medical Center

Stephen Crane Hauser, MD

Assistant Professor of Medicine
Consultant, Division of Gastroenterology and Hepatology
Mayo Clinic

Helen Karakelides

Senior Associate Consultant
Division of Endocrinology, Diabetes, Metabolism and Nutrition
Mayo Clinic

Kyle W. Klarich, MD

Consultant
Cardiovascular Diseases
Mayo Clinic

Robert M. McCarron, DO

Program Director
Internal Medicine / Psychiatry Residency
Department of Psychiatry and Behavioral Sciences
Department of Internal Medicine
University of California, Davis

Lauren McGovern, MD

Professor
Department of Pediatric and Adolescent Medicine
Mayo Clinic

Jason Napolitano, MD

Clinical Instructor
Department of General Internal Medicine
University of California, Los Angeles

Ravi D. Rao, MBBS

Assistant Professor
Department of Oncology
Mayo Clinic

Nicholas Stollenwerk, MD

Clinical Fellow
Division of Pulmonary and Critical Care
University of California, Davis Medical Center

David Taylor, MD

Associate Physician Diplomate
Division of Nephrology
Department of General Internal Medicine
University of California, Los Angeles

Pritish K. Tosh, MD

Fellow
Division of Infection Diseases
Mayo Clinic

Shaji K. Kumar, MD

Associate Professor of Medicine
Division of Hematology
Mayo Clinic

Liza H. Kunz, MD

Division of Maternal Fetal Medicine
Santa Clara Valley Medical Center
San Jose, California

L. Elaine Waetjen, MD

Associate Professor
Department of Obstetrics and Gynecology
UC Davis Medical Center

Christopher M. Wittich, PharmD, MD

Chief Resident
Department of Medicine
Mayo Clinic

PREFACE

With *First Aid for the USMLE Step 3*, we continue our commitment to providing residents and international medical graduates with the most useful and up-to-date preparation guides for the USMLE exams. This second edition represents a thorough review in many ways and includes the following:

- An exam preparation guide for the computerized USMLE Step 3 with test-taking strategies for the FRED format.
- A high-yield guide to the CCS that includes invaluable tips and shortcuts.
- A review of hundreds of high-yield Step 3 topics with an emphasis on management.
- One hundred minicases with presentations and management similar to CCS cases.

We invite you to share your thoughts and ideas to help us improve *First Aid for the USMLE Step 3*. See How to Contribute, p. xv.

Louisville	Tao Le
Los Angeles	Vikas Bhushan
Rochester	Robert W. Grow
Sacramento	Véronique Taché

ACKNOWLEDGMENTS

This has been a collaborative project from the start. We gratefully acknowledge the thoughtful comments, corrections, and advice of the residents, international medical graduates, and faculty who have supported the authors in the development of *First Aid for the USMLE Step 3*.

Thanks to William Shakespeare; Matthew Thompson; Ravi Gada; Linda Dao; Jeremy Cooke, MD and Mark Mansour, MD for their support to the authors during the manuscript preparation process.

For support and encouragement throughout the process, we are grateful to Thao Pham, Selina Bush, and Louise Petersen.

Thanks to our publisher, McGraw-Hill, for the valuable assistance of their staff. For enthusiasm, support, and commitment to this challenging project, thanks to our editor, Catherine Johnson. For outstanding editorial work, we thank Andrea Fellows. A special thanks to David Hommel (Rainbow Graphics) for remarkable production work.

Louisville	Tao Le
Los Angeles	Vikas Bhushan
Rochester	Robert W. Grow
Sacramento	Véronique Taché

HOW TO CONTRIBUTE

To continue to produce a high-yield review source for the USMLE Step 3 exam, you are invited to submit any suggestions or corrections. We also offer **paid internships** in medical education and publishing ranging from three months to one year (see next page for details).

Please send us your suggestions for

- Study and test-taking strategies for the computerized USMLE Step 3.
- New facts, mnemonics, diagrams, and illustrations.
- CCS-style cases.
- Low-yield topics to remove.

For each entry incorporated into the next edition, you will receive a $10 gift certificate, as well as personal acknowledgment in the next edition. Diagrams, tables, partial entries, updates, corrections, and study hints are also appreciated, and significant contributions will be compensated at the discretion of the authors. Also let us know about material in this edition that you feel is low yield and should be deleted.

The preferred way to submit entries, suggestions, or corrections is via the First Aid Team's blog at **www.firstaidteam.com**. Please include name, address, school affiliation, phone number, and e-mail address (if different from the address of origin).

NOTE TO CONTRIBUTORS

All entries become property of the authors and are subject to editing and reviewing. Please verify all data and spellings carefully. In the event that similar or duplicate entries are received, only the first entry received will be used. Include a reference to a standard textbook to facilitate verification of the fact. Please follow the style, punctuation, and format of this edition if possible.

INTERNSHIP OPPORTUNITIES

The author team is pleased to offer part-time and full-time paid internships in medical education and publishing to motivated physicians. Internships may range from three months (e.g., a summer) up to a full year. Participants will have an opportunity to author, edit, and earn academic credit on a wide variety of projects, including the popular First Aid series. Writing/editing experience, familiarity with Microsoft Word, and Internet access are desired. For more information, e-mail a résumé or a short description of your experience along with a cover letter to the authors at **www.firstaidteam.com**.

Guide to the USMLE Step 3

▶ Introduction

▶ USMLE Step 3—
Computer-Based
Testing Basics

▶ USMLE/NBME
Resources

▶ Testing Agencies

For house officers, the USMLE Step 3 constitutes the last step one must take toward becoming a licensed physician. For international medical graduates (IMGs) applying for residency training in the United States, it represents an opportunity to strengthen the residency application and to obtain an H1B visa. Regardless of who you are, however, do **not** make the mistake of assuming that the Step 3 exam is just like Step 2. Whereas Step 2 focuses on clinical diagnosis, disease pathogenesis, and basic management, Step 3 emphasizes initial and **long-term** management of **common** clinical problems in **outpatient** settings. Indeed, part of the exam includes **computerized patient simulations** in addition to the traditional multiple-choice questions.

In this section, we will provide an overview of the Step 3 exam and will offer you proven approaches toward conquering the exam. For a high-yield guide to the Computer-Based Clinical Simulations (CCS), go to **Section I Supplement: Guide to the CCS.** For a detailed description of Step 3, visit **www.usmle.org** or refer to the *USMLE Step 3 Content Description and Sample Test Materials* booklet that you will receive upon registering for the exam.

Step 3 is not a retread of Step 2.

How Is Step 3 Structured?

The Step 3 exam is a two-day computer-based test (CBT) administered by Prometric, Inc. The USMLE is now using new testing software called **FRED.** FRED allows you to **highlight** and **strike out** test choices as well as make **brief notes** to yourself.

Day 1 of Step 3 consists of seven 60-minute blocks of 48 multiple-choice questions for a total of 336 questions over seven hours. You get a minimum of 45 minutes of break time and 15 minutes for an optional tutorial. During the time allotted for each block, you can answer test questions in any order as well as review responses and change answers. Examinees cannot, however, go back and change answers from previous blocks. Once an examinee finishes a block, he or she must click on a screen icon to continue to the next block. Time not used during a testing block will be added to your overall break time, but it cannot be used to complete other testing blocks. Expect to spend up to nine hours at the test center.

Day 2 consists of four 45-minute blocks of 36 multiple-choice questions for a total of 144 questions over three hours. This is followed by **nine interactive case simulations** over four hours using the Primum CCS format. There is a 15-minute CCS tutorial as well as 45 minutes of allotted break time.

What Is Step 3 Like?

Even if you're familiar with the CBT and the Prometric test centers, FRED is a relatively new testing format that you should access from the USMLE CD-ROM or Web site and try out prior to the exam. In addition, the CCS format definitely requires practice.

If you familiarize yourself with the FRED testing interface ahead of time, you can skip the 15-minute tutorial offered on exam day and add those minutes to your allotted break time of 45 minutes.

For security reasons, examinees are not allowed to bring personal electronic equipment into the testing area, including digital watches, watches with computer communication and/or memory capability, cellular telephones, and electronic paging devices. Food and beverages are also prohibited in the testing area. For note-taking purposes, examinees are given laminated writing surfaces that must be returned after the examination. The testing centers are monitored by audio and video surveillance equipment.

You should become familiar with a typical question screen (see Figure 1). A window to the left displays all the questions in the block and shows you the incomplete questions (marked with an "*i*"). Some questions will contain figures or color illustrations adjacent to the question. Although the contrast and brightness of the screen can be adjusted, there are no other ways to manipulate the picture (e.g., zooming or panning). Larger images are accessed with an "**exhibit**" button. You can also call up a window displaying normal **lab** values. You may mark questions to review at a later time by clicking the check mark at the top of the screen. The **annotation** feature functions like the provided erasable dryboards and allows you to jot down notes during the exam. Play with the **highlighting/strike-through** and annotation features with the vignettes and multiple choices.

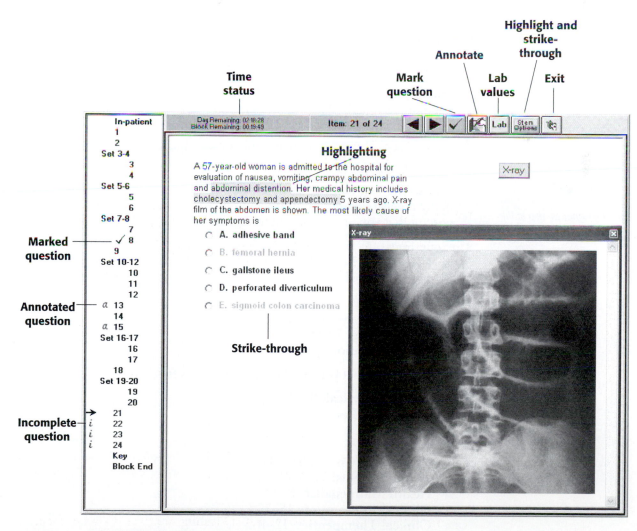

FIGURE 1. Typical FRED question screen.

Keyboard shortcuts:

A–E–Letter choices.

Enter or Spacebar–Move to the next question.

Esc–Exit pop-up Lab and Exhibit windows.

Alt-T–Countdown and time-elapsed clocks for current session and overall test.

If you find that you are not using the marking, annotation, or highlighting tools, the available keyboard shortcuts can save you time over using the mouse.

The Primum CCS software is a patient simulation in which you are **completely** in charge of the patient's management regardless of the setting. You obtain a selected history and physical, develop a short differential, order diagnostics, and implement treatment and monitoring. CSS features simulated time (the case can play out over hours, days, or months), **different locations** from outpatient to ER to ICU settings, free-text entry of orders (no multiple choice here!), and patient response to your actions over simulated time (patients can get well, worsen, or even die depending on your actions or inaction). Please see **Section I Supplement: Guide to the CCS** for a practical guide to acing the CCS.

The USMLE also offers an opportunity to take a simulated test, or "Practice Session," at a Prometric center in the United States or Canada for about $50. You may register for a practice session online at the USMLE Web site.

What Types of Questions Are Asked?

Virtually all questions on Step 3 are vignette based. A substantial amount of extraneous information may be given, or a clinical scenario may be followed by a question that could be answered without actually necessitating that you read the case. It is your job to determine which information is superfluous and which is pertinent to the case at hand. There are three question formats:

Single items. This is the **most frequent** question type. It consists of the traditional single-best-answer question with four to five choices.

For long vignettes, skip to the question stem first, and then read the case.

Multiple-item sets. This consists of a clinical vignette followed by two to three questions regarding that case. These questions can be answered **independently** of each other. Again, there is only one best answer.

Cases. This is a clinical vignette followed by two to five questions. You actually receive additional information as you answer questions, so it is important that you answer questions sequentially without skipping.

The questions are organized by clinical **settings,** including an outpatient clinic, an inpatient hospital, and an emergency department. According to the USMLE, the clinical care **situations** you will encounter in these settings include the following:

- **Initial Workup:** 20–30%.
- **Continued Care:** 50–60%.
- **Urgent Intervention:** 15–25%.

The clinical tasks that you will be tested on are as follows:

- **History and Physical:** 8–12%.
- **Diagnostic Studies:** 8–12%.
- **Diagnosis:** 8–12%.
- **Prognosis:** 8–12%.
- **Applying Basic Concepts:** 8–12%.
- **Managing Patients:** 39–55%.
  - **Health Maintenance:** 5–9%.
  - **Clinical Intervention:** 18–22%.
  - **Clinical Therapeutics:** 12–16%.
  - **Legal and Ethical Issues:** 4–8%.

When approaching the vignette questions, you should keep a few things in mind:

- Note the age and race of the patient in each clinical scenario. When ethnicity is given, it is often relevant. Know these associations well (see high-yield facts), especially for more common diagnoses.
- Be able to recognize key facts that distinguish major diagnoses.
- Questions often describe clinical findings rather than naming eponyms (e.g., they cite "audible hip click" instead of "positive Ortolani's sign").

Remember that Step 3 tends to focus on outpatient continuing management scenarios.

How Are the Scores Reported?

Like the Step 1 and 2 score reports, your Step 3 report includes your pass/fail status, two numeric scores, and a performance profile organized by discipline and disease process. The first score is a three-digit scaled score based on a predefined proficiency standard. A three-digit score of **184** is required for passing. The second score scale, the two-digit score, defines 75 as the minimum passing score (equivalent to a score of 184 on the first scale). This score is not a percentile. A score of 82 is equivalent to a score of 200 on the first scale. Approximately **95%** of graduates from U.S. and Canadian medical schools pass Step 3 on their first try (see Table 1). Approximately **two-thirds of IMGs** pass on their first attempt.

Check the USMLE Web site for the latest passing requirements.

TABLE 1. Recent Step 2 Examination Results

	2004		2005[a]	
	# TESTED	**% PASSING**	**# TESTED**	**% PASSING**
Examinees from U.S./Canadian schools				
MD degree	17,600	94	16,934	94
First-time takers	16,446	96	15,868	96
Repeaters	1,154	69	1,066	69
DO degree	85	93	58	95
First-time takers	81	93	54	94
Repeaters	4	Not reported	4	Not reported
Total U.S./Canadian	17,685	94	16,992	94
Examinees from non-U.S./Canadian schools				
First-time takers	7,668	74	8,307	75
Repeaters	4,791	57	3,712	52
Total non-U.S./Canadian	12,459	68	12,019	68

[a] Source: www.usmle.org/scores/2005perf.htm.

How Do I Register to Take the Exam?

To register for the Step 3 exam in the United States and Canada, apply online at the Federation of State Medical Boards (FSMB) Web site (**www.fsmb.org**). A printable version of the application is also available on this site. Note that some states require you to apply for licensure when you register for Step 3. A list of those states can be found on the FSMB Web site. The registration fee varies and was $655 in 2007.

In a recent change, the USMLE is no longer mailing a hard copy of your scheduling permit. Instead, the scheduling permit is sent via e-mail to the e-mail address provided on the application materials. Once you have received your scheduling permit, it is your responsibility to print it and decide when and where you would like to take the exam. For a list of Prometric locations nearest you, visit **www.prometric.com.** Call Prometric's toll-free number or visit www.prometric.com to arrange a time to take the exam.

Your electronic scheduling permit will contain the following important information:

- Your USMLE identification number.
- The eligibility period in which you may take the exam.
- Your "scheduling number," which you will need to make your exam appointment with Prometric.
- Your "Candidate Identification Number," or CIN, which you must enter at your Prometric workstation in order to access the exam.

Prometric has no access to these codes or your scheduling permit and will not be able to supply these for you. You will not be allowed to take Step 3 unless you present your permit, printed by you ahead of time, along with an unexpired, government-issued photo identification that contains your signature (e.g., driver's license or passport). Make sure the name on your photo ID exactly matches the name that appears on your scheduling permit.

Because the exam is scheduled on a "first-come, first-served" basis, you should contact Prometric as soon as you receive your scheduling permit!

What If I Need to Reschedule the Exam?

You can change your date and/or center within your three-month period without charge by contacting Prometric. If space is available, you may reschedule up to five days before your test date. If you reschedule within five days of your test date, Prometric will charge a rescheduling fee. If you need to reschedule outside your initial three-month period, you can apply for a single three-month extension (e.g., April/May/June can be extended through July/August/September) after your eligibility period has begun (go to **www.nbme.org** for more information). For other rescheduling needs, you must submit a new application along with another application fee.

Never, ever leave a question blank! You can always mark it and come back later.

What About Time?

Time is of special interest on the CBT exam. The computer will keep track of how much time has elapsed. However, the computer will show you only how much time you have remaining in a given block (unless you look at the full clock with **Alt-T**). Therefore, it is up to you to determine if you are pacing yourself properly. Note that on both day 1 and day 2 of testing, you have approximately **75 seconds** per multiple-choice question. If you recognize that a question is not solvable in a reasonable period of time, move on after making an educated guess; there are **no penalties** for wrong answers.

It should be noted that 45 minutes is allowed for break time. However, you can elect not to use all of your break time, or you can gain extra break time either by skipping the tutorial or by finishing a block ahead of the allotted time. The computer **will not warn you** if you are spending more than your allotted break time.

If I Leave During the Exam, What Happens to My Score?

You are considered to have started the exam once you have entered your CIN onto the computer screen. In order to receive an official score, however, you must finish the entire exam. This means that you must start and either finish or run out of time for each block of the exam. If you do **not** complete all the blocks, your exam will be documented on your USMLE score transcript as an incomplete attempt, but no actual score will be reported.

The exam ends when all blocks have been completed or time has expired. As you leave the testing center, you will receive a written test-completion notice to document your completion of the exam.

How Long Will I Have to Wait Before I Get My Scores?

The USMLE typically reports scores three to four weeks after the examinee's test date. During peak periods, however, it may take **up to six weeks** for scores to be made available. Official information concerning the time required for score reporting is posted on the USMLE Web site.

Use USMLE practice tests to identify concepts and areas of weakness, not just facts that you missed.

USMLE/NBME RESOURCES

We strongly encourage you to use the free materials provided by the testing agencies and to study the following NBME publications:

- **USMLE Bulletin of Information.** This publication provides you with nuts-and-bolts details about the exam (included on the USMLE Web site; free to all examinees).
- **USMLE Step 3 Content Description and Sample Test Materials.** This is a hard copy of test questions and test content also found on the CD-ROM.
- **NBME Test Delivery Software (FRED) and Tutorial.** This includes 168 valuable practice questions. The questions are available on the USMLE CD-ROM and Web site. Make sure you are using the new FRED version and not the older Prometric version.
- **USMLE Web site (www.usmle.org).** In addition to allowing you to become familiar with the CBT format, the sample items on the USMLE Web site provide the only questions that are available directly from the test makers. Student feedback varies as to the similarity of these questions to those on the actual exam, but they are nonetheless worthwhile to know.

National Board of Medical Examiners (NBME)
Department of Licensing Examination Services
3750 Market Street
Philadelphia, PA 19104-3102
215-590-9500
www.nbme.org

Educational Commission for Foreign Medical Graduates (ECFMG)
3624 Market Street, Fourth Floor
Philadelphia, PA 19104-2685
215-386-5900
Fax: 215-386-9196
www.ecfmg.org

Federation of State Medical Boards (FSMB)
P.O. Box 619850
Dallas, TX 75261-9850
817-868-4000
Fax: 817-868-4099
www.fsmb.org

USMLE Secretariat
3750 Market Street
Philadelphia, PA 19104-3190
215-590-9700
www.usmle.org

Guide to the CCS

The focus is management, management, management. You will see few diagnostic zebras in the CCS.

Do all the sample CCS cases prior to the actual exam.

The orders require free-text entry. There is no multiple choice here!

INTRODUCTION

The Primum CCS is a computerized patient simulation that is administered on the second day of Step 3. You will be given nine cases over four hours and will have up to 25 minutes per case. Like the rest of the Step 3 exam, the CCS is meant to test your ability to properly diagnose and manage common conditions in various patient-care settings. Many of the conditions are obvious or easily diagnosed. Clinical problems range from acute to chronic and from mundane to life-threatening. A case may last from a few minutes to a few months in terms of **simulated time,** even though you have only 25 minutes of real time per case. Cases can, and frequently do, end in less than 25 minutes. Regardless of where the patient is during the case (i.e., office, ER, or ICU), you are the patient's **primary** physician and have **complete** responsibility for care.

WHAT IS THE CCS LIKE?

For the CCS, there is **no substitute** for trying out the cases on the USMLE CD-ROM or downloading the software from the USMLE Web site. If you spend at least a few hours doing the sample cases and familiarizing yourself with the interface, you **will do better** on the actual exam, regardless of your prior computer experience.

For each case, you will be presented with a chief complaint, vital signs, and the history of present illness (HPI). At that point, you will initiate patient management, continue care, and advance the case taking one of the following four types of actions that are represented on the computer screen.

1. Get Interval History or Physical Exam

You can get a focused or full physical exam. You can also get interval history to see how a patient is doing. Getting interval history or doing a physical exam will **automatically** advance the clock in simulated time.

Quick tips and shortcuts:

- If the vital signs are unstable, you may be forced to write some orders (e.g., IV fluids, oxygen, type and crossmatch) even **before** doing the exam.
- Keep the physical exam **focused.** A full physical and exam is often wasteful and can cost you valuable simulated time in an emergency situation. You can always do additional physical exam components as necessary.

2. Write Order or Review Chart

You can manage the patient by typing orders. You can order tests, monitoring, treatments, procedures, consultations, and counseling in your management of the patient. The order sheet format is free-text entry, so you need to type whatever you want. The computer has a 12,000-term vocabulary for approximately 2,500 orders or actions. If you order a medication, you also need to specify the **route** and **frequency.** If the patient comes into the case with preexisting medications, they will appear on the order sheet with an order time of "Day 1 @00:00." The medications will continue unless you decide to cancel them. Unlike interval history or PE, you must **manually** advance simulated time to see the results or your orders (see the next page).

Quick tips and shortcuts:

- As long as the computer can recognize the **first three characters** of your order, it can provide a list of orders to choose from.
- Simply type the test, therapy, or procedure you want. Don't type any verbs like "get," "administer," or "do."
- Do the sample cases to get a sense of the common abbreviations the computer will recognize (e.g., CBC, CXR, ECG).
- Familiarize yourself with routes and dosing frequencies for common medications. You do not need to know dosages or drip rates.
- Don't ever assume that other health care staff or consultants will write orders for you. Even routine actions such as IV fluids, oxygen, monitoring, and diabetic diet have to be ordered by you. If a patient is preop, don't forget NPO, type and crossmatch, and antibiotics.
- You can always change your mind and cancel an order as long as the clock has not been advanced.
- Review any preexisting medications on the order sheet. Sometimes the patient's problem is due to a preexisting medication **side effect** or a drug-drug interaction!

3. Obtain Results or See Patient Later

To see how the case evolves after you have entered your orders, you have to advance the clock. You can specify a time to see the patient either in the future or when the next results become available. When you advance the clock, you may receive messages from the patient, the patient's family, or the health care staff updating you on the patient's status prior to the specified time or result availability. If you stop a clock advance to a future time (such as a follow-up appointment) to review results from previous orders, that future time appointment will be canceled.

Quick tips and shortcuts:

- Before advancing the clock, ask yourself whether the patient should be okay during that time period.
- Before advancing the clock, ask yourself whether the patient is in the appropriate location or should be transferred to a new location.
- If you receive an update while the clock is advancing, especially if the patient is **worsening,** you should review your current management.

4. Change Location

According to the USMLE, you have an outpatient office with admitting privileges to a 400-bed tertiary-care facility. As in real life, the patient typically presents to you in an office or ER setting. Once you've done all you can, you can transfer the patient to another setting to receive appropriate care. This may include the **ward** or **ICU**. Note that the ICU represents all types of ICUs, including medical, surgical, pediatric, obstetrics, neonatal, and so on. When appropriate, the patient may be discharged **home** with follow-up.

Quick tips and shortcuts:

- Always ask yourself if the patient is in the right location for optimal management.
- Remember that you remain the **primary physician** wherever the patient goes.

- When changing locations (and especially when discharging the patient), discontinue any orders that are no longer needed.
- Anyone discharged home requires a follow-up appointment.
- Before discharging a patient, think about whether the patient needs any health maintenance or counseling.

Finishing the Case

The case ends when you have used your allotted 25 minutes. If the measurement objectives for the case have been met, the computer may ask you to exit it early. Toward the end of a case, you will be given a warning that the case will end. You are given an opportunity to cancel orders as well as write some short-term orders. You will be asked for a final diagnosis before exiting.

HOW IS THE CCS GRADED?

You will be graded by a scoring algorithm based on generally accepted practices of care. It allows for wide variation and recognizes that there may be more than one appropriate way to approach a case. In general, you **gain** points for appropriate management actions and **lose** points for actions that are not indicated or that can harm your patient. These actions are worth **different** points such that key actions (e.g., emergent needle thoracostomy for a patient with tension pneumothorax) will earn you big points, and very inappropriate actions (e.g., liver biopsy for a patient with an ear infection) will lose you big points. Note that you may not get full credit for correct actions if you perform them **out of sequence** or **after an inappropriate delay** in simulated time. **Unnecessary and excessive orders** (even if there is no risk to the patient) will cost you points. The bottom line is that the CCS tends to reward **thorough but efficient** medicine.

HIGH-YIELD STRATEGIES FOR THE CCS

As mentioned before, it is essential to do the available practice CCS cases prior to the exam. Make sure that you do both outpatient and inpatient cases. Try different abbreviations to get a feel for the vocabulary when you write orders. Try using different approaches to the same case to see how the computer reacts. Read through the 100 cases in **Section III: High-Yield Cases.** They will show you how clinical conditions can present and play out as a CCS case. Remember that the computer wants you to do the **right things** at the **right times** with **minimum waste** and **unnecessary risk** to the patient. When taking the exam, also keep the following in mind:

- **Read through the HPI carefully.** Use it to develop a short differential that will direct your physical exam and initial management. Often, the diagnosis is apparent before you even do the physical. Jot down pertinent positives and negative so that you don't have to come back and review the chart. Keep in mind any drug allergies.
- **Any unstable patient needs immediate management.** If the vital signs are unstable, you may want to do some basic management such as IV fluids and oxygen before doing your physical exam. With unstable patients, you should be ordering tests that will give you fast results in identifying and managing the underlying condition.
- **Consultants are rarely helpful.** You will get some points for calling a consultant for an indicated procedure (e.g., a surgeon for an appendectomy).

Otherwise, consultants will offer little in the way of diagnostic or management help.

- **Don't forget health maintenance, education, and counseling.** After treating a patient's tension pneumothorax, counsel the patient about smoking cessation if the HPI mentions that he is an active smoker.
- **Don't treat just the patient.** The computer will not let you treat a patient's family or sexual partner, but it does allow you to provide education or counseling. If a female patient is of childbearing age, check a pregnancy test prior to starting a potentially teratogenic treatment.
- **Sometimes the patient will worsen despite good care.** And sometimes the patient will improve with poor management. If the case is not going your way, reassess your approach to make sure you're not missing anything. If you are confident about your diagnosis and management, then stop second-guessing. Sometimes the computer tests your ability to handle difficult clinical situations.

NOTES

SECTION II

Database of High-Yield Facts

▶ Ambulatory Medicine

▶ Cardiovascular

▶ Emergency Medicine

▶ Endocrinology

▶ Ethics and Statistics

▶ Gastroenterology

▶ Hematology

▶ Oncology

▶ Infectious Disease

▶ Musculoskeletal

▶ Nephrology

▶ Neurology

▶ Obstetrics

▶ Gynecology

▶ Pediatrics

▶ Psychiatry

▶ Pulmonary

SECTION II

Ambulatory Medicine

Glaucoma

Optic neuropathy caused by elevated intraocular pressure (defined as > 20 mmHg) that results in progressive loss of peripheral vision.

OPEN-ANGLE GLAUCOMA

- The most common type of glaucoma. More common in African-Americans.
- **Sx/Dx:** Diagnosis is made in patients who are **losing peripheral vision** and who have high intraocular pressures and an abnormal cup-disk ratio (> 50%).
- Tx: Treat with the following:
    - Nonselective β-blockers (e.g., timolol, levobunolol).
    - Adrenergic agonists (e.g., epinephrine).
    - Cholinergic agonists (e.g., pilocarpine, carbachol).
    - Carbonic anhydrase inhibitors (e.g., dorzolamide, brinzolamide).

CLOSED-ANGLE GLAUCOMA

- **An emergency!**
- Most common in those of Asian descent.
- **Sx/Exam:** Presents with eye pain, headache, nausea, conjunctival injection, halos around lights, and fixed, moderately dilated pupils. Check intraocular pressure.
- **Tx:**
    - Contact an ophthalmologist immediately.
    - Treatment consists of topical pilocarpine for pupillary constriction, timolol and acetazolamide to ↓ intraocular pressure, and laser iridotomy.

Do not confuse closed-angle glaucoma with a simple headache!

Hearing Loss

Common in the elderly. Principal causes are as follows:

- **External canal:** Cerumen impaction, foreign bodies in the ear canal, otitis externa, new growth/mass.
- **Internal canal:** Otitis media, barotrauma, perforation of the tympanic membrane.
- **Other:**
    - **Presbycusis:** Age-related hearing loss.
    - **Otosclerosis:** Progressive fixation of the stapes → bilateral progressive conductive hearing loss. Begins in the second or third decade of life and may advance in pregnancy. Exam is normal; surgery with stapedectomy or stapedotomy yields excellent results.
    - Drug-induced loss (e.g., from aminoglycosides); noise-induced loss.
- **Dx:** Distinguish conductive from sensorineural hearing loss:
    - **Weber test:** Press a vibrating tuning fork in the middle of the patient's forehead and ask in which ear it sounds louder.
        - **Conductive hearing loss:** The sound will be louder in the affected ear.

- **Sensorineural hearing loss:** The sound will be louder in the normal ear.
  - **Rinne test:** Place a vibrating tuning fork against the patient's mastoid bone, and once it is no longer audible, immediately reposition it near the external meatus.
    - **Conductive hearing loss:** Bone conduction is audible longer than air conduction.
    - **Sensorineural hearing loss:** Air conduction is audible longer than bone conduction.

Otosclerosis is the most common cause of conductive hearing loss in young adults.

Allergic Rhinitis

Affects up to 20% of the adult population. Patients may also have asthma and atopic dermatitis.

SYMPTOMS/EXAM

- Presents with congestion, rhinorrhea, sneezing, eye irritation, and postnasal drip.
- Generally, one can readily identify exposure to environmental allergens such as pollens, animal dander, dust mites, and mold spores. May be seasonal.
- Exam reveals edematous, pale mucosa.

DIAGNOSIS

- Often based on clinical impression given the signs and symptoms.
- Skin testing to a standard panel of antigens can be performed, or blood testing can be conducted to look for specific IgE antibodies via radioallergosorbent testing (RAST).

TREATMENT

- **Allergen avoidance:** Use dust-mite-proof covers on bedding and remove carpeting. Keep the home dry and avoid pets.
- **Drugs:**
  - **Antihistamines (diphenhydramine, fexofenadine):** Block the effects of histamine released by mast cells.
  - **Intranasal corticosteroids:** Anti-inflammatory properties → excellent symptom control.
  - **Sympathomimetics (pseudoephedrine):** α-adrenergic agonist effects → vasoconstriction.
  - **Intranasal anticholinergics (ipratropium):** ↓ mucous membrane secretions.
  - **Immunotherapy ("allergy shots"):** Slow to take effect, but useful for difficult-to-control symptoms.

Epistaxis

Bleeding from the nose or nasopharynx. Roughly 90% of cases are anterior nasal septum bleeds (at Kiesselbach's plexus). The most common etiology is local trauma 2° to digital manipulation. Other causes include dryness of the nasal mucosa, nasal septal deviation, use of antiplatelet medications, bone abnormalities in the nares, rhinitis, and bleeding diatheses.

SYMPTOMS/EXAM

- **Posterior bleeds:** More brisk and less common; blood is swallowed and may not be seen.
- **Anterior bleeds:** Usually less severe; bleeding is visible as it exits the nares.

TREATMENT

- Treat with direct pressure and topical nasal vasoconstrictors (phenylephrine or oxymetazoline).
- If bleeding does not stop, cauterize with silver nitrate or insert nasal packing (with antibiotics to prevent toxic shock syndrome, covering for *S. aureus*).
- If severe, type and screen, obtain IV access, and consult an ENT surgeon.

Leukoplakia

White patches or plaques in the oral mucosa that are considered precancerous. Cannot be removed by rubbing the mucosal surface. If easily removed, think of *Candida*. Can occur in response to chronic irritation and can represent either dysplasia or early invasive squamous cell carcinoma. Common in smokeless tobacco users.

DERMATOLOGY

Atopic Dermatitis (Eczema)

Pruritic, lichenified eruptions that are classically found in the antecubital fossa but may also appear on the neck, face, wrists, and upper trunk.

- Has a chronic course with remissions.
- Characterized by an early age of onset (often in childhood).
- Associated with a ⊕ family history of atopy.
- Patients tend to have ↑ serum IgE and repeated skin infections.

SYMPTOMS/EXAM

Presents with severe pruritus, with distribution generally in the face, neck, upper trunk, and bends of the elbows and knees. The skin is dry, leathery, and lichenified (see Figure 2.1-1). The condition usually worsens in the winter and in low-humidity environments.

DIFFERENTIAL

Seborrheic dermatitis, contact dermatitis, impetigo.

DIAGNOSIS

Diagnosis is clinical.

TREATMENT

Keep skin moisturized. **Topical steroid creams should be used sparingly** and should be tapered off once flares resolve. The first-line steroid-sparing agent is tacrolimus ointment.

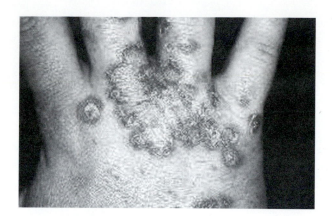

FIGURE 2.1-1. Atopic dermatitis.

Note the lichenified plaques, erosions, and fissures, which are characteristic of the condition. (Courtesy of James J. Nordlund, MD.)

Contact Dermatitis

Caused by exposure to certain substances in the environment. Allergens may → acute, subacute, or chronic eczematous inflammation.

SYMPTOMS

Patients present with itching, burning, and an intensely pruritic rash.

EXAM

- **Acute:** Presents with vesicles, weeping erosions where vesicles have ruptured, crusting, and excoriations. The pattern of lesions often reflects the mechanism of exposure (e.g., a line of vesicles or lesions under a watchband; see Figure 2.1-2).
- **Chronic:** Characterized by hyperkeratosis and lichenification.

DIAGNOSIS

- Usually a clinical diagnosis that is made in the setting of a possible exposure.
- A detailed history for exposures is essential.
- In the case of leather, patch testing can be used to elicit the reaction with the exact agent that caused the dermatitis.
- Consider the occupation of the individual and the exposure area of the body to determine if they suggest a diagnosis.

TREATMENT

- Avoid causative agents.
- Cold compresses and oatmeal baths help soothe the area.
- Administer topical steroids. A short course of oral steroids may be needed if a large region of the body is involved.

Common causes of contact dermatitis include leather, nickel (earrings, watches, necklaces), and poison ivy.

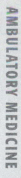

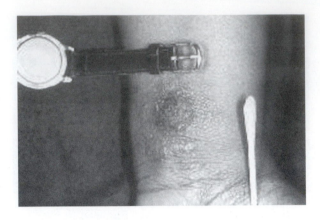

FIGURE 2.1-2.   Contact dermatitis.

The erythematous, edematous base of the eruption corresponds to the posterior surface of the watch. (Courtesy of the Department of Dermatology, Wilford Hall USAF Medical Center and Brooke Army Medical Center, San Antonio, TX.)

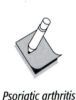

Psoriatic arthritis characteristically involves the DIP joints.

Psoriasis

An idiopathic, benign skin disease characterized by silver plaques with an erythematous base and sharply defined margins. The condition is common and is generally chronic with a probable genetic predisposition.

SYMPTOMS/EXAM

Presents with well-demarcated silvery, scaly plaques (the most common type) on the knees, elbows, and scalp (see Figure 2.1-3). **Nails may show pitting and onycholysis.**

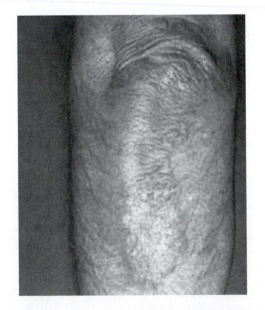

FIGURE 2.1-3.   Psoriasis.

A scaly, erythematous, silvery plaque can be seen on the elbow. (Reproduced, with permission, from Bondi EE, Jegasothy BV, Lazarus GS [editors]: *Dermatology: Diagnosis & Treatment.* Orginally published by Appleton & Lange. Copyright © 1991 by The McGraw-Hill Companies, Inc.)

TREATMENT

- **Limited disease:** Topical steroids, occlusive dressings, topical vitamin D analogs, topical retinoids.
- **Generalized disease (involving > 30% of the body):** UVB light exposure three times per week; PUVA (psoralen and UVA) if UVB is not effective. Methotrexate may also be used for severe cases.

Erythema Nodosum

An inflammatory lesion that is characterized by red or violet nodules and is more common in women than in men. Although the condition is often idiopathic, it may also occur 2° to sarcoidosis, IBD, or infections such as streptococcus, coccidioidomycosis, or TB.

SYMPTOMS/EXAM

- Lesions are painful and may be preceded by fever, malaise, and arthralgia. Recent URI or diarrheal illness may suggest a cause.
- Exam reveals deep-seated, poorly demarcated, painful red nodules without ulceration on the extensor surfaces of the lower legs (see Figure 2.1-4).

DIFFERENTIAL

Cellulitis, trauma, thrombophlebitis.

TREATMENT

Treat the underlying disease. The condition is usually self-limited, but NSAIDs are helpful for pain. In more persistent cases, potassium iodide drops and corticosteroids may be of benefit.

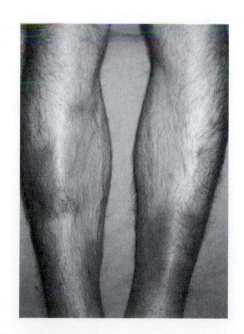

FIGURE 2.1-4. Erythema nodosum.

Panniculitis characterized by tender deep-seated nodules and plaques usually located on the lower extremities. (Reproduced, with permission, from Kasper DL et al. *Harrison's Principles of Internal Medicine*, 16th ed. New York: McGraw-Hill, 2005: 2019.)

Rosacea

A chronic condition that occurs in patients 30–60 years of age. More commonly affects people with fair skin, those with light hair and eyes, and those who have frequent flushing.

SYMPTOMS/EXAM

- Presents with erythema and with inflammatory papules that mimic acne and appear on the cheeks, forehead, nose, and chin.
- Open and closed comedones (whiteheads and blackheads) are not present.
- Recurrent flushing may be elicited by spicy foods, alcohol, or emotional reactions.
- Rhinophyma (thickened, lumpy skin on the nose) occurs late in the course of the disease and is a result of sebaceous gland hyperplasia (see Figure 2.1-5).

DIFFERENTIAL

The absence of comedones in rosacea and the patient's age help distinguish the condition from acne vulgaris.

TREATMENT

- **Initial therapy:** The goal is to control rather than cure the chronic disease. Use mild cleansers (Dove, Cetaphil), benzoyl peroxide, and/or metronidazole topical gel with or without oral antibiotics as initial therapy.
- **Persistent symptoms:** Treat with oral antibiotics (tetracycline, minocycline) and tretinoin cream.
- **Maintenance therapy:**
  - Topical metronidazole may be used once daily.
  - Clonidine or α-blockers are effective in the management of flushing, and patients should avoid triggers.
  - Consider referral for surgical evaluation if rhinophyma is present and is not responding to treatment.

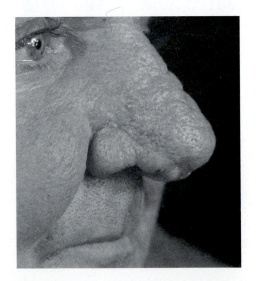

FIGURE 2.1-5.   Rhinophyma.

(Reproduced, with permission, from Wolff K, Johnson RA, Suurmond D. *Fitzpatrick's Color Atlas & Synopsis of Clinical Dermatology*, 5th ed. New York: McGraw-Hill, 2005: 11.)

Erythema Multiforme (EM)

An acute inflammatory disease that is sometimes recurrent. EM is probably a distinct disease entity from Stevens-Johnson syndrome and toxic epidermal necrolysis. **Many causative factors** are linked with EM, such as infectious agents (especially HSV and *Mycoplasma*), drugs, connective tissue disorders, physical agents, radiotherapy, pregnancy, and internal malignancies. Many cases are idiopathic and sometimes recurrent idiopathic.

SYMPTOMS/EXAM

- May be preceded by malaise, fever, or itching and burning at the site where the eruptions will occur.
- Sudden onset of rapidly progressive, symmetrical lesions.
- Target lesions and papules are typically located on the back of the hands and on the palms, soles, and limbs but can be found anywhere (see Figure 2.1-6). Lesions recur in crops for 2–3 weeks.

DIAGNOSIS

Typically a clinical diagnosis. Biopsy can help in uncertain cases.

TREATMENT

- Mild cases can be treated symptomatically with histamine blockers for pruritus.

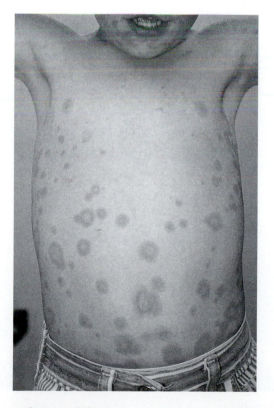

FIGURE 2.1-6. **Erythema multiforme.**

Note the symmetric distribution of target macules. (Courtesy of Michael Redman, PA-C.)

- If many target lesions are present, patients usually respond well to prednisone for 1–3 weeks.
- Azathioprine has been helpful in cases that are unresponsive to other treatments. Levamisole has also been successfully used in patients with chronic or recurrent oral lesions.
- When HSV causes recurrent EM, maintenance acyclovir or valacyclovir can ↓ recurrences of both.

Pemphigus Vulgaris

A rare autoimmune disease in which blisters are formed as **autoantibodies destroy intracellular adhesions between epithelial cells** in the skin. Pemphigus vulgaris is the most common subtype of pemphigus.

SYMPTOMS/EXAM

- Presents with **flaccid bullae** and with **erosions** where bullae have been unroofed (see Figure 2.1-7). Oral lesions usually precede skin lesions.
- If it is not treated early, the disease usually generalizes and can affect the esophagus. Nikolsky's sign is elicited when gentle lateral traction on the skin separates the epidermis from underlying tissue.

DIAGNOSIS

Skin biopsy shows acantholysis (separation of epidermal cells from each other); immunofluorescence reveals antibodies in the epidermis.

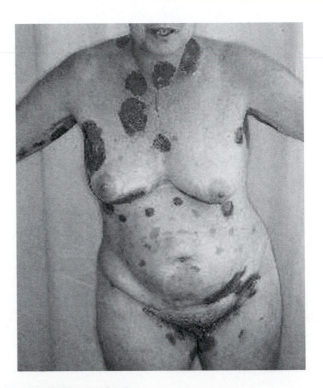

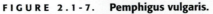

FIGURE 2.1-7.   Pemphigus vulgaris.

Vesiculobullous lesions and erosions of pemphigus vulgaris are seen throughout the chest and abdomen. (Courtesy of James J. Nordlund, MD.)

Corticosteroids and immunosuppressive agents.

Bullous Pemphigoid

- An autoimmune disease characterized by **antibodies against basement membrane → subepidermal bullae.** More common than pemphigus vulgaris and typically occurs in those > 60 years of age.
- **Sx/Exam:** Presents as large, tense bullae with few other symptoms.
- **DDx:** Pemphigus vulgaris, dermatitis herpetiformis.
- **Dx:** Diagnosis is clinical, with confirmation via immuno- and histopathology.
- **Tx:** Corticosteroids.

Acne Vulgaris (Common Acne)

A common skin disease that primarily affects adolescents. Results from ↑ pilosebaceous gland activity, *Propionibacterium acnes*, and plugging of follicles.

SYMPTOMS/EXAM

Various lesions are seen, including closed comedones (whiteheads), open comedones (blackheads), papules, nodules, and scars. Lesions typically appear over the face, back, and chest.

DIFFERENTIAL

Rosacea, folliculitis.

DIAGNOSIS

Diagnosis is clinical.

TREATMENT

- Begin with topical antibiotics such as erythromycin, benzoyl peroxide gels, and topical retinoids.
- A 2° line of treatment includes addition of oral antibiotics such as minocycline and tetracycline.
- Isotretinoin (Accutane) can be used but is teratogenic and should be prescribed with caution in women of childbearing age. Concomitant contraception and pregnancy tests are necessary.

Herpes Zoster

A disease caused by reactivated varicella-zoster virus (VZV), which lives dormant in the dorsal roots of nerves. Risk factors include increasing age and immunosuppression. Patients can develop postherpetic neuralgia, a painful disorder, after the eruption.

SYMPTOMS/EXAM

Presents with the cutaneous finding of **painful vesicles evolving into crusted lesions in a dermatomal distribution.** Lesions are typically preceded by paresthesias in the area of distribution.

DIFFERENTIAL

Contact dermatitis.

DIAGNOSIS

Diagnosis is largely clinical. Giant cells may be seen on Tzanck smear of fluid.

TREATMENT

- Pain management.
- If initiated within 72 hours of symptom onset, antiviral treatment with acyclovir, valacyclovir, or famciclovir can ↓ the duration of illness and may also ↓ the occurrence of postherpetic neuralgia.
- Vaccination to help prevent recurrence is becoming more popular in select patients.

GENITOURINARY DISORDERS

Erectile Dysfunction (ED)

Inability to achieve or maintain an erection sufficient to effect penetration and ejaculation. Affects 30 million men. Associated with age; some degree of ED is seen in 40% of 40-year-olds and in 70% of 70-year-olds. Etiologies are as follows:

- **Psychological:**
  - Symptoms often have a sudden onset.
  - Patients are unable to sustain or sometimes even obtain an erection.
  - Patients have normal nocturnal penile tumescence (those with organic causes do not).
- **Organic:**
  - **Endocrine:** Diabetes mellitus (DM), hypothyroidism or thyrotoxicosis, pituitary or gonadal disorders, ↑ prolactin.
  - **Vascular disease:** Atherosclerosis of penile arteries or venous leaks.
  - **Neurologic disease:** Stroke, temporal lobe seizure, MS, spinal surgery, neuropathy.
- **Exogenous:** Drugs that cause ED include α-blockers, clonidine, CNS depressants, anticholinergics, and TCAs.

DM may → both vascular and neurologic causes of ED.

EXAM

Look for exam findings suggesting an organic cause—e.g., small testes, evidence of Peyronie's disease, perineal sensation/cremaster reflex, evidence of peripheral neuropathy, or galactorrhea. Assess peripheral pulses; look for skin atrophy, hair loss, and low skin temperature.

DIAGNOSIS

Assess TSH, prolactin, and testosterone; order a fasting glucose to assess for diabetes.

TREATMENT

- PDE-5a inhibitors (sildenafil [Viagra], tadalafil, vardenafil) inhibit cGMP-specific phosphodiesterase type 5a, thereby improving relaxation of

smooth muscle in the corpora cavernosa. Side effects include flushing, headache, and ↓ BP. Patients cannot be on nitrates or α-blockers.
- Testosterone for hypogonadism; behavioral treatment for depression and anxiety.
- Vascular surgery may be an option if indicated.

Benign Prostatic Hyperplasia (BPH)

Hyperplasia of the prostate → bladder outlet obstruction. Incidence ↑ with age. Common in patients > 45 years of age.

SYMPTOMS/EXAM

- Patients complain of frequency, urgency, nocturia, ↓ force and size of stream, and incomplete emptying → overflow incontinence.
- Exam reveals a firm, rubbery, smooth prostatic surface (vs. the rock-hard areas that suggest prostate cancer).

DIAGNOSIS

Diagnosed by an appropriate history and exam. Check a UA for infection or hematuria, both of which should prompt further evaluation. PSA is elevated in up to 50% of patients but is not diagnostically useful.

TREATMENT

- α-blockers (terazosin), 5α-reductase inhibitors (finasteride).
- Avoid anticholinergics, antihistamines, or narcotics.
- If the condition is refractory to medications, consider surgical options such as transurethral resection of the prostate (TURP). An open procedure is appropriate if gland size is > 75 g.

COMPLICATIONS

Acute urinary retention 2° to necrosis and edema of a small part of the prostate; UTIs resulting from incomplete emptying.

Workup of Prostatic Nodules and Abnormal PSA

- Significant controversy surrounds prostate cancer screening, with different groups offering varying recommendations ranging from no screening at all to a yearly rectal exam and PSA testing (see Table 2.1-1).
- If an abnormality is found on exam, proceed to prostatic biopsy.
- The PSA may be used as a marker to follow the response to prostate cancer treatment.

CANCER SCREENING

Table 2.1-1 outlines recommended guidelines for the screening of common forms of cancer.

TABLE 2.1-1. Recommended Cancer Screening Guidelines

TYPE OF CANCER	RECOMMENDATIONS
Cervical cancer	An annual Pap smear is recommended starting at age 18 or at the onset of sexual activity. After three normal Pap smears, the screening interval can be ↑ to every three years.
Breast cancer	Monthly self-examination and an annual exam by a physician. Mammography should be conducted every year after age 40–50 (may start earlier if there is a ⊕ family history at a young age).
Colon cancer	Hemoccult annually (especially in patients > 50 years old); flex sigmoidoscopy (every 3–5 years in those > 50) or colonoscopy (every 10 years in those > 50). If a first-degree relative has colon cancer, begin screening at age 40 or when the patient is 10 years younger than the age at which that relative was diagnosed, whichever comes first.
Prostate cancer	Controversial. Some groups recommend no screening; others recommend a yearly rectal exam and PSA beginning at age 45 for African-Americans and for patients with a strong family history, and beginning at age 50 for all others.

IMMUNIZATIONS

Table 2.1-2 lists indications for adult immunizations.

TABLE 2.1-2. Indications for Immunization in Adults

IMMUNIZATION	INDICATION/RECOMMENDATION
Tetanus	Give 1° series in childhood, then boosters every 10 years.
Hepatitis B	Administer to all young adults and to patients at ↑ risk (e.g., IV drug users, health care providers, those with chronic liver disease).
Pneumococcal	Give to those > 65 years or to any patient at ↑ risk (e.g., splenectomy, HIV, or immunocompromised patients on chemo or posttransplant).
Influenza	Give annually for all patients > 50 years and to high-risk patients.
Hepatitis A	Give to those traveling to endemic areas, those with chronic liver disease (hepatitis B or C), and IV drug abusers.
Smallpox	Currently recommended only for individuals working in laboratories in which they are exposed to the virus.
Meningococcal	Not recommended for routine use. Used in outbreaks. There is an ↑ risk of disease in college students, but the vaccine is only suggested and is not mandatory in this group.

SECTION II

Cardiovascular

The 1° cause of ischemic heart disease is atherosclerotic occlusion of the coronary arteries. **Major risk factors** include age, family history, smoking, diabetes, hypertension, and hyperlipidemia.

SYMPTOMS

- **May be asymptomatic.**
- **Stable angina** presents with chest tightness/pain or shortness of breath with a consistent amount of exertion; relief is obtained with rest or nitroglycerin. Reflects a stable, flow-limiting plaque.
- **Unstable angina (acute coronary syndrome)** presents with chest tightness/pain and/or shortness of breath, typically at rest, that does not totally improve with nitroglycerin or recurs soon after nitroglycerin. Reflects plaque rupture with formation of a clot in the lumen of the blood vessel.

EXAM

- Exam can be normal when the patient is asymptomatic. During episodes of angina, an S4 or a mitral regurgitation murmur may occasionally be heard.
- Look for signs of heart failure (e.g., ↑ JVD, bibasilar crackles, lower extremity edema) from prior MI.
- Look for vascular disease elsewhere—e.g., bruits, asymmetric pulses, and lower extremity ischemic ulcers.

DIFFERENTIAL

Consider pericarditis, pulmonary embolism, pneumothorax, aortic dissection, peptic ulcer, and musculoskeletal causes.

DIAGNOSIS

- **Stress testing:** Exercise or dobutamine to ↑ heart rate; ECG, echocardiogram, or radionuclide imaging to assess perfusion (see the discussion of advanced cardiac evaluation below).
- **Cardiac catheterization:** Defines the location and severity of lesions.

TREATMENT

- **To slow progression:** Control diabetes, ↓ BP, ↓ cholesterol (**goal for low-density cholesterol < 70**), and encourage **smoking cessation.**
- **To prevent angina:** β-blockers ↓ BP and ↓ cardiac workload, which ↓ exertional angina. If symptoms arise on a β-blocker, a long-acting nitrate or calcium channel blocker can be added.
- **To prevent MI: Aspirin;** clopidogrel can be given to aspirin-sensitive patients.

Table 2.2-1 describes the clinical characteristics and treatment of common valvular lesions.

TABLE 2.2-1. **Presentation and Treatment of Select Valvular Lesions**

LESION	SYMPTOMS	EXAM	TREATMENT	COMMENTS
Mitral stenosis	Symptoms of heart failure; hemoptysis.	Diastolic murmur; opening snap.	HR control, balloon valvuloplasty, valve replacement.	Usually caused by **rheumatic fever.**
Mitral regurgitation	Long asymptomatic period; when severe or acute, presents with symptoms of heart failure.	**Blowing** systolic murmur at the apex, **radiating to the axilla.** Posterior leaflet may lead to a murmur along the sternal border.	If acute, surgery is usually required. For chronic mitral regurgitation, repair or replace the valve when symptomatic or if the ejection fraction (EF) is falling.	Long-standing regurgitation dilates the atrium, ↑ the chance of atrial fibrillation (AF).
Mitral valve prolapse	Asymptomatic.	Midsystolic click; also murmur if mitral regurgitation is present.	Endocarditis prophylaxis not required.	Questionable association with palpitations and panic attacks.
Aortic stenosis	Chest pain, syncope, heart failure.	Harsh systolic murmur radiating to the carotids. **A small and slow carotid upstroke** (parvus et tardus) is seen with severe stenosis.	**Avoid overdiuresis; avoid vasodilators** such as nitrates and ACEIs. Surgery for all symptomatic patients.	Once symptoms appear, mortality is 50% at three years.
Aortic regurgitation	Usually asymptomatic until advanced; then presents with symptoms of heart failure.	**Wide pulse pressure;** soft, high-pitched diastolic murmur along the sternal border.	**Afterload reduction** with ACEIs, hydralazine; valve replacement if symptomatic or in the setting of a ↓ EF.	Many cases are associated with aortic root disease, dissection, syphilis, ankylosing spondylitis, and Marfan's.

HIGH-YIELD FACTS

CARDIOVASCULAR

HEART FAILURE (CONGESTIVE HEART FAILURE)

Defined as inability of the heart to pump adequate blood to meet the needs of the body. Can be categorized in different ways. One such categorization scheme includes the following:

- Systolic dysfunction
- Diastolic dysfunction
- Valvular dysfunction
- Arrhythmia causing heart failure

Active ischemia can acutely worsen diastolic dysfunction, so treat any coexisting CAD!

Ventricular tachycardia is a common cause of death in patients with a ↓ ejection fraction.

ACEIs, ARBs, and spironolactone all cause hyperkalemia.

Systolic Heart Failure

Weakened pumping function of the heart. Common causes include **ischemic heart disease, long-standing hypertension,** and viral or idiopathic cardiomyopathy in younger patients.

SYMPTOMS

- Patients present with poor exercise tolerance, exertional dyspnea, and easy fatigability.
- If patients are volume overloaded, they may present with **orthopnea,** paroxysmal nocturnal dyspnea, and ankle swelling.

EXAM

Exam reveals bibasilar crackles, a diffuse PMI that is displaced to the left (reflects cardiomegaly), an **S3 gallop,** JVD (normal is about 0–2 cm vertical elevation above the sternomanubrial junction), and lower extremity edema.

DIFFERENTIAL

Deconditioning, lung disease (e.g., COPD), heart failure of other types (e.g., diastolic dysfunction), other causes of edema (e.g., vascular incompetence, low albumin, and nephrotic syndrome).

DIAGNOSIS

- The history and exam are suggestive, but determination of the EF via an imaging study (e.g., **echocardiography,** sestamibi radionuclide imaging) confirms the diagnosis.
- **Look for the cause of the low EF:**
  - Perform a stress test or cardiac catheterization to look for CAD; obtain TSH levels.
  - Look for a history of alcohol use or exposure to offending medications such as **doxorubicin.**
  - A myocardial biopsy may be performed in selected cases.

TREATMENT

- **Maintenance medications** include the following:
  - β-blockers: Metoprolol, atenolol, **carvedilol.**
  - **Afterload reduction:** Ideally an **ACEI** or an angiotensin receptor blocker (ARB).
  - **Other:** Give spironolactone if the potassium level is not high. Digoxin may be used to lower the frequency of hospitalizations but does not ↓ mortality.
- **Exacerbations:** Give **loop diuretics** such as furosemide when the patient is volume overloaded.
- **Automatic implantable cardiac defibrillators (AICDs)** are associated with ↓ mortality from VT/VF, especially when the EF is < 35%.
- Treat the cause of the systolic heart failure (e.g., CAD).

Diastolic Heart Failure

During diastole, the heart is **stiff** and does not relax well, resulting in ↑ diastolic filling pressure. **Hypertension with left ventricular hypertrophy** is the most common cause; other causes include hypertrophic cardiomyopathy and infiltrative diseases such as amyloidosis and sarcoidosis.

- Symptoms are the same as those of systolic heart failure.
- Exam findings are similar to those of systolic failure. Listen for an **S4** rather than an S3.

DIFFERENTIAL

The same as that for systolic heart failure.

DIAGNOSIS

- Presents with symptoms of heart failure with a normal EF on echocardiogram.
- Echocardiography usually shows ventricular hypertrophy. Biopsy may be needed to establish the underlying diagnosis.

TREATMENT

- Control hypertension.
- Give diuretics to control volume overload, but **avoid overdiuresis**, which ↓ preload and cardiac output.

Valvular Causes of Heart Failure

- Right-sided valvular lesions do not typically cause heart failure but can cause profound edema that is refractory to diuresis.
- Left-sided valvular lesions can produce heart failure.

Arrhythmia Causing Heart Failure

- This cause of heart failure is generally apparent from palpitations or ECG.
- Rhythms that can cause symptoms of heart failure include **AF** and bradyarrhythmias. Others present abruptly with palpitations, shortness of breath, or even syncope.
- There is an entity known as **tachycardia-induced cardiomyopathy** that reverses with rate control.

PERICARDIAL DISEASE

Pericarditis

Inflammation of the pericardial sac. May be acute (< 6 weeks; most common), subacute (6 weeks to 6 months) or chronic (> 6 months). Causes include viral infection (especially enterovirus), mediastinal radiation, post-MI (Dressler's syndrome), cancer, rheumatologic diseases (SLE, RA), and idiopathic pericarditis.

SYMPTOMS/EXAM

- Presents with **chest pain** that is often improved by sitting up or leaning forward. The pain may radiate to the back and to the left trapezius ridge.
- If a large effusion is present, the patient may be short of breath.
- Exam may reveal a pericardial friction rub (a leathery sound that is inconstant).

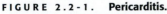

DIFFERENTIAL

Myocardial ischemia, aortic dissection, pneumonia, pulmonary embolism, pneumothorax.

DIAGNOSIS

- Look for diffuse ST-segment elevation (often with upward concavity) on ECG (see Figure 2.2-1) and PR-segment depression. ECG changes in pericarditis tend to be more generalized. Sequential ECGs are helpful in distinguishing pericarditis from MI, as in the latter, ECG changes tend to normalize more rapidly.
- Echocardiography may reveal an associated effusion.
- Search for an underlying cause—i.e., take a history for viral illness, radiation exposure, and malignancy. Check ANA, PPD, blood cultures if febrile, and renal function.
- In North America, TB is an uncommon cause of chronic constrictive pericarditis that presents with ascites, hepatomegaly, and distended neck veins. A chest CT will be needed for diagnosis, and pericardial resection may be required.

TREATMENT

- Where possible, treat the underlying disorder, such as SLE or advanced renal failure.
- For viral or idiopathic pericarditis, give NSAIDs or aspirin. Avoid NSAIDs in post-MI pericarditis, as they may interfere with scar formation.

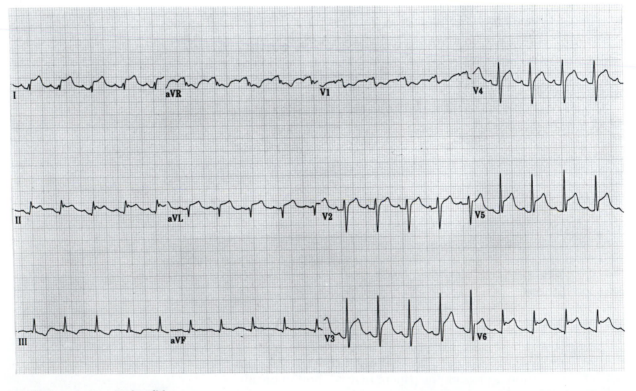

FIGURE 2.2-1. **Pericarditis.**

(Reproduced, with permission, from Stobo J et al. *The Principles and Practice of Medicine*, 23rd ed. Stamford, CT: Appleton & Lange, 1996: 20.)

COMPLICATIONS

Patients may develop a clinically significant pericardial effusion and **tamponade** (see below).

Pericardial Effusion and Cardiac Tamponade

Accumulation of fluid (usually chronic) or blood (usually acute and post-traumatic) in the pericardial cavity surrounding the heart.

SYMPTOMS/EXAM

- If **acute**, patients may present with **shock**. If **chronic**, patients may present with **shortness of breath and heart failure. One to two liters of fluid may gradually accumulate.**
- Exam reveals distant heart sounds, elevated JVP, and pulsus paradoxus (more than a 10-mmHg drop in systolic BP during inspiration).

DIFFERENTIAL

Pneumothorax, MI, cardiac failure.

DIAGNOSIS

Echocardiography is needed to confirm the diagnosis. CXR may show a large cardiac silhouette, and ECG may show low voltages.

TREATMENT

Consider emergent pericardiocentesis for patients with post–chest trauma shock as well as for those in whom echocardiography shows evidence of tamponade physiology.

ADVANCED CARDIAC EVALUATION

- **Indications for stress testing** include the following (not exhaustive):
  - **Diagnosis** of CAD/evaluation of symptoms
  - Preoperative evaluation
  - Risk assessment in patients with known disease
  - Decision making about the need for revascularization
- **Contraindications** include severe aortic stenosis, acute coronary syndrome, and decompensated heart failure.
- Testing consists of a stressing modality and an evaluating modality (see Tables 2.2-2 and 2.2-3).
  - The stressor can be walking on a treadmill or IV dobutamine.
  - Evaluating modalities are ECG, echocardiogram, and nuclear imaging such as thallium.
- An additional testing method is adenosine or dipyridamole with nuclear imaging.
  - These agents dilate the coronary arteries, but areas with plaque cannot vasodilate.
  - Such agents thus ↑ blood flow in healthy arteries but cause no change in diseased arteries, thereby creating a differential flow that is detected on nuclear imaging.

TABLE 2.2-2. Stressing Modalities in Cardiac Testing

STRESSING MODALITY	PROS	CONS
Treadmill	Good for patients who can walk.	
Dobutamine	Good for patients who cannot exercise.	
Adenosine or dipyridamole (with nuclear imaging)	Good for patients who cannot exercise.	Can cause bronchospasm—be cautious in patients with COPD.

HYPERTENSION

A major contributor to cardiovascular disease; more common with increasing age and among African-Americans.

SYMPTOMS

Asymptomatic unless severe. If severe, patients may complain of chest tightness, shortness of breath, headache, or visual disturbances.

EXAM

- BP > 140/90.
- A displaced PMI or an S4 indicates LVH.
- Fundi show **AV nipping** and "copper-wire" changes to the arterioles. Listen for bruits, which indicate peripheral vascular disease.
- In severe hypertension, look for papilledema and retinal hemorrhages.

TABLE 2.2-3. Evaluating Modalities in Cardiac Testing

EVALUATING MODALITY	PROS	CONS
ECG	Inexpensive.	Cannot localize the lesion; cannot use with baseline ST-segment abnormalities or left bundle branch block.
Echocardiogram	Good in patients with left bundle branch block; cheaper than nuclear imaging.	Technically limited echo images or resting wall motion abnormalities can limit usefulness.
Radionuclide tracer (thallium or technetium)	Localizes ischemia; localizes infarcted tissue.	Expensive.

DIFFERENTIAL

Most cases are essential hypertension, but consider causes of 2° hypertension:

- **Endocrine causes:** Cushing's syndrome, Conn's syndrome (aldosterone-producing tumor), hyperthyroidism.
- **Renal causes:** Chronic renal failure; renal artery stenosis (listen for abdominal bruit).
- **Young patients:** Fibromuscular dysplasia of the renal arteries; aortic coarctation.
- **Medications:** OCPs, NSAIDs.

DIAGNOSIS

- Diagnosed in the setting of **BP > 140/90** on two separate occasions (elevation of either systolic or diastolic BP).
- A systolic BP of 120–139 or a diastolic BP of 80–89 is considered "prehypertension" and predicts the development of hypertension.

TREATMENT

- The **goal BP** is < 140/90. In diabetics and those with renal insufficiency, the goal is < 130/80.
- **Interventions** include the following:
  - **Step 1—lifestyle modification:** Weight loss, exercise, ↓ sodium intake.
  - **Step 2—medications: Begin with a thiazide diuretic** unless there is an indication for another class (see Table 2.2-4). Consider starting two drugs initially if systolic BP is > 160 mmHg.
- Control other cardiovascular risk factors, such as diabetes, smoking, and high cholesterol.

COMPLICATIONS

Long-standing hypertension contributes to renal failure, heart failure (both systolic and diastolic), CAD, peripheral vascular disease, and stroke.

TABLE 2.2-4. Antihypertensive Medications

COMMONLY USED CLASSES	OPTIMAL USE	MAIN SIDE EFFECTS
Thiazide diuretics	First-line treatment if no indication for other agents.	↓ excretion of calcium and uric acid.
β-blockers	Low EF, **angina.**	Bradycardia, erectile dysfunction, bronchospasm in asthmatics.
ACEIs	Low EF, chronic kidney disease, diabetes with **microalbuminuria.**	**Cough,** angioedema, hyperkalemia.
ARBs	Same as ACEIs; cough with ACEI.	Hyperkalemia.
Calcium channel blockers	Second-line agent.	Lower extremity edema.

Always think about dissection

in patients with chest pain!

AORTIC DISSECTION

Most common in patients with a history of long-standing hypertension, cocaine use, or aortic root disease such as Marfan's syndrome or Takayasu's arteritis.

SYMPTOMS/ EXAM

- Presents with sudden onset of severe chest pain that sometimes radiates to the back. May also present with neurologic symptoms from occlusion of vessels supplying the brain or spinal cord.
- On exam, look for aortic regurgitation, **asymmetric pulses,** and neurologic findings.

DIFFERENTIAL

MI, pulmonary embolus, pneumothorax.

DIAGNOSIS

- Requires a high index of suspicion.
- CXR has low sensitivity but may show a widened mediastinum or a hazy aortic knob.
- **CT scan with IV contrast** is diagnostic and shows the extent of dissection.
- Transesophageal echocardiography (TEE) is highly sensitive and specific.

TREATMENT

- **Initial medical stabilization:** Aggressive **HR and BP control,** first with β-blockers (typically IV esmolol) and then with IV nitroprusside if needed.
- **Ascending dissection (involves the ascending aorta): Emergent surgical repair.**
- **Descending dissection (distal to the left subclavian artery):** Medical management unless there is intractable pain, progressive dissection in patients with chest pain, or vascular occlusion of aortic branches.

COMPLICATIONS

Aortic rupture, acute aortic regurgitation, tamponade, neurologic impairment, limb or mesenteric ischemia, renal ischemia.

PERIPHERAL VASCULAR DISEASE

Atherosclerotic disease of vessels other than the coronary arteries. Risk factors are similar to those for CAD and include **smoking,** diabetes, hypercholesterolemia, hypertension, and increasing age.

SYMPTOMS

Presentation depends on the organ affected:

- **Mesenteric ischemia:** Postprandial abdominal pain and food avoidance.
- **Lower extremities:** Claudication, ulceration.
- **Kidneys:** Usually asymptomatic, but may present with difficult-to-control hypertension.
- **CNS:** Stroke and TIA (see the Neurology chapter).

- **Mesenteric disease:** No specific findings. The patient may be thin because of weight loss from avoidance of food.
- **Lower extremity disease:** Exam reveals ulcers, diminished pulses, skin atrophy and loss of hair, and **bruits** over affected vessels (abdominal, femoral, popliteal).
- **Renal artery stenosis:** Listen for a **bruit during systole and diastole** (highly specific).

Acute vessel occlusion from an embolus or an in situ thrombus presents with sudden pain (abdominal or extremity) and is an emergency.

DIFFERENTIAL

- **Abdominal pain:** Stable symptoms can mimic PUD or biliary colic. If the colon is predominantly involved, episodes of pain and bloody stool can look like infectious colitis.
- **Lower extremities: Spinal stenosis** can produce lower extremity discomfort similar to claudication. Claudication improves with standing still, but spinal stenosis classically improves with **sitting** (lumbar flexion improves spinal stenosis symptoms).

DIAGNOSIS

- **Mesenteric disease:** A diagnosis of exclusion. Angiography reveals lesions.
- **Lower extremity disease:** Diagnosed via the **ankle-brachial index** (compares BP in the lower and upper extremities) and Doppler ultrasound. Angiography or MRA is used in preparation for revascularization but is generally not used for diagnosis.
- **Renal artery stenosis:** Angiography, MRA, or ultrasound with Doppler flow (technically difficult).

TREATMENT

- Control risk factors, especially smoking.
- **Mesenteric disease:** Treat with surgical revascularization or angioplasty.
- **Lower extremity disease:** Treat with exercise to improve functional capacity, surgical revascularization, and sometimes angioplasty. Cilostazol is moderately useful (improves pain-free walking distance 50%), whereas pentoxifylline is of marginal benefit.
- **Renal artery stenosis:** Surgery or angioplasty may be of benefit.

HYPERCHOLESTEROLEMIA

One of the principal factors contributing to atherosclerotic vascular disease. An ↑ LDL and a low concentration of HDL are the 1° contributors. Hypercholesterolemia can be idiopathic, genetic, or 2° to other diseases, such as diabetes, nephrotic syndrome, and hypothyroidism.

SYMPTOMS

Asymptomatic unless the patient develops ischemia (e.g., angina, stroke, claudication) or unless severe hypertriglyceridemia → pancreatitis.

EXAM

- Look for evidence of atherosclerosis—e.g., carotid, subclavian, and other bruits; diminished pulses; or ischemic foot ulcers.
- Look for **xanthomas** (lipid depositions) over the tendons, above the upper eyelid, and on the palms.

DIAGNOSIS

- Diagnosis is based on a lipid panel. A full fasting lipid panel consists of total cholesterol, HDL, LDL, and triglycerides.
    - Because triglycerides rise following a meal, only total cholesterol and HDL can be measured after a meal. Triglycerides and LDL can be measured only when fasting.
    - LDL is not measured directly; it is **calculated** on the basis of total cholesterol, HDL, and triglycerides. **High triglycerides (> 400)** make LDL calculation unreliable.
- Look for other contributing conditions. **Check glucose and TSH;** check body weight; and consider nephrotic syndrome.
- In patients with a family history of early heart disease, consider novel risk factors such as homocysteine, Lp(a), and C-reactive protein. These are treated with folic acid supplementation, niacin, and statins, respectively.

TREATMENT

Treatment is aimed at preventing pancreatitis when triglycerides are very high as well as preventing atherosclerotic disease (see Table 2.2-5).

- **Triglycerides:** If > 500, recommend dietary modification (↓ total fat and ↓ saturated fat) and aerobic exercise, and begin medication (fibrate or nicotinic acid). At lower levels, treatment can begin with diet and exercise, and medication can be added as needed. **Treat diabetes** if present.
- **LDL:** In patients with **diabetes or CAD, the goal LDL is < 70.** The mainstay of treatment is diet, exercise, and a statin. LDL control is the 1° cholesterol-related goal in patients with CAD or diabetes.
- **HDL:** Can be modestly ↑ with fibrate or nicotinic acid.

INFECTIVE ENDOCARDITIS

Inflammation of the heart valves. Can be infectious or noninfectious. Infectious endocarditis is commonly seen in IV drug abusers and in those with valvular lesions or prosthetic heart valves.

TABLE 2.2-5. Mechanisms and Side Effects of Cholesterol-Lowering Medications

MEDICATION	PRIMARY EFFECT	SIDE EFFECT	COMMENTS
HMG-CoA reductase inhibitors ("statins")	↓ LDL	Hepatitis, myositis.	A potent LDL-lowering medication.
Cholesterol absorption inhibitors (ezetimibe)	↓ LDL	Generally well tolerated; side effects are the same as those of placebo.	Introduced in 2003; its role in therapy is being defined.
Fibrates (gemfibrozil)	↓ triglycerides, slightly ↑ HDL	Potentiates myositis with statins.	
Bile acid–binding resins	↓ LDL	Bloating and cramping.	Most patients cannot tolerate GI side effects.
Nicotinic acid (niacin)	↓ LDL, ↑ HDL	Hepatitis, flushing.	Aspirin before doses ↓ flushing.

SYMPTOMS

- **Acute endocarditis:** Presents with fever, rigors, heart failure from valve destruction, and symptoms related to systemic emboli (neurologic impairment, back pain, pulmonary symptoms).
- **Subacute bacterial endocarditis:** Characterized by weeks to months of fever, malaise, and weight loss. Also presents with symptoms of systemic emboli.
- **Noninfectious endocarditis:** Generally asymptomatic. Can cause heart failure by destroying valves.

EXAM

- Look for a new **murmur.**
- Findings associated with emboli include focal neurologic deficits and tenderness to percussion over the spine.
- With infectious endocarditis, look at the fingers and toes for deep-seated, painful nodules (**Osler's nodes,** or "Ouchler's nodes") and small skin infarctions (**Janeway lesions**). Retinal exudates are called **Roth's spots.**

DIFFERENTIAL

The differential diagnosis of endocarditis is outlined below and in Table 2.2-6.

- **Differential of a vegetation found on echocardiography:** Infectious endocarditis, nonbacterial thrombotic endocarditis (NBTE, also known as marantic endocarditis), verrucous endocarditis (Libman-Sacks endocarditis), valve degeneration.
- **Differential of bacteremia:** Infectious endocarditis, infected hardware (e.g., from a central line), abscess, osteomyelitis.

DIAGNOSIS

- The discovery of noninfectious endocarditis is usually an incidental finding on echocardiography. It may be found during the workup of systemic emboli.
- Infectious endocarditis is diagnosed by a combination of lab and clinical data. If suspicious, obtain **three sets of blood cultures** and an echocardiogram. If the transthoracic echocardiogram is $\ominus$, proceed to **TEE** (more sensitive). $\oplus$ blood cultures and echocardiogram findings diagnose endocarditis. The Duke criteria are often used for diagnosis.

TABLE 2.2-6. Causes of Endocarditis

ACUTE	SUBACUTE	CULTURE NEGATIVE	NBTE (MARANTIC ENDOCARDITIS)	VERRUCOUS ENDOCARDITIS (LIBMAN-SACKS)
Most commonly *S. aureus.*	Viridans streptococci, *Enterococcus, S. epidermidis*, gram-negative rods, *Candida.*	HACEK organisms,[a] *Coxiella burnetii,* noncandidal fungi.	Thrombus formation on the valve is seen in many cancers.	Seen in lupus; vegetation is composed of fibrin, platelets, immune complexes, and inflammatory cells.

[a]**HACEK = H**aemophilus aphrophilus and **H.** parainfluenzae, **A**ctinobacillus actinomycetemcomitans, **C**ardiobacterium hominis, **E**ikenella corrodens, **K**ingella kingae.

Any patient with S. aureus bacteremia should be evaluated for endocarditis with echocardiography.

TREATMENT

- Treat with **prolonged antibiotic therapy,** generally for 4–6 weeks. Begin empiric therapy with gentamicin and antistaphylococcal penicillin (**oxacillin or nafcillin**). If there is a risk of methicillin-resistant *S. aureus*, use vancomycin instead of oxacillin/nafcillin.
- **Valve replacement** is appropriate for fungal endocarditis, **heart failure** from valve destruction, valve ring abscess, or systemic emboli despite adequate antibiotic therapy.
- Following treatment for infectious endocarditis, patients should receive endocarditis prophylaxis.
- For **NBTE,** treat the underlying disorder (often malignancy). Heparin is useful in the short term.
- For **verrucous endocarditis,** no treatment is required. Patients should receive endocarditis prophylaxis (see below).

PREVENTION

- Administer endocarditis prophylaxis only to patients whose cardiac conditions are associated with the **highest risk of an adverse outcome from endocarditis.** These include the following:
  - **Congenital cardiac disease:**
    - Patients with unrepaired cyanotic disease, including those with palliative shunts and devices.
    - Patients with congenital cardiac defects that have been completely repaired through use of prosthetic material/devices, whether surgically or percutaneously, during the first six months after the repair procedure (endothelialization occurs after six months).
    - Patients with repaired congenital cardiac disease who have residual defects at or adjacent to the site of a patch device that may inhibit endothelialization.
  - **Other:** Patients with prosthetic heart valves, those with previous infective endocarditis, and cardiac transplant patients with cardiac valvulopathy.
- Guidelines for prophylaxis are as follows:
  - **Dental procedures:** Prophylaxis is appropriate for all dental procedures that involve the manipulation of gingival tissue or the periapical region of teeth, or for procedures involving perforation of the oral mucosa (but **not** for routine anesthetic infections through noninfected tissue, dental radiographs, bleeding from trauma, adjustment of orthodontic devices, or shedding of deciduous teeth).
  - **Respiratory tract procedures:** Prophylaxis is indicated for any of the above-mentioned cardiac patients who are undergoing an invasive procedure of the respiratory tract that involves incision or biopsy of the respiratory mucosa (but **not** for bronchoscopy if no biopsy is performed).
  - **Skin procedures:** Prophylaxis is appropriate for any of the above-mentioned cardiac patients who are undergoing procedures involving infected skin, skin structures, or musculoskeletal tissue.
  - **GI and GU procedures:** Prophylaxis is not recommended but may be considered in special scenarios involving the above-mentioned cardiac patients.
- **Prophylactic regimens:** Amoxicillin (or clindamycin/azithromycin for those with penicillin allergy) 30–60 minutes before the procedure.

COMPLICATIONS

Spinal osteomyelitis, valve destruction and heart failure, embolic stroke.

SECTION II

Emergency Medicine

In dealing with a patient who has been exposed to a toxin, begin by determining which toxin was involved and the means by which the patient was exposed—e.g., through ingestion (most common), inhalation, injection, or absorption. Also determine the time and extent of the exposure, and ascertain if any other substances were involved. Ask about symptoms and determine if the exposure was intentional.

SYMPTOMS/EXAM/DIAGNOSIS

Vital signs may yield clues to the type of ingestion:

- **Hyperthermia:** Thyroid medication, nicotine, aspirin, anticholinergics, amphetamines, PCP, cocaine, SSRIs, neuroleptics.
- **Hypothermia:** Carbon monoxide, alcohol, sedative-hypnotics, barbiturates.
- **Tachycardia:** Cocaine, amphetamines, PCP, thyroid medication, anticholinergics, TCAs.
- **Bradycardia:** β-blockers, calcium channel blockers (CCBs), clonidine, digitalis, opioids.
- **Tachypnea:** Salicylates, organophosphates (e.g., pesticides).
- **Hypertension:** Amphetamines, cocaine, PCP, anticholinergics.
- **Hypotension:** Sedative-hypnotics, organophosphates, alcohols, opioids, digitalis, β-blockers, CCBs, TCAs.

Other diagnostic clues derived from physical findings include the following:

- **Breath odor:**
    - **Bitter almonds:** Cyanide.
    - **Violets:** Turpentine.
    - **Mothballs:** Camphor, naphthalene.
    - **Garlic:** Organophosphates.
    - **Pear:** Chloral hydrate.
- **Pupils:**
    - **Constricted:** Follow the mnemonic **COPS**—Clonidine, Opiates, Pontine bleed, Sedative-hypnotics.
    - **Dilated:** Amphetamines, anticholinergics, cocaine.
- **Pulmonary edema:** Opioids, salicylates, toxic inhalations (chlorine, nitric oxide, phosgene), cocaine, organophosphates, ethylene glycol.
- **Bowel sounds:**
    - **Increased:** Sympathomimetics, opiate withdrawal.
    - **Decreased:** Anticholinergics, opiate toxicity.
- **Skin findings:**
    - **Needle tracks:** Opioids.
    - **Diaphoresis:** Salicylates, organophosphates, sympathomimetics.
    - **Jaundice:** Acetaminophen (after liver failure), mushroom poisoning.
    - **Alopecia:** Arsenic, thallium, chemotherapeutic agents.
    - **Cyanosis:** Drugs causing methemoglobinemia (e.g., nitrates/nitrites, "caine" anesthetics, aniline dyes, chlorates, dapsone, sulfonamides).

Table 2.3-1 lists symptoms and signs associated with common toxin-induced syndromes (toxidromes).

TABLE 2.3-1. Common "Toxidromes"

	SYMPTOMS/SIGNS	EXAMPLES
Cholinergics	**DUMBBELS:** **D**iarrhea, **U**rination, **M**iosis, **B**radycardia, **B**ronchospasm, **E**mesis, **L**acrimation, **S**alivation.	Organophosphates, pilocarpine, pyridostigmine, muscarine-containing mushrooms.
Anticholinergics	"Hot as a stove, red as a beet, dry as a bone, mad as a hatter": fever, skin flushing, dry mucous membranes, psychosis, mydriasis, tachycardia, urinary retention.	TCAs, atropine, scopolamine, antihistamines, Jimson weed.
Opioids	Triad of coma, respiratory depression, and miosis.	Morphine, oxycodone, heroin.
Sedative-hypnotics	CNS depression, respiratory depression, and coma.	Alcohol, barbiturates, benzodiazepines.
Extrapyramidal	Parkinsonian symptoms: tremor, torticollis, trismus, rigidity, oculogyric crisis, opisthotonos, dysphonia, and dysphagia.	Phenothiazines, haloperidol, metoclopramide.

TREATMENT

Treatment options are as follows:

- **Elimination:**
  - **Activated charcoal:** First-line treatment. Administer in a dose of 1 g/kg. Avoid multiple doses of cathartics (e.g., sorbitol), especially in young children.
  - **Whole bowel irrigation** (e.g., polyethylene glycol with electrolytes to wash toxins from the GI tract): Useful for ingestions of lithium, iron, heavy metals, sustained-released drugs, and body packers (e.g., cocaine).
- **Removal of unabsorbed toxin:**
  - **Emesis:** Ipecac in adults (30 cc) and children (15 cc).
    - **Indications:** The patient is awake; the ingestion was recent (< 30–60 minutes); the ingestion was moderately or highly toxic.
    - **Contraindications:** Altered mental status, ↓ or absent gag reflex, caustic agents (to prevent reinjury of the esophagus on emesis), agents that are easily aspirated, nontoxic ingestion.
  - **Gastric lavage:**
    - **Indications:** The ingestion is known or suspected to be serious; the ingestion was recent (< 30–60 minutes before presentation); the patient is awake and cooperative or is intubated; the patient can be placed in the left lateral decubitus position.
    - **Contraindications:** The same as those for emetics (see above).
- **Removal of absorbed toxin:**
  - **Alkalization methods:** Involve mixing D_5W with 2–3 amps of $NaHCO_3$.
    - Alkalinization of blood improves clearance of TCAs.
    - Alkalinization of urine to a pH > 8 ionizes weak acids into ionized molecules, thereby increasing the excretion of salicylates, phenobarbital, and chlorpropamide.

- **Charcoal hemoperfusion:** ↑ absorption of toxic substances in the blood by filtering blood from a shunt through a column of activated charcoal. Particularly useful for aminophylline, barbiturates, carbamazepine, and digoxin.
- **Hemodialysis:** Filters **small, ionized molecules** such as salicylates, theophylline, methanol, lithium, barbiturates, and ethylene glycol.

Substance-specific antidotes are outlined in Table 2.3-2. Drug withdrawal treatments are delineated in Table 2.3-3.

TABLE 2.3-2. Specific Antidotes

TOXIN	ANTIDOTE
Acetaminophen	*N*-acetylcysteine
Anticholinesterases/ organophosphates	Atropine, pralidoxime
Antimuscarinics, anticholinergics	Physostigmine (crosses the blood-brain barrier)
Arsenic, mercury, lead	British anti-Lewisite (BAL): dimercaprol + 2,3-dimercaptosuccinic acid
Atropine	Physostigmine
Benzodiazepine	Flumazenil
β-blockers	Glucagon
Carbon monoxide	O_2
Cyanide	Amyl nitrite pearls, sodium nitrite, sodium thiosulfate
Digoxin	Digitalis Fab fragments
Ethylene glycol, methanol	Fomepizole; alternatively, ethanol drip
Heparin	Protamine sulfate
Iron	Deferoxamine
Isoniazid (INH)	Pyridoxine (vitamin B_6)
Lead	Calcium disodium edetate (EDTA)
Nitrites	Methylene blue
Opioids	Naloxone
Phenothiazines	Diphenhydramine, benztropine

(continues)

TABLE 2.3-2. Specific Antidotes *(continued)*

Toxin	Antidote
Salicylates	Sodium bicarbonate, dialysis
TCAs	Sodium bicarbonate
Warfarin	Vitamin K, fresh frozen plasma

SEXUAL ASSAULT

In dealing with a victim of sexual assault, begin by diagnosing and treating the victim's physical and emotional injuries. It is also critical to collect legal evidence as well as to document that evidence carefully and completely. Information sought should include the following:

- **Where and when** did the assault occur?
- What happened **during the assault?** Determine the following:
  - **Number** of assailants.
  - Use of force, weapons, objects, or restraints.
  - **Orifices** penetrated.
  - Use of alcohol or drugs.

TABLE 2.3-3. **Drug Withdrawal Syndromes and Treatment**

Drug	Withdrawal Symptoms	Treatment
Alcohol	Tremor, tachycardia, hypertension, agitation, seizures, hallucinations, **DTs** (autonomic instability, including tachycardia, hypertension, and delirium) within 2–7 days. Mortality is 15–20%.	Benzodiazepines; haloperidol for hallucinations. Thiamine, folate, and multivitamin replacement—i.e., **banana bag** (does not affect withdrawal but may prevent Wernicke's encephalopathy). Give thiamine before glucose.
Barbiturates	Anxiety, seizures, delirium, tremor, cardiac and respiratory depression.	Benzodiazepines.
Benzodiazepines	Rebound anxiety, seizures, tremor. May lead to **DTs.**	Benzodiazepines.
Cocaine and amphetamines	Depression, hyperphagia, hypersomnolence.	Supportive treatment. Avoid β-blockers in cocaine users (→ uninhibited α-cardiac stimulation with cocaine use).
Opioids	Anxiety, insomnia, **flulike symptoms,** sweating, piloerection, fever, rhinorrhea, nausea, stomach cramps, diarrhea, mydriasis.	Symptom management. Clonidine and/or buprenorphine for moderate withdrawal; methadone for severe symptoms.

- What happened **after the assault?**
  - Did the patient bathe, defecate, urinate, brush teeth, or change clothes?
  - Are there any specific symptoms or pains?
- Has the patient had **sexual intercourse in the last 72 hours?**
- Determine the **risk of pregnancy.** Last menstrual period? Any birth control?

EXAM

Conduct a general trauma and pelvic exam (see the discussion of trauma on the following page).

DIAGNOSIS

- Medically indicated tests include the following:
  - Pregnancy test.
  - Culture for gonorrhea and chlamydia.
  - Serology for syphilis.
  - HBV and HCV testing.
  - HIV testing.
- **Evidence collection:** The following must pass through an unbroken **chain of evidence:**
  - Debris and dried secretions from skin.
  - Combed and plucked head and pubic hairs.
  - Fingernail scraping and clipped fingernails.
  - Saliva sample.
  - Oral, anal, and vaginal smears.
  - Blood sample.
  - Nasal mucus sample.

TREATMENT

- Treat traumatic injuries.
- **Infection prevention:**
  - Where appropriate, treat gonorrhea, chlamydia, trichomoniasis, and bacterial vaginosis.
  - Institute HBV and HIV prophylaxis.
- **Pregnancy prevention:** Administer two Ovral tablets PO stat and in 12 hours.
- Offer counseling.

TRAUMA

Always do the trauma algorithm in order.

In dealing with trauma patients, begin with the ABCs and **1° survey** and then progress to resuscitation and the **2° survey.**

ABCs and 1° Survey

Initiate trauma treatment as follows:

- **A: A**irway maintenance with cervical spine control.
- **B: B**reathing with ventilation.
- **C: C**irculation with hemorrhage control.
- **D: D**isability—brief neurologic examination:
  - **AVPU system: A**—Alert; **V**—responds to Vocal stimuli; **P**—responds to Painful stimuli; **U**—Unresponsive.

- **Glasgow Coma Scale (GCS):** Based on the **best** response of E + V + M (see Figure 2.3-1).
- **Other neurologic exam:** Examine for unequal pupils, depressed skull fracture, focal weakness, and posturing.
- **E: Exposure/Environmental control**—completely undress the patient, but prevent hypothermia.
- **Resuscitation:**
  - **IV access:** Think **short and fat** IV lines—e.g., two large-bore, 18-gauge antecubital lines.
  - Estimate and replace fluid and blood losses.

The maximum score on the GCS is 15; the lowest score is 3.

2° Survey

The **2° survey**—total patient evaluation—proceeds as follows:

- **AMPLE history:** Inquire about **A**llergies, **M**edications, **P**ast medical history, **L**ast meal eaten, and **E**vents/Environment related to the injury.
- **Organ system assessment and management:**
  - **Head and skull:**
    - **Assessment:** Inspect for trauma, pupils, and loss of consciousness. Examine for hemorrhage around the mastoid (**Battle's sign**), eyes (**raccoon eyes**), and tympanic membrane (all are indicative of a basilar skull fracture). Inspect the nose for CSF leakage and for an unstable airway due to facial fractures.
    - **Management:** Maintain the airway; continue oxygenation and ventilation. Obtain a CT scan of the head and face if indicated; intubate if necessary. **If the GCS is < 8, intubate!**
  - **Neck:**
    - **Assessment:** Look for trauma; palpate for midline tenderness/deformity and tracheal deformity.
    - **Management:** Maintain in-line immobilization and protection with a hard cervical collar. Obtain cervical spine radiographs as needed.
  - **Chest:**
    - **Assessment:** Inspect for irregular or paradoxical breathing patterns resulting from multiple rib fractures—i.e., **flail chest.** Listen for equal and bilateral breath sounds (if not found, suspect **pneumothorax**) and for clear heart sounds (if muffled and accompanied by JVD, suspect **cardiac tamponade**).
    - **Management:** Tube thoracostomy for pneumothorax (needle thoracostomy for tension pneumothorax); pericardiocentesis for cardiac tamponade.

GCS < 8—intubate!

Eye Opening (E)	Verbal Response (V)	Motor Response (M)
4 Spontaneous	**5** Oriented	**6** Obeys commands
3 Responds to voice	**4** Confused speech	**5** Localizes pain
2 Responds to pain	**3** Inappropriate speech	**4** Withdraws to pain
1 No response	**2** Incomprehensible	**3** Abnormal flexion
	1 No response	**2** Abnormal extension
		1 No response

FIGURE 2.3-1. **Scoring of the Glasgow Coma Scale.**

The spleen is the most commonly injured solid organ in blunt abdominal trauma.

- **Abdomen:**
  - **Assessment:** Inspect the anterior and posterior abdomen for signs of trauma. Palpate the pelvis for tenderness or instability. Obtain a pelvic x-ray; arrange for an abdominal ultrasound/abdominal CT if indicated.
  - **Management:** Transfer to an OR in the presence of a penetrating wound to the abdomen deeper than the fascia or with any significant bleeding or bowel injury.
- **Perineum/rectum/vagina:** Assess for trauma, including urethral bleeding. Check for prostate position, rectal tone, and rectal blood. In female patients, check for vaginal trauma and blood in the vaginal vault.
- **Musculoskeletal system:**
  - **Assessment:** Look for evidence of trauma, including contusions, lacerations, and deformities. Inspect the extremities for tenderness, crepitus, abnormal range of motion, and sensation.
  - **Management:** Obtain radiographs as needed. Maintain immobilization of the patient's thoracic and lumbar spine; apply a splint as indicated. Open fractures and suspected compartment syndromes require urgent orthopedic consultation. Administer tetanus immunization as required.

COMMON DYSRHYTHMIAS

Figures 2.3-2 through 2.3-13 illustrate a variety of board-testable dysrhythmias.

ADVANCED CARDIAC LIFE SUPPORT (ACLS)

Start with CPR and determine rhythm. Then proceed as outlined below.

ACLS steps—ABCDEF

Airway
Breathing
Circulation
Drugs
Electricity (shock)
Fluids

Ventricular Fibrillation (VF)/Pulseless Ventricular Tachycardia (VT)

- **Shock** once (up to 360 J if monophasic and 250 J if biphasic).
- Then administer **epinephrine** (up to three times) → shock → vasopressin → shock.
- Amiodarone, lidocaine, magnesium, or procainamide may be tried. Shock after each dose.

Pulseless Electrical Activity (PEA)

- Identify and treat underlying causes:
  - **The 5 H's**—Hypovolemia, Hypoxia, H$^+$ acidosis, Hyper-/Hypokalemia, Hypothermia.
  - **The 5 T's**—Tablets (drug OD), cardiac Tamponade, Tension pneumothorax, Thrombosis (coronary), Thrombosis (pulmonary embolism).
- Epinephrine q 3–5 minutes × 3.
- Atropine q 3–5 minutes × 3 in the setting of a slow PEA rate.

Asystole

- Identify and treat underlying causes.
- Consider a transcutaneous pacemaker.
- Epinephrine q 3–5 minutes × 3 or vasopressin × 1.
- Atropine q 3–5 minutes × 3.

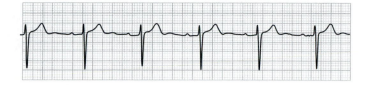

FIGURE 2.3-2. First-degree AV block.

(Reproduced, with permission, from Gomella LG, Haist SA. *Clinician's Pocket Reference*, 10th ed. New York: McGraw-Hill, 2004: 394.)

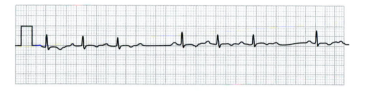

FIGURE 2.3-3. Second-degree AV block, Mobitz I/Wenckebach: progressive PR widening.

(Reproduced, with permission, from Gomella LG, Haist SA. *Clinician's Pocket Reference*, 10th ed. New York: McGraw-Hill, 2004: 394.)

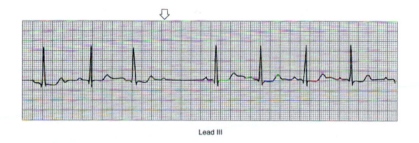

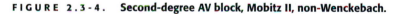

Lead III

FIGURE 2.3-4. Second-degree AV block, Mobitz II, non-Wenckebach.

(Reproduced, with permission, from Hay W et al. *Current Pediatric Diagnosis and Treatment*, 17th ed. New York: McGraw-Hill, 2005: 623.)

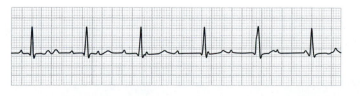

FIGURE 2.3-5. Third-degree AV block.

(Reproduced, with permission, from Gomella LG, Haist SA. *Clinician's Pocket Reference*, 10th ed. New York: McGraw-Hill, 2004: 395.)

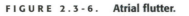

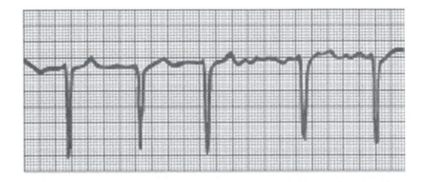

FIGURE 2.3-6.   Atrial flutter.

(Reproduced, with permission, from Gomella LG, Haist SA. *Clinician's Pocket Reference*, 10th ed. New York: McGraw-Hill, 2004: 391.)

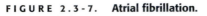

FIGURE 2.3-7.   Atrial fibrillation.

(Reproduced, with permission, from Kasper DL et al. *Harrison's Principles of Internal Medicine*, 16th ed. New York: McGraw-Hill, 2005: 1344.)

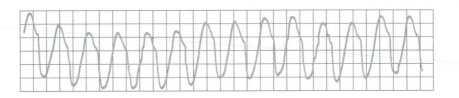

FIGURE 2.3-8.   Ventricular tachycardia.

(Reproduced, with permission, from Katzung BG. *Basic & Clinical Pharmacology*, 8th ed. New York: McGraw-Hill, 2001: 1016.)

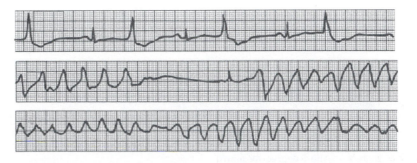

FIGURE 2.3-9.   Torsades de pointes.

(Reproduced, with permission, from Kasper DL et al. *Harrison's Principles of Internal Medicine*, 16th ed. New York: McGraw-Hill, 2005: 1353.)

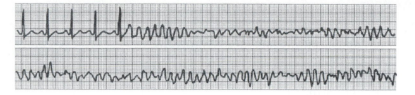

FIGURE 2.3-10. Ventricular fibrillation.

(Reproduced, with permission, from Kasper DL et al. *Harrison's Principles of Internal Medicine,* 16th ed. New York: McGraw-Hill, 2005: 1354.)

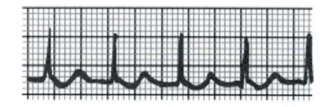

FIGURE 2.3-11. AV nodal reentrant tachycardia.

(Reproduced, with permission, from Kasper DL et al. *Harrison's Principles of Internal Medicine,* 16th ed. New York: McGraw-Hill, 2005: 1349.)

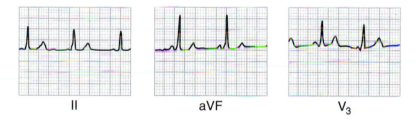

| II | aVF | V3 |

FIGURE 2.3-12. Wolff-Parkinson-White syndrome (slurred upstroke – delta wave).

(Reproduced, with permission, from Gomella LG, Haist SA. *Clinician's Pocket Reference,* 10th ed. New York: McGraw-Hill, 2004: 402.)

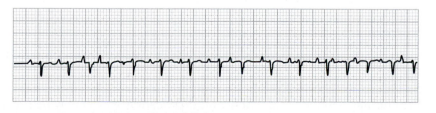

FIGURE 2.3-13. Multifocal atrial tachycardia.

(Reproduced, with permission, from Gomella LG, Haist SA. *Clinician's Pocket Reference,* 10th ed. New York: McGraw-Hill, 2004: 390.)

Bradycardia

- Atropine q 3–5 minutes × 3 prn.
- Transcutaneous pacemaker (also appropriate with 2° or 3° **AV block**).
- Dopamine drip.
- Epinephrine drip.
- Isoproterenol drip.

Unstable Tachycardia

Synchronized cardioversion.

Stable Supraventricular Tachycardia (SVT)

- Vagal stimulation.
- Adenosine 6 mg IV push (both diagnostic and therapeutic).
- Adenosine 12 mg IV push.
- IV diltiazem if no CHF.
- Adenosine 12 mg IV push.

Stable Monomorphic Ventricular Tachycardia

- Procainamide or sotalol.
- Amiodarone or lidocaine.
- In the setting of CHF, amiodarone or lidocaine followed by DC cardioversion.

Stable Wide-Complex Tachycardia

- If no CHF, treat with DC cardioversion, procainamide, or amiodarone.
- In the setting of CHF, treat with DC cardioversion or amiodarone.

HEAT EMERGENCIES

Heat Exhaustion

- Extreme fatigue with **profuse sweating**. Also presents with nausea/vomiting and a dull headache.
- **Sx/Exam:** Body temperature is **normal** or **slightly elevated.** Patients are tachypneic, tachycardic, and hypotensive.
- **Tx:** Treat with IV NS and a cool environment.

Heat Stroke

- Elevation of body temperature above normal due to temperature dysregulation. Constitutes a **true emergency.**
- **Sx/Exam:** Presents with ↑ **body temperature** and altered mental status. Patients have hot, dry skin, often with no sweating. Ataxia may be seen.
- **Tx:** Treat with **aggressive cooling.** Remove from the heat source and undress. Use an atomized tepid water spray; apply ice packs to the groin/axillae.

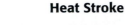

Heat stroke presents with altered mental status and ↑ temperature, often with no sweating.

Frostbite

- Cold injury with pallor and loss of cold sensation. Results from exposure to cold air **or** direct contact with cold materials. Nonviable structures demarcate and slough off. Subtypes are as follows:
  - **Superficial:** Injury to cutaneous and subcutaneous tissue. Skin is soft under a frozen surface. Large, clear, fluid-filled vesicles develop within two days (indicating a good prognosis); sloughing leaves new skin that is pink and hypersensitive.
  - **Deep:** Injury to the above tissues plus deep structures (muscle, bone). Skin is hard under a frozen surface.
- **Tx:** Rapidly rewarm once refreezing can be prevented. Circulating water at 40°C; wound care; tetanus prophylaxis.

Do not rewarm frostbite until refreezing can be prevented.

Hypothermia

- Defined as a core body temperature < 35°C (< 95°F).
- Causes include environmental exposure, **alcohol ingestion,** drugs (barbiturates, benzodiazepines, narcotics), hypoglycemia, CNS or hypothalamic dysfunction (via loss of stimulus of shivering response and adrenal activity), hypothyroidism, skin disorders, and sepsis.
- **Dx:** Look for **Osborn/J waves** on ECG.
- **Tx:**
  - ABCs, CPR, and stabilization.
  - **Rewarming:**
    - **Passive external:** Blankets.
    - **Active external:** Warmed blankets; hot water bottles.
    - **Active internal:** Warm humidified O$_2$; heated IV fluids; gastric, colonic, bladder, or peritoneal lavage; extracorporeal rewarming.
    - Do not pronounce patients until they have been rewarmed to 35°C; full recovery is not uncommon.
- **Cx:** Associated with a risk of dysrhythmias, especially VF at core temperatures < 30°C. **Bretylium** is generally the drug of choice.

"No one is dead until they're warm and dead."

In dealing with burn patients, begin by determining if the victim is in an enclosed or an open space. Are there any toxic products of combustion? Any respiratory symptoms? Consider carbon monoxide poisoning.

EXAM

- Gauge the body surface area (BSA) involved. Observe the **rule of 9's: 9%** BSA for the head and each arm; **18%** BSA for the back torso, the front torso, and each leg. In **children,** the rule is 9% BSA for each arm; 18% BSA for the head, back torso, and front torso; and 14% BSA for each leg.
- Determine the **depth of the burn** (see Table 2.3-4).

TREATMENT

- **Prehospital treatment:**
  - Administer IV fluids and high-flow O$_2$.
  - Remove the patient's clothes and cover with clean sheets or dressings.
  - Administer pain medications.

TABLE 2.3-4. Burn Classification

	TISSUE INVOLVEMENT	FINDINGS
First degree	Epidermis only.	Red and painful.
Second degree (superficial)	Epidermis and superficial dermis.	Red, wet, and painful with **blisters.**
Second degree (deep)	Epidermis and deep dermis.	White, dry, and tender.
Third degree	Epidermis and **entire dermis.**	Charred, pearly white, and **nontender.**
Fourth degree	Below the dermis to bone, muscle, and fascia.	

- **In-hospital treatment:**
  - **ABCs: Early airway control** is critical. Intubate if:
    - The patient is unconscious or obtunded.
    - The patient is in respiratory distress with facial burns, soot in the airway, singed nasal hairs, and carbonaceous sputum.
  - **Fluid resuscitation:** Appropriate for patients with > 20% BSA second-degree burns.
    - Give 4 cc/kg per % total BSA (**Parkland formula**) over 24 hours—the first half over the first 8 hours and the second half over the next 16 hours.
    - Maintain a urine output of 1 cc/kg/hr.
  - Additional treatment: Tetanus prophylaxis; pain control.
- **Disposition:**
  - **Minor burns:** Discharge with pain medications.
  - **Moderate burns** (partial thickness 15–25% BSA or full thickness < 10% BSA): Admit to the hospital.
  - **Major burns** (partial thickness > 25% BSA or full thickness > 10% BSA; burns to the face, hands, joints, feet, or perineum; electrical or circumferential burns): Refer to a burn center.

ELECTRICAL INJURIES

Electrical current flows most easily through tissues of low resistance (e.g., nerves, blood vessels, mucous membranes, muscles). The current pathway determines which organs are affected.

SYMPTOMS/EXAM

Symptoms vary according to the nature of the current:

- **Alternating current (household and commercial):**
  - Associated with explosive exit wounds.
  - Effects are worse with AC than with DC current at the same voltage.
  - VF is common.
- **Direct current (industrial, batteries, lightning):**
  - Causes discrete exit wounds.
  - Asystole is common.

TREATMENT

- ABCs; IV fluids for severe burns.
- Administer pain medications and treat burns.
- Treat **myoglobinuria** with IV fluids to maintain a urine output of 1.5–2.0 cc/kg/hr.
- Tetanus prophylaxis.
- Asymptomatic low-voltage (< 1000-V) burn victims can be discharged.

TETANUS

Presents with trismus (i.e., lockjaw), glottal spasm, and convulsive spasms. High-risk patients include the elderly (due to inadequate immunization), IV drug users, and ulcer patients.

TREATMENT

- Benzodiazepine to control muscle spasms; neuromuscular blockade if needed to control the airway.
- **Metronidazole** is the antibiotic of choice.
- Administer tetanus immune globulin (TIG) and/or adsorbed tetanus and diphtheria toxoid (Td) vaccine as indicated in Table 2.3-5.

ANIMAL BITES

- The treatment protocol for animal bites is as follows:
  - If the bite is from a domestic animal that can be captured/secured and its behavior observed as normal for 10 days, no treatment is necessary.
  - If the bite is from a domestic animal that exhibits abnormal behavior or becomes ill, the animal should be sacrificed and its head/brain tested for rabies via a direct immunofluorescent antibody study. If that study is ⊖, no treatment is necessary. If it is ⊕, immediate treatment is indicated.
  - If the animal is wild, immediate treatment is indicated.
- Treatment options include the following:
  - **Active immunization** with human diploid cell vaccine (HDCV).
  - **Passive immunization** with **human rabies immune globulin (HRIG)**.
- Table 2.3-6 summarizes bite types (including human), associated infecting organisms, and appropriate treatment.

TABLE 2.3-5.   Tetanus Prophylaxis Schedule

HISTORY OF ADSORBED TETANUS TOXOID (DOSES)	NON-TETANUS-PRONE WOUNDS	TETANUS-PRONE WOUNDS[a]	
	Td	Td	TIG
Unknown or < 3 doses	✓	✓	✓
Three doses:			
Last dose > 5 years		✓	
Last dose > 10 years	✓	✓	

[a]Tetanus-prone wounds are those that are present > 6 hours; are nonlinear; are > 1 cm deep; and show signs of infection, devitalized tissue, and contamination.

TABLE 2.3-6. Bite Types, Infecting Organisms, and Treatment

BITE TYPE	LIKELY ORGANISMS	TREATMENT
Dog	α-hemolytic streptococci, *S. aureus,* and *Pasteurella multocida.*	**Amoxicillin/clavulanate** or a first-generation cephalosporin +/– tetanus and rabies prophylaxis.
Cat	**P. multocida** (high rate of infection).	**Amoxicillin/clavulanate** +/– tetanus.
Human	Polymicrobial. Viridans streptococci are most frequently implicated.	Second- or third-generation cephalosporins, dicloxacillin + penicillin, **amoxicillin/clavulanate,** or clarithromycin +/– tetanus prophylaxis, HBV vaccine HBIG, and postexposure HIV prophylaxis.

EYE CONDITIONS

Corneal Abrasion

- **Sx/Exam:** Presents with **pain out of proportion to the exam** as well as with foreign-body sensation and photophobia.
- **Dx:** Fluorescein staining (cobalt blue light source via slit-lamp or Wood's lamp examination) reveals an abraded area.
- **Tx:** Treat with topical broad-spectrum antibiotics (e.g., gentamicin, sulfacetamide, bacitracin), tetanus prophylaxis, and oral analgesics.

Viral Conjunctivitis

- **Sx/Exam:** Presents as a painful, itchy, red eye with watery discharge. The condition is **frequently bilateral** and often occurs in conjunction with cold symptoms (e.g., rhinorrhea, sore throat, cough).
- **Dx:** Look for diffuse conjunctival injection with normal vision and **preauricular lymphadenopathy.** Multiple superficial punctate corneal lesions are seen on fluorescein staining.
- **Tx:** Treat with topical antibiotics to prevent bacterial superinfection.

Bacterial Conjunctivitis

- Painful, red eye that is **usually unilateral.** Causative organisms include *Staphylococcus, Streptococcus, Neisseria gonorrhoeae,* and *Chlamydia trachomatis* (in newborns and sexually active adults).
- **Sx/Exam:** Presents with photophobia, a gritty foreign-body sensation, and purulent exudate.
- **Dx:** Diffuse conjunctival injection with normal visual acuity. Bacteria can be seen on Gram stain.
- **Tx:**
  - Treat staphylococcal and streptococcal infection with topical **10% sulfacetamide** or aminoglycoside; treat suspected *N. gonorrhoeae* with IV ceftriaxone and topical erythromycin or tetracycline.
  - IV and topical erythromycin are appropriate for *Chlamydia.*
  - Warm compresses and frequent flushes are also of benefit.

Allergic Conjunctivitis

- Intensely pruritic, watery eyes. Most commonly affects males with a family history of atopy.
- **Sx/Exam/Dx:** Look for diffuse conjunctival injection with normal visual acuity. Lid edema and cobblestone papillae under the upper lid may also be seen.
- **Tx:** Treat with topical antihistamine/vasoconstrictor preparations such as **naphazoline/pheniramine** or mast cell stabilizers such as **cromolyn** or **olopatadine.** Cool compresses are also of benefit.

Chemical Conjunctivitis

- Caused by acid or alkali exposure.
- **Dx:** Determine pH from litmus paper. **Coagulation necrosis** is associated with acid burns; **liquefaction necrosis** is seen in alkali burns.
- **Tx:** Treat with copious irrigation with a Morgan lens until pH is neutral; provide tetanus prophylaxis.

Alkali burns do far more damage than acid burns.

Ruptured Globe

- **Sx/Exam:** Patients present with trauma and loss of vision. Exam may reveal a vitreous humor leak → a teardrop-shaped pupil as well as a marked ↓ in visual acuity.
- **Dx:** Order a CT scan. Diagnosis can often be made only by clinical means.
- **Tx:** Manage with a rigid eye shield to prevent pressure on the globe. An immediate ophthalmologic consultation is necessary.

SECTION II

Endocrinology

The 3 P's of DM type 1:

Polydipsia
Polyphagia
Polyuria

The "honeymoon period" is a remission phase that is seen in type 1 diabetics days after the initiation of insulin therapy. During this phase, which may last several months, patients often have ↓ insulin requirements.

Type 1 Diabetes Mellitus

Destruction of the pancreatic beta cells → insulin deficiency (see Table 2.4-1). Generally immune mediated.

SYMPTOMS/EXAM

Presents with the classic symptoms of Polyuria (including nocturia), Polydipsia, and Polyphagia (**the 3 P's**). Patients may also have rapid or unexplained weight loss, blurry vision, or recurrent infections (e.g., candidiasis).

DIFFERENTIAL

Pancreatic disease (e.g., chronic pancreatitis), glucagonoma, Cushing's disease, iatrogenic factors (e.g., corticosteroids), gestational diabetes, diabetes insipidus.

DIAGNOSIS

At least one of the following is required to make the diagnosis:

- A random plasma glucose concentration of ≥ 200 mg/dL with classic symptoms of diabetes.
- A fasting plasma glucose of ≥ 126 mg/dL on two separate occasions.
- A two-hour postprandial glucose of ≥ 200 mg/dL after a 75-g oral glucose tolerance test on two separate occasions.

TABLE 2.4-1.   Type 1 vs. Type 2 DM

	TYPE 1 (INSULIN-DEPENDENT DM)	TYPE 2 (NON-INSULIN-DEPENDENT DM)
Pathophysiology	Failure of the pancreas to secrete insulin as a result of autoimmune destruction of beta cells.	Insulin resistance and inadequate insulin secretion by the pancreas to compensate.
Incidence	15%.	85%.
Age (exceptions are common)	< 30 years of age.	> 40 years of age.
Association with obesity	No.	Yes.
"Classic symptoms"	Common.	Sometimes.
Diabetic ketoacidosis (DKA)	Common.	Rare.
Genetic predisposition	Weak, polygenic.	Strong, polygenic.
Association with HLA system	Yes (HLA-DR3 and -DR4).	No.
Serum C-peptide	↓; can be normal during the "honeymoon period."	↓ late in the disease.

- Type 1 diabetics should be started on insulin (see Table 2.4-2). Both basal and bolus insulin is required. Oral hypoglycemic agents are not effective.
- Most people with type 1 diabetes are on a multiple-daily-injection (MDI) regimen consisting of pre-meal short-acting insulin (e.g., Lispro or Aspart) and bedtime glargine. Others are on insulin pumps consisting of short-acting insulin.
- Long-term management should include the following:
  - Check a **hemoglobin A_{1c} (HbA$_{1c}$)** level every three months. Maintain HbA$_{1c}$ < 7.
  - Maintain a low-fat, reduced-carbohydrate diet, and refer patients to a dietitian.
  - Manage **CAD risk factors** (hypertension, smoking, obesity, hyperlipidemia).
  - Obtain a baseline ECG if the patient has heart disease or is > 35 years of age.
  - Check eyes annually for retinopathy or cataracts. An eye exam is also indicated if the patient is planning a pregnancy.
  - Screen newly diagnosed type 1 diabetics for **thyroid disease.**
  - Order an annual BUN/creatinine and UA for **microalbuminuria** to screen for diabetic nephropathy.
  - Check the **feet** annually for neuropathy, ulcers, and peripheral vascular disease. Patients should inspect their feet daily and wear comfortable shoes.
  - Administer an annual flu shot and keep pneumococcal vaccinations up to date.

Type 2 Diabetes Mellitus

Patients with type 2 DM have two defects: insufficient insulin secretion and ↑ insulin resistance (see Table 2.4-1).

TABLE 2.4-2. Types of Insulin[a]

INSULIN	ONSET	PEAK EFFECT	DURATION
Regular	30–60 minutes	2–4 hours	5–8 hours
Humalog (lispro)	5–10 minutes	0.5–1.5 hours	6–8 hours
NovoLog (aspart)	10–20 minutes	1–3 hours	3–5 hours
Apidra (glulisine)	5–15 minutes	1.0–1.5 hours	1.0–2.5 hours
Exubera (inhaled)	10–12 minutes	0.5–1.5 hours	6 hours
NPH	2–4 hours	6–10 hours	18–28 hours
Levemir (detemir)	2 hours	No discernible peak	20 hours
Lantus (glargine)	1–4 hours	No discernible peak	20–24 hours

[a]Combination preparations mix longer-acting and shorter-acting types of insulin together to provide immediate and extended coverage in the same injection, e.g., 70 NPH/30 regular = 70% NPH + 30% regular.

Reproduced, with permission, from Le T et al. *First Aid for the USMLE Step 2,* 6th ed. New York: McGraw-Hill, 2007: 108.

SYMPTOMS/EXAM

The 3 P's (see above), recurrent blurred vision, paresthesias, and fatigue are common to both forms of diabetes. Because of the insidious onset of hyperglycemia, however, type 2 DM patients may be asymptomatic at the time of diagnosis.

DIFFERENTIAL

Similar to that of type 1 DM.

DIAGNOSIS

Similar to that of type 1 DM.

TREATMENT

- Diet and exercise are critical. Type 2 diabetics should be started on an oral antidiabetic medication (see Table 2.4-3).
- Typical stepwise pharmacologic management includes metformin, a "glitazone," and a sulfonylurea (e.g., glyburide).
- If the patient continues to have inadequate control on three oral antidiabetic drugs, glyburide should be replaced with NPH or glargine insulin at bedtime.
- For those who require more intense therapy, a split/mixed regimen of regular and NPH insulin may be used.
    - **Pre-breakfast glucose level:** Reflects pre-dinner NPH dose.
    - **Pre-lunch glucose level:** Reflects pre-breakfast regular insulin dose.

TABLE 2.4-3. Oral Antidiabetic Medications

MEDICATION	EXAMPLES	MECHANISM OF ACTION	SIDE EFFECTS	CONTRAINDICATIONS
Sulfonylureas	**First generation:** Chlorpropamide **Second generation:** Glipizide, glyburide	↑ insulin secretion.	Hypoglycemia.	Renal/liver disease.
Meglitinides	Repaglinide	↑ insulin secretion.	Hypoglycemia.	Renal/liver disease.
Biguanides	Metformin	Inhibit hepatic gluconeogenesis; ↑ glucose utilization; ↓ insulin resistance.	Lactic acidosis, diarrhea, GI discomfort, metallic taste, weight loss.	Renal insufficiency, any form of acidosis, liver disease, severe hypoxia.
α-glucosidase inhibitors	Acarbose	↓ glucose absorption.	↑ flatulence, GI discomfort, elevated LFTs.	Renal/liver disease.
Thiazolinediones ("glitazones")	Rosiglitazone, pioglitazone	↓ insulin resistance; ↑ glucose utilization.	Hepatocellular injury, anemia, pedal edema, CHF.	Liver disease, CHF (class III/IV), LFTs > 2 times normal.
Glucagon-like peptide-1 (GLP-1) agonists	Exenatide	↑ postprandial glucose utilization	Nausea, vomiting, weight loss, pain at injection site, hypoglycemia.	Renal disease.

- **Pre-dinner glucose level:** Reflects pre-breakfast NPH dose.
- **Bedtime glucose level:** Reflects pre-dinner regular insulin dose.
- Long-term management includes **monitoring blood glucose** (see Table 2.4-4) and checking a fasting glucose level once a day. Otherwise, management is similar to that of type 1.

Complications of Diabetes Mellitus

DIABETIC KETOACIDOSIS (DKA)

DKA may be the initial manifestation of **type 1 DM** and is usually precipitated by a stressor (e.g., infection, surgery). $\uparrow$ catabolism due to lack of insulin action plus $\uparrow$ counterregulatory hormones $\rightarrow$ life-threatening metabolic acidosis. Hyperkalemia is due to $\downarrow$ insulin and hyperosmolality, **not** H^+-K^+ shifts.

SYMPTOMS/EXAM

Symptoms and signs of DKA include a "fruity" breath odor, Kussmaul hyperpnea, dehydration, abdominal pain, an $\uparrow$ anion gap, hyperkalemia, hyperglycemia, and ketones in the blood and urine.

DIAGNOSIS

- Order a CBC, electrolytes, BUN/creatinine, glucose, ABG, serum ketones, CXR, blood culture, UA/urine cultures, and an ECG.
- Labs reveal hyperglycemia (blood glucose > 250 mg/dL), acidosis with blood pH < 7.3, serum bicarbonate < 15 mEq/L, and $\uparrow$ serum/urine ketones.

TREATMENT

- Admission to the ICU/floor may be necessary depending on the patient's clinical status.
- Fluid resuscitation (3–4 L in eight hours) with NS and IV insulin.
- Sodium, potassium, phosphate, and glucose must be monitored and repleted every two hours (change NS fluids to D5NS when glucose < 250 mg/L).
- Change IV insulin to a SQ insulin sliding scale once the anion gap normalizes.

HYPERGLYCEMIC HYPEROSMOLAR NONKETOTIC STATE (HHNK)

Typically occurs in **type 2 DM.** Can be precipitated by dehydration, infection, or medications (e.g., β-blockers, steroids, thiazides).

SYMPTOMS/EXAM

Patients are acutely ill and are dehydrated with altered mental status.

> **Symptoms and signs of DKA:**
>
> "**F**ruity" breath
> **K**ussmaul hyperpnea
> **D**ehydration
> **A**bdominal pain
> $\uparrow$ anion gap
> **H**yperkalemia
> **H**yperglycemia
> **K**etones in blood/urine

TABLE 2.4-4. Target Glucose Levels in Diabetics

	NORMAL GLUCOSE LEVEL (mg/dL)	TARGET GLUCOSE LEVEL WITH DRUG TREATMENT (mg/dL)	ADJUST DOSAGE OF DRUG WHEN GLUCOSE LEVEL IS:
Preprandial glucose	< 110	80–120	< 80 or > 140
Bedtime glucose	< 120	100–140	< 100 or > 160

DIAGNOSIS

Diagnostic criteria for HHNK are as follows:

- Serum glucose > 600 mg/dL (hyperglycemia)
- Serum pH > 7.3
- Serum bicarbonate > 15 mEq/L
- Anion gap < 14 mEq/L (normal)
- Serum osmolality > 310 mOsm/kg

TREATMENT

- Fluid resuscitate with 4–6 L NS within the first eight hours.
- Identify the precipitating cause and treat.
- Monitor and replete sodium, potassium, phosphate, and glucose every two hours. Give IV insulin only if glucose levels remain elevated after sufficient fluid resuscitation.

OTHER COMPLICATIONS

Both type 1 and type 2 diabetics are at ↑ risk for macro- and microvascular disease and infections. The three most common microvascular complications are as follows:

- **Retinopathy:**
  - Correlates with the duration of DM and the degree of glycemic control.
  - **Sx/Exam:** Classified as nonproliferative or proliferative.
    - **Nonproliferative diabetic retinopathy:** Characterized by retinal vascular microaneurysms, blot hemorrhages, and cotton wool spots. Macular edema may be seen.
    - **Proliferative diabetic retinopathy:** Neovascularization in response to retinal hypoxia is the hallmark.
  - **Tx:** Prevention, regular eye exams, and laser therapy are the mainstays of therapy.
- **Nephropathy:**
  - **Sx/Exam:** Usually asymptomatic, but can present with bilateral lower extremity edema (from nephrotic syndrome).
  - **Dx:**
    - Kimmelstiel-Wilson lesions (nodular glomerulosclerosis) may be seen on kidney biopsy.
    - Look for **coexisting retinopathy.**
  - **Tx:**
    - Patients with microalbuminuria or proteinuria should be started on an ACEI to keep their BP < 125/75.
    - End-stage nephropathy requires chronic hemodialysis or transplantation.
- **Neuropathy:**
  - **Sx/Exam:** Can present as polyneuropathy, mononeuropathy, and/or autonomic neuropathy.
  - **Tx:**
    - Strict glycemic control improves nerve conduction.
    - TCAs and carbamazepine are used to treat sensory dysfunction.

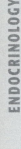

Diabetics have ↑ susceptibility to the following:

- *Pseudomonal external otitis*
- *Mucormycosis facial infection*
- *Pyelonephritis*
- *Emphysematous cholangitis*

Classified as hyperthyroidism or hypothyroidism. **Myxedema coma** is a form of severe hypothyroidism characterized by altered mental status and hypothermia. **Thyroid storm** is a form of severe hyperthyroidism that is characterized by high fever, dehydration, tachycardia, coma, and high-output cardiac failure.

SYMPTOMS/EXAM

Table 2.4-5 lists distinguishing features of hypo- and hyperthyroidism.

DIAGNOSIS

- Order a TSH and a free T_4 to distinguish hyperthyroidism from hypothyroidism.
  - **Hyperthyroid patients ($\downarrow$ TSH):** Order a radioactive iodine uptake scan as well as thyroglobulin antibody and thyroid-stimulating immunoglobulin assays.
  - **Hypothyroid patients ($\uparrow$ TSH):** Order anti–thyroid peroxidase (anti-TPO) antibody assay.
- Figure 2.4-1 and Table 2.4-6 outline the workup, differential, and treatment of functional thyroid disease.

TREATMENT

- **Symptomatic hyperthyroidism:**
  - Treat with **propranolol,** hydration, rest, and adequate nutrition. Cooling measures are required for severe hyperthermia.

TABLE 2.4-5. Clinical Presentation of Functional Thyroid Disease

	HYPOTHYROIDISM	HYPERTHYROIDISM
General	Fatigue, lethargy.	Hyperactivity, nervousness, fatigue.
Temperature	Cold intolerance.	Heat intolerance.
GI	Constipation → ileus; weight gain despite poor appetite.	Diarrhea; weight loss despite good appetite.
Cardiac	Bradycardia, pericardial effusion, hyperlipidemia.	Tachycardia, atrial fibrillation, CHF; systolic hypertension, $\uparrow$ pulse pressure.
Neurologic	Delayed DTRs.	Fine resting tremor; apathetic hyperthyroidism (elderly).
Menstruation	Heavy.	Irregular.
Dermatologic	Dry, coarse skin; thinning hair; thin, brittle nails; myxedema.	Warm, sweaty skin; fine, oily hair; nail separation from matrix.
Other	Arthralgias/myalgias.	**Osteoporosis,** proptosis.

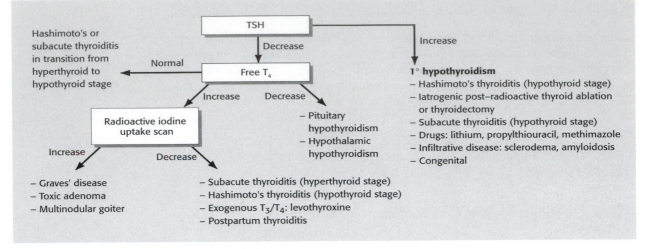

FIGURE 2.4-1. **Workup of functional thyroid disease.**

- Mild cases of hyperthyroidism can then be treated with **propylthiouracil** or **methimazole**. More severe cases require radioactive ^{131}I thyroid ablation.
- **Thyroidectomy** is indicated for large goiters, pregnant patients, or obstruction of the trachea. Patients who have undergone radioactive abla-

TABLE 2.4-6. **Differential and Treatment of Thyroid Disease**

	GRAVES' DISEASE	SUBACUTE THYROIDITIS	HASHIMOTO'S THYROIDITIS
Etiology/ pathophysiology	Antibody directed at TSH receptor. More prevalent in females.	Viral (possibly mumps or coxsackievirus).	Autoimmune disorder.
Symptoms/exam	Hyperthyroidism; diffuse, painless goiter. Proptosis, lid lag, diplopia, conjunctival injection. Pretibial myxedema.	Hyperthyroidism → hypothyroidism. Tender thyroid. Malaise, upper respiratory tract symptoms, fever early on.	Hyperthyroidism. Painless thyroid enlargement.
Diagnosis	↓ radioactive uptake scan, ⊕ thyroid-stimulating immunoglobulin, ⊕ thyroglobulin antibody.	↑ radioactive uptake scan ⊕ thyroglobulin antibody, high ESR.	⊕ anti-TPO antibody.
Disease-specific treatment	Propylthiouracil, methimazole, thyroid ablation with ^{131}I. Ophthalmopathy may require surgical decompression, steroids, or orbital radiation.	NSAIDs for pain control; steroids for severe pain. Self-limited.	Levothyroxine.

tion or thyroidectomy become hypothyroid and are treated with levothyroxine.

- **Hypothyroidism:**
    - Treat with **levothyroxine.** Patients with myxedema coma require IV levothyroxine and IV hydrocortisone.
    - Mechanical ventilation and warming blankets are required for hypoventilation and hypothermia, respectively.

*Methimazole should **not** be given during pregnancy because it can cause aplasia cutis in the fetus.*

HYPERCALCEMIA

Most cases of 1° hyperparathyroidism are caused by a parathyroid adenoma. Initial treatment is focused on correcting the hypercalcemia. Table 2.4-7 lists the clinical characteristics of 1° hyperparathyroidism and other causes of hypercalcemia.

OSTEOPOROSIS

A common metabolic bone disease characterized by ↓ bone strength and abnormal bone density. More common among inactive, **postmenopausal Caucasian women.**

SYMPTOMS/EXAM

Commonly asymptomatic. Patients may present with **hip fractures, vertebral compression fractures** (resulting in loss of height and progressive thoracic kyphosis), and/or distal radius fractures following minimal trauma.

DIFFERENTIAL

Osteomalacia (inadequate bone mineralization), hyperparathyroidism, multiple myeloma, metastatic carcinoma (pathologic fracture).

TABLE 2.4-7. Clinical Characteristics of Hypercalcemia

	1° HYPERPARATHYROIDISM	OTHER
Etiology	Adenoma. Multiglandular disease.	Malignancy that produces PTH-related peptide, multiple myeloma, sarcoidosis, vitamin D excess, vitamin A excess, thiazide diuretics, lithium.
Symptoms/exam	Fatigue, constipation, polyuria, polydipsia, bone pain, nausea.	Presentation is the same as that of 1° disease.
Diagnosis	↑ calcium and PTH; low PO_4.	↑ calcium; normal or low PTH; sometime ↑ PO_4.
Treatment	Surgical removal of the parathyroid glands. Hydrate with IV fluids; give furosemide after volume deficit is corrected; bisphosphonate for severe hypercalcemia.	Sarcoidosis, multiple myeloma: steroids. Low-calcium diet. Hydrate with IV fluids; give furosemide after volume deficit is corrected; bisphosphonate for severe hypercalcemia.
Complications	Nephrolithiasis, nephrocalcinosis, osteopenia, osteoporosis, pancreatitis, cardiac valve calcifications.	Same as those for 1° disease.

HIGH-YIELD FACTS

ENDOCRINOLOGY

DIAGNOSIS

- All patients > 65 years of age, as well as patients 40–60 years of age with at least one risk factor for osteoporotic fractures after menopause, should be screened with a DEXA scan of the spine and hip.
- Take the lowest **T-score** between the hip and the spine:
  - **T-score −1 to −2.5:** Osteopenia.
  - **T-score ≤ −2.5:** Osteoporosis.
- Rule out 2° causes, including smoking, alcoholism, renal failure, hyperthyroidism, multiple myeloma, 1° hyperparathyroidism, vitamin D deficiency, hypercortisolism, heparin use, and chronic steroid use.

TREATMENT

- Treat when a T-score is < −2 or when a T-score is < −1.5 in a patient with risk factors for osteoporotic fractures.
- Drugs of choice, in order of efficacy, include **bisphosphonates** (alendronate, etidronate, ibandronate), teriparatide, selective estrogen receptor modulators (SERMs) such as raloxifene, and intranasal calcitonin.
- Eliminate or treat 2° causes, and add weight-bearing exercises and calcium/vitamin D supplementation.
- A DEXA scan should be repeated 1–2 years after the initiation of drug therapy. If the T-score is found to have worsened, combination therapy (e.g., a SERM and a bisphosphonate) or a change in therapy should be initiated with consideration given to ruling out 2° causes.

Avoid HRT in osteoporotic patients in view of the risk of cardiovascular mortality and breast cancer.

CUSHING'S SYNDROME (HYPERCORTISOLISM)

Cushing's disease is Cushing's syndrome caused by hypersecretion of ACTH from a pituitary adenoma. Etiologies of hypercortisolism include adrenal (adenoma, carcinoma), pituitary (adenoma), ectopic (lung cancer), or exogenous (corticosteroid administration).

SYMPTOMS/EXAM

- Look for truncal obesity with moon facies and a **"buffalo hump."**
- Psychiatric disturbances, hypertension, impotence, oligomenorrhea, growth retardation, hirsutism (excessive hair growth, acne), easy bruisability, and purple striae can also be seen.
- Table 2.4-8 lists the laboratory characteristics of Cushing's syndrome according to etiology.

DIFFERENTIAL

Chronic alcoholism, depression, DM, chronic steroid use, adrenogenital syndrome, acute stress, obesity.

DIAGNOSIS

- ↑ 24-hour urine cortisol is diagnostic for Cushing's syndrome.
- Check A.M. serum ACTH.
  - **A.M. serum ACTH < 5 pg/mL:** Give exogenous steroids or obtain an adrenal CT scan or MRI to look for adrenal adenoma or carcinoma (unilateral) or adrenal hyperplasia (bilateral).
  - **A.M. serum ACTH > 5 pg/mL:** Administer a high-dose dexamethasone suppression test.
    - **Suppressed cortisol response:** Cushing's disease (e.g., ACTH-secreting pituitary adenoma). Confirm with a pituitary MRI.

	ACTH DEPENDENT	**ACTH INDEPENDENT**
Plasma cortisol	↑	↑
Urinary cortisol	↑	↑
ACTH	↑	↓
Source	Pituitary (suppressible) Ectopic (nonsuppressible)	Adenoma (↓ DHEA) Carcinoma (↑ DHEA)

- **Nonsuppressed cortisol response:** Ectopic ACTH-producing tumor such as carcinoid tumors and small cell lung cancer. Can be seen on octreotide scan and/or MRI/CT of the chest. If ⊖, do a pituitary MRI.
- DHEA is most elevated in adrenal carcinoma.

TREATMENT

- **Ectopic secreting ACTH tumor:** Surgical resection of the tumor.
- **Adrenal carcinoma, adenoma, or hyperplasia:** Adrenalectomy.
- **ACTH-secreting pituitary adenoma:** Transsphenoidal resection or radiation treatment.
- **Exogenous steroids:** Minimize use.

ADRENAL INSUFFICIENCY

Adrenocortical hypofunction can stem from adrenal failure (1° adrenal insufficiency, also known as **Addison's disease**) or from ↓ ACTH production from the pituitary (2° adrenal insufficiency). Etiologies are as follows:

- **1° adrenal insufficiency:** Autoimmune (idiopathic), metastatic tumor, hemorrhagic infarction (from coagulopathy or septicemia), adrenalectomy, granulomatous disease (TB, sarcoid).
- **2° adrenal insufficiency:** Withdrawal of exogenous steroids, hypothalamic or pituitary pathology (tumor, infarct, trauma, infection, iatrogenic).

> **A**ddison's **D**isease is due to **A**drenocortical **D**eficiency.

SYMPTOMS/EXAM

Symptoms include weakness, anorexia, weight loss, nausea, vomiting, postural hypotension, diarrhea, abdominal pain, myalgias, and arthralgias. Infection, surgery, or other stressors can trigger an **addisonian crisis** with symptomatic adrenal insufficiency, confusion, and vasodilatory shock.

DIAGNOSIS

An A.M. serum cortisol < 5 μg/dL or < 20 μg/dL serum cortisol after an ACTH stimulation test or < 9 μg/dL serum cortisol increase after the same test are diagnostic. Nonspecific findings include hyponatremia, hyperkalemia, and eosinophilia. Check A.M. serum ACTH to distinguish 1° from 2° adrenal insufficiency (see Table 2.4-9).

Hyperpigmentation, dehydration, hyponatremia, hyperkalemia, and salt craving are specific to 1° adrenal insufficiency.

TABLE 2.4-9. 1° vs. 2° Adrenal Insufficiency

	ADDISON'S DISEASE	2° ADRENAL INSUFFICIENCY
ACTH	↑	↓
Cortisol after ACTH challenge	↓	↑

Reproduced, with permission, from Le T et al. *First Aid for the USMLE Step 2,* 4th ed. New York: McGraw-Hill, 2004: 121.

TREATMENT

- Treat with glucocorticoids and mineralocorticoids. **Hydrocortisone** is the drug of choice. Add **fludrocortisone** for orthostatic hypotension, hyponatremia, or hyperkalemia. Glucocorticoid doses should be ↑ in times of illness, trauma, or surgery.
- Patients in **adrenal crisis** need immediate fluid resuscitation and IV hydrocortisone.

PROLACTINOMA

The most common functional pituitary tumor.

SYMPTOMS/EXAM

Women typically present with galactorrhea and amenorrhea. Men may develop impotence and, later in the disease, symptoms related to mass effect (e.g., CN III palsy, diplopia, temporal field visual loss, headache).

DIAGNOSIS

↑ prolactin levels; ↓ LH and FSH. Order an MRI to confirm the tumor.

TREATMENT

Treat medically with a dopamine agonist such as bromocriptine or cabergoline. If medical therapy is not tolerated or if the tumor is large, transsphenoidal surgery followed by irradiation is indicated.

MULTIPLE ENDOCRINE NEOPLASIA (MEN)

A group of familial, autosomal-dominant syndromes (see Table 2.4-10).

TABLE 2.4-10. Characteristics of MEN Syndromes

SYNDROME	TYPE	CHARACTERISTICS
Wermer's syndrome	I	**P**arathyroid hyperplasia **P**ancreatic islet cell tumor **P**ituitary adenoma
Sipple's syndrome	IIa	Parathyroid hyperplasia Thyroid medullary cancer Pheochromocytoma
	IIb	Thyroid medullary cancer Pheochromocytoma Mucocutaneous neuromas Ganglioneuromatosis of the colon Marfan-like habitus

The 3 P's of primary MEN:

Parathyroid hyperplasia
Pancreatic islet cell tumor
Pituitary adenoma

MEN IIa and IIb— two common characteristics:

Thyroid medullary cancer
Pheochromocytoma

SECTION II

Ethics

Be familiar with the following principles:

- **Autonomy:** The right to make decisions for oneself according to one's own system of morals and beliefs.
- **Paternalism:** Providing for patients' needs without their input.
- **Beneficence:** Action intended to bring about a good outcome.
- **Nonmaleficence:** Action not intended to bring about harm.
- **Truth telling:** Revealing all pertinent information to patients.
- **Proportionality:** Ensuring that a medical treatment or plan is commensurate with the illness and with the goals of treatment.
- **Distributive justice:** Allocation of resources in a manner that is fair and just, though not necessarily equal.

AUTONOMY

Informed Consent

Involves discussing diagnoses and prognoses with patients as well as any proposed treatment, its risks and benefits, and its alternatives. Only with such information can a patient reach an informed decision. **Do not conceal a diagnosis from a patient;** doing so violates the principle of truth telling. However, respect your patients' wishes if they tell you to share only certain things with them.

Rights of Minors

Treatment of patients < 18 years of age requires parental consent unless:

- They are emancipated (i.e., financially independent, married, raising children, living on their own, or serving in the armed forces).
- They are requesting contraception or treatment of pregnancy, STDs, or psychiatric illness. Note: Many states require parental consent or notice for termination of pregnancy in a minor.

Most questions on the Step 3 test regarding parental consent will deal with situations such as those cited above. In general, this means that for the Step 3 test, the governing principle should be to let minors make their own decisions.

COMPETENCY

Competency vs. Capacity

It is a mistake to use the terms **competency** and **capacity** interchangeably. Competency is a **legal** determination made only by a court, whereas capacity is a **clinical** assessment. Each involves the assessment of a patient's ability to think and act rationally (not necessarily wisely). Incompetence is permanent (e.g., severe dementia), and incompetent patients are generally assigned a surrogate by the court. Incapacity may be temporary (e.g., delirium), and careful decision making is important when considering therapeutic interventions for patients with questionable capacity.

HIGH-YIELD FACTS

ETHICS

Detention and Use of Restraints

Psychiatric patients may be held against their will only if they are a danger to themselves or to others (in accordance with the principle of beneficence). The use of restraints can be considered if a patient is at risk of doing harm to self or others, but such use must be evaluated on at least a daily basis.

Durable Power of Attorney (DPoA) for Health Care

DPoA has two related meanings. First, it can refer to a document signed by the patient assigning a surrogate decision maker in the event that he or she becomes incapacitated. Second, it can refer to the person to whom that authority has been granted.

Surrogate/Proxy

Defined as an alternate decision maker, designated by the patient (DPoA), by law, or by convention. If no person has been formally designated to represent the patient, surrogacy falls to relatives in accordance with a hierarchy that may vary from state to state (typically, a spouse is at the top of this hierarchy).

CONFIDENTIALITY

Importance of Confidentiality (and HIPAA)

Maintaining the confidentiality of patient information is critical. Violations are unethical, can result in legal troubles, and may irreparably harm the patient-doctor relationship. The Health Insurance Portability and Accountability Act (HIPAA) outlines rules and guidelines for preserving patient privacy.

When to Violate Confidentiality

If a physician learns about a threat to an individual's life or well-being (i.e., a danger to self or to others), violating confidentiality is mandatory. In a similar manner, information about child abuse or elder abuse must be reported.

Reportable Conditions

Most contagious, rare, and incurable infections, as well as other threats to public health, are reportable. The list of reportable infections varies by state but often includes syphilis, gonorrhea, chlamydia, TB, mumps, measles, rubella, smallpox, and suspected bioterrorist events. Such reporting is mandatory and does not constitute a violation of confidentiality.

Asking Follow-up Questions

Follow-up questions should be used to clarify unclear issues regarding questions such as which family members can be included in discussions of care, who is the primary surrogate, and what patients want to know about their own conditions.

Patients in the end stages of a terminal illness have the right to obtain medical treatment that is intended to preserve human dignity in dying. The best means of reaching an agreement with the patient and his or her family regarding end-of-life care is to continue to talk about the patient's condition and to resolve decision-making conflicts. Ultimately, this is the same task that an ethics consultant would attempt to perform for the physician and the patient.

Advance Directives

Defined as oral or written statements regarding what a patient would want in the event that intensive resuscitative intervention becomes necessary to sustain life. These instructions can be detailed—which is obviously preferable—or they can be broad. Oral statements are ethically binding but are not legally binding in all states. Remember that an informed, competent adult can refuse treatment even if it means that doing so would lead to death; such instructions must be honored.

Do Not Resuscitate (DNR) Orders/Code Status

The express wishes of a patient (e.g., "I do not want to be intubated") supersede the wishes of family members or surrogates. Physicians should inquire about and follow DNR orders during each hospitalization. If code status has not been addressed and the matter becomes relevant, defer to the surrogate.

Pain in Terminally Ill Patients

Terminally ill patients are often inadequately treated for pain. Prescribe as much narcotic medication as is needed to relieve patients' pain and suffering. Do not worry about addiction in this setting. Two-thirds of patients in their last three days of life stated that they felt moderate to severe pain.

The Principle of "Double Effect"

Actions can have more than one consequence, some intended, others not. Unintended medical consequences are acceptable if the intended consequences are legitimate and the harm proportionately smaller than the benefit. For example, a dying patient can be given high doses of analgesics even if it may unintentionally shorten life.

Persistent Vegetative State (PVS)

Defined as a state in which the brain stem is intact and the patient has sleep-wake cycles, but there is no consciousness, voluntary activity, or ability to interact with the environment. Reflexes may be normal or abnormal. Some patients survive this way for five years or more, with the aggregate annual cost reaching into the billions of dollars.

Quality of Life

Defined as a subjective evaluation of a patient's current physical, emotional, and social well-being. This must be evaluated from the perspective of the patient.

Euthanasia

Euthanasia (physician-assisted suicide) is assisting an informed, competent, terminally ill patient to end life, usually by prescription or administration of a lethal dose of medication. It is not the same as withdrawal of care. Currently, euthanasia is illegal in all states except Oregon.

Palliation and Hospice

These related concepts involve the provision of end-of-life care within (palliation) or outside (hospice) a traditional medical system. Each is an attempt to manage psychosocial and physical well-being in a manner that preserves dignity and maximizes comfort. Both involve interdisciplinary collaboration (MD, RN, chaplain, social worker, aide), focusing on patient-defined goals of care.

Withdrawal of Treatment

Withdrawal of treatment is the removal of life-sustaining treatment and is legally and ethically no different from never starting treatment. The decision to withdraw treatment may come from the patient, an advance directive, a DPoA, or, absent any of these, the closest relative and/or a physician. It is easiest when all parties are in agreement, although this is not required. When there is conflict, the patient's wishes take precedence. In futile cases or those involving extreme suffering, a physician may withdraw or withhold treatment; if the family disagrees, the physician should seek input from an ethics committee or a court's approval.

BIOSTATISTICS

Not everyone with a given disease will test positive for that disease, and not everyone with a positive test result has the disease.

Sensitivity and Specificity

Sense (sensitivity) who does have a disease. Specify (specificity) who does not.

Sensitivity is the probability that a person with a disease will have a positive result on a given test. High sensitivity is useful in a screening test, as the goal is to identify everyone with a given disease. **Specificity** is the probability that a person without a disease will have a negative result on a test. High specificity is desirable for a confirmatory test.

Ideally a test will be highly sensitive and specific, but this is rare. A test that is highly sensitive but not specific will have many false positives, whereas one that is highly specific but not sensitive will have many false negatives.

Predictive Values

Positive predictive value (PPV) is the probability that a person with a positive test result has the disease (true positives/all positives; see Table 2.5-1). If a disease has a greater prevalence, then the PPV is higher. **Negative predictive value (NPV)** is the probability that a person with a negative test result is disease free (see Table 2.5-1). A test has a higher NPV value when a disease has a lower prevalence.

Incidence

Defined as the number of **new** cases of a given disease per year; for example, 4 cases of X per year.

Prevalence

Defined as the total number of **existing** cases of a given disease in the entire population; for example, 20 people have X (right now).

Absolute Risk

The **probability** of an event in a given time period; for example, 0.1% chance of developing X in 10 years.

Relative Risk (RR)

Used to evaluate the results of cohort (prospective) studies. The RR compares the incidence of a disease in a group exposed to a particular risk factor with the incidence in those not exposed to the risk factor (see Table 2.5-2). An RR < 1 means that the event is less likely in the exposed group; conversely, an RR > 1 signifies that the event is more likely in that group.

Odds Ratio (OR)

Used in case-control (retrospective) studies. The OR compares the rate of exposure among those with and without a disease (see Table 2.5-2). It is considered less accurate than RR, but in rare diseases the OR approximates the RR.

Absolute Risk Reduction (ARR) or Attributable Risk

Measures the risk accounted for by exposure to a given factor, taking into account the background of the disease. Useful in randomized controlled trials.

TABLE 2.5-1. Determination of PPV and NPV

	DISEASE PRESENT	NO DISEASE	
Positive test	a	b	PPV = a/(a + b)
Negative test	c	d	NPV = d/(c + d)
	Sensitivity = a/(a + c)	Specificity = d/(b + d)	

TABLE 2.5-2. Determination of RR and OR

	DISEASE DEVELOPS	NO DISEASE	
Exposure	a	b	RR = [a/(a + b)]/[c/(c + d)]
No exposure	c	d	OR = ad/bc

Numerically, ARR = the absolute risk (rate of adverse events) in the placebo group minus the absolute risk in treated patients.

Relative Risk Reduction (RRR)

Also used in randomized controlled trials, this is the ratio between two risks. Numerically, RRR = [the event rate in control patients minus the event rate in experimental patients] ÷ the event rate in control patients.

RRR can be deceptive and is clinically far less important than ARR. Consider a costly intervention that reduces the risk of an adverse event from 0.01% to 0.004%. ARR is 0.01 − 0.004 = 0.006%, but RRR is (0.01 − 0.004)/0.01 = 0.6, or 60%! Would you order this intervention?

Number Needed to Treat (NNT)

The number of patients that would need to be treated to prevent one event. NNT = 1/ARR. In the example above, the NNT is 167.

Statistical Significance/*p*-Value

The *p*-value expresses the likelihood that an observed outcome was due to random chance. A *p*-value < 0.05 is generally accepted as indicating that an outcome is statistically significant.

Confidence Interval (CI)

Like the *p*-value, the CI expresses the certainty that the observation is real or is a product of random chance. Used with ORs and RR, the 95% CI says the observed risk or odds have a 95% chance of being within the interval. Thus, in Figure 2.5-1, the relative risk of cancer with smoking is 2.0 with a 95% CI of 1.3–3.5 — meaning that the **observed** RR of cancer was 2.0, and that there is a 95% certainty that the **actual** RR of cancer from smoking falls somewhere between 1.3 and 3.5.

ARR and RRR give very different values and should not be confused. ARR is a much better measure of benefit; because it is a ratio, RRR can look deceptively large. Watch out for drug advertising that touts RRR.

If a 95% CI includes 1.0, the results are not significant. So if an RR is 1.9 but the 95% CI is 0.8–3.0, the RR is not significant.

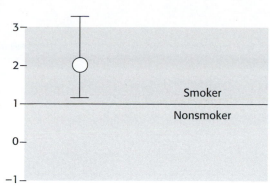

FIGURE 2.5-1. Relative risk of cancer.

Statistical analyses are used as a means of assessing relationships between events and outcomes. They do not prove irrefutably that a relationship exists but point to the likelihood. The validity of the results depends on the strength of the design.

Surveys

These are self-reporting of symptoms, exposures, feelings, and other subjective data. They are scientifically unreliable.

Prospective and Retrospective Studies

Prospective studies assess future outcomes relating to present or future events; this enables the study designer to control for biases and to modify inputs/exposures. Retrospective studies relate to outcomes from past events. They are limited in scope and are less reliable than prospective studies.

Cohort Study

In a **cohort study,** a population is observed over time, grouped based on exposure to a particular factor, and watched for a specific outcome. Such studies are not good for rare conditions. Studies can be prospective or retrospective. Use RR to interpret results. Examples include the Nurses' Health Study and the Framingham Heart Study.

Case-Control Study

A retrospective study involving a group of people with a given disease and an otherwise similar group of people without the disease who are compared for exposure to risk factors. Good for rare diseases. Use OR to interpret results.

Randomized Controlled Trial (RCT)

The most valid study design; a prospective study that randomly assigns participants to a treatment group or to a placebo group. The placebo group and the treatment group are then compared to determine if the treatment made a difference. The double-blind RCT is the gold standard of experimental design.

HIGH-YIELD FACTS

ETHICS

Gastroenterology

Obstruction of passage of food or liquid through the esophagus.

SYMPTOMS/EXAM

Patients note difficulty swallowing (dysphagia) or state that food "sticks" or "hangs up." Distinguish from **odynophagia,** or pain with swallowing that is typically caused by *Candida*, CMV, or HSV infection, usually in immunocompromised patients (e.g., HIV patients or those on chemotherapy).

DIAGNOSIS

Think cancer in older patients with worsening dysphagia, weight loss, and heme-⊕ stools.

- Workup includes barium swallow and/or EGD.
- If difficulty is with **solids alone,** consider the following:
    - **Lower esophageal ring:** Characterized by intermittent symptoms or sudden obstruction with a food bolus (**"steakhouse syndrome"**). The ring is located at the gastroesophageal junction.
    - **Zenker's diverticulum:** Outpouching of the upper esophagus. Presents with foul-smelling breath and food regurgitation as well as with difficulty initiating swallowing.
    - **Plummer-Vinson syndrome:** Cervical esophageal web and iron-deficiency anemia. Associated with esophageal cancer.
    - **Peptic stricture:** Progressive symptoms with long-standing heartburn.
    - **Esophagitis:** Inflammation 2° to gastroesophageal reflux or eosinophilic esophagitis.
    - **Carcinoma:** Progressive symptoms in an older patient.
- If difficulty is with **both solids and liquids,** consider the following:
    - **Esophageal spasm:** Intermittent symptoms with chest pain. Triggered by acid, stress, and hot and cold liquids. Presents with **"corkscrew esophagus"** on barium swallow.
    - **Achalasia:** Progressive symptoms that worsen at night with no heartburn (see Figure 2.6-1). Presents with a **"bird's beak"** on barium swallow.
    - **Scleroderma:** Progressive symptoms with heartburn and Raynaud's phenomenon (**CREST** syndrome: **C**alcinosis cutis, **R**aynaud's phenomenon, **E**sophageal dysmotility, **S**clerodactyly, and **T**elangiectasia).

GASTROESOPHAGEAL REFLUX DISEASE (GERD)

Risk factors include hiatal hernia, obesity, collagen vascular disease, alcohol, caffeine, nicotine, chocolate, fatty foods, and pregnancy.

SYMPTOMS/EXAM

- Presents with an uncomfortable hot and burning sensation beneath the sternum.
- Symptoms usually worsen after meals, on reclining, and with use of tight clothes.

DIFFERENTIAL

Angina pectoris, esophageal motility disorders, peptic ulcer.

DIAGNOSIS

GERD is a common cause of hoarseness and chronic cough, and can exacerbate or mimic asthma.

Barium swallow, endoscopy, esophageal biopsy, and ambulatory pH monitoring.

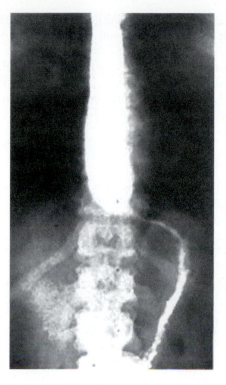

FIGURE 2.6-1. Achalasia of the esophagus.

Moderately advanced achalasia. Note the dilated body of the esophagus and the smoothly tapered lower portion. (Reproduced, with permission, from Way LW, Doherty GM [eds]. *Current Surgical Diagnosis & Treatment*, 11th ed. New York: McGraw-Hill, 2003: 478.)

TREATMENT

- **Lifestyle modification:** Elevate the head of the bed; avoid bedtime snacks, trigger foods (fatty foods, chocolate, mint, alcohol), cigarettes, and NSAIDs; and promote weight loss.
- **Drugs:** Antacids, H_2 blockers, PPIs. If symptomatic relief is achieved with an H_2 blocker or a PPI, an attempt to discontinue treatment after 8–12 weeks may be successful.
- **Other:**
    - If the disorder is refractory to medical therapy, consider evaluation for Nissen fundoplication or other hiatal hernia repair.
    - Consider endoscopy to screen for Barrett's esophagus, especially in patients with long-standing or severe GERD.

PEPTIC ULCER DISEASE (PUD)

The most common sites of PUD are the **stomach** and **duodenum**. *H. pylori* infection and **NSAID/aspirin use** are the major causes; Zollinger-Ellison syndrome, HSV infection, CMV, and cocaine use are less common etiologies.

SYMPTOMS/EXAM

- Presents with **epigastric** abdominal pain that patients describe as a **"gnawing"** or **"aching"** sensation that comes in waves. May also present with dyspepsia and upper GI bleed.

- Symptoms are often further distinguished by disease site:
  - **Duodenal ulcers:** Pain is relieved by food and comes on **postprandially.**
  - **Stomach ulcers:** Pain worsens with food **(pain with eating).**
- **Red flags:** With diarrhea, weight loss, and excessive gastric acid (elevated basal acid output), think of the rare causes (Zollinger-Ellison syndrome, systemic mastocytosis, hyperparathyroidism, extensive small bowel resection).

DIAGNOSIS

- **Detect the ulcer:** Perform **endoscopy** with rapid urease testing for *H.pylori*; biopsy any gastric ulcers to rule out malignancy.
- **Look for *H. pylori* infection:**
  - **Urease testing** of the biopsy sample.
  - **Serum antibody** is easy to obtain, but a ⊕ antibody may not necessarily indicate active infection. Antibody remains ⊕ even after treatment.
  - A **urea breath test** is good for detecting active infection, but patients must be off PPIs for two weeks and off antibiotics and bismuth for four weeks.
  - Fecal antigen test for *H. pylori*, with patients off antibiotics, PPIs, and bismuth.

Warning signs of more serious disease than PUD include age > 45, weight loss, anemia, and heme-⊕ stools.

TREATMENT

- **Discontinue aspirin/NSAIDs;** promote smoking cessation.
- Give PPIs to control symptoms, ↓ acid secretion, and heal the ulcer (4 weeks for duodenal ulcers; 8–12 weeks for gastric ulcers).
- For *H. pylori* infection, initiate multidrug therapy. Two of the following three drugs may be used—**amoxicillin 1 g BID, clarithromycin 500 mg BID,** or **metronidazole 500 mg BID**—along with a PPI (**omeprazole, lansoprazole**) for 10–14 days.
- Indications for surgery include recurrent/refractory upper GI bleed, gastric outlet obstruction, recurrent/refractory ulcers, perforation, and Zollinger-Ellison syndrome.

INFLAMMATORY BOWEL DISEASE (IBD)

Describes two distinct chronic inflammatory diseases: **Crohn's disease** and **ulcerative colitis.** IBD clusters in families and is more common among **Jewish persons** and four times more common in **Caucasians but can occur in anyone, including young children and older adults.**

Crohn's Disease

Transmural inflammation anywhere from the mouth to the anus (**skip lesions**). Most often affects the **terminal ileum,** small bowel, and colon. Has a bimodal distribution with peaks in the 20s and 50s–70s.

SYMPTOMS/EXAM

- Patients may be pale or thin with temporal wasting and often have RLQ tenderness/fullness; some present with perianal fistula.
- Symptoms include the following:
  - **GI: Colicky RLQ pain,** diarrhea (mucus-containing, nonbloody stools), weight loss, anorexia, low-grade fever, **perirectal abscess/fistula,** and, less often, GI blood loss, fecal incontinence, and oral ulcers.

- **Other: Low-grade fever,** erythema nodosum, pyoderma gangrenosum (see Figure 2.6-2), iritis and episcleritis, gallstones, kidney stones, and peripheral arthritis.

DIAGNOSIS

- Obtain a CBC, iron, folate, B_{12}, ESR, LFTs, stool WBC, RBC, and O&P.
  - Look for normocytic anemia of chronic disease or anemia due to iron, vitamin B_{12}, or folate deficiency.
  - ESR or CRP may be ↑; ⊕ ASCA.
  - O&P is ⊖, but fecal leukocytes and occult blood may be ⊕.
  - LFTs should be normal or mildly elevated.
- **Skip lesions** are seen on colonoscopy; **cobblestoning** is seen on barium enema. Biopsy may show noncaseating granuloma with mononuclear cell infiltrate. Stricture formation, pseudodiverticula, abscesses, and fistulas (to the skin, bladder, vagina, other bowel loops) may be seen on imaging (see Figure 2.6-3).

TREATMENT

- **Mild cases: 5-ASA** compounds.
- **Moderate cases:** Oral corticosteroids +/− azathioprine, 6-mercaptopurine (6-MP), or methotrexate.
- **Refractory disease:** IV steroids +/− other immunomodulators (anti-TNF). Imaging (CT, MRI, CT enterography) is important to rule out perforation, megacolon, fistula, or abscess formation. In some cases, stricturoplasty +/− resection may be needed.
- **Follow-up:** Surveillance colonoscopy with multiple biopsies to look for dysplasia in patients with a large extent of colonic involvement 8–10 years after diagnosis and biannually or annually thereafter.

Ulcerative Colitis

Continuous colonic mucosal inflammation extending proximally for variable distances from the anal verge. Usually occurs in a bimodal distribution (ages 15–30 and 60–80). Can → **toxic megacolon.**

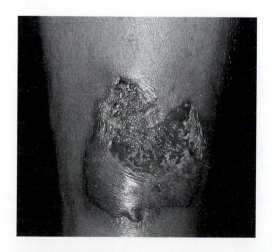

FIGURE 2.6-2.   Pyoderma gangrenosum.

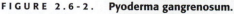

(Reproduced, with permission, from Wolff K, Johnson RA, Suurmond D. *Fitzpatrick's Color Atlas & Synopsis of Clinical Dermatology,* 5th ed. New York: McGraw-Hill, 2005: 153.)

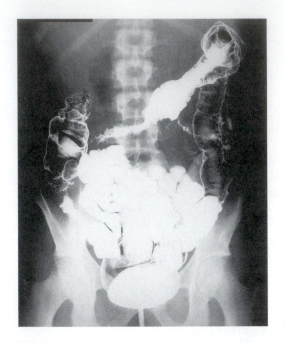

FIGURE 2.6-3. **Crohn's disease of the colon.**

The lumen of the terminal ileum is narrowed and separated by the thickened wall of the small bowel. Cobblestone-appearing skip lesions are present in the colon. (Adapted, with permission, from Brunicardi FC et al. [eds]. *Schwartz's Principles of Surgery*, 8th ed., www.Access Medicine.com, ©2007 McGraw-Hill Companies.)

SYMPTOMS/EXAM

Presents with **cramping** abdominal pain, **urgency, bloody diarrhea,** weight loss, and fatigue. Exam reveals low-grade fever, tachycardia, orthostatic hypotension, heme-⊕ stools, and mild tenderness in the lower abdomen.

DIAGNOSIS

- **Labs:** Laboratory studies reveal **normocytic, normochromic anemia or iron-deficiency anemia;** low albumin; ⊕ **p-ANCA;** and ⊖ stool cultures.
- **Imaging:**
    - Colonoscopy shows **friable mucosa** with ulcerations and erosions along with inflammation that is continuous from the anus up.
    - Barium enema shows a **lead-pipe colon** and loss of haustra (see Figure 2.6-4).
- Biopsy reveals crypt abscess and microulcerations but no granuloma.

TREATMENT

- **Mild cases: 5-ASA** compounds.
- **Moderate cases:** Oral corticosteroids +/− azathioprine, 6-MP, or methotrexate.
- **Refractory disease:** IV steroids +/− cyclosporine, +/− anti-TNF antibody. Serial imaging to rule out perforation or toxic megacolon. In some cases resection may be needed, especially if complications arise or if the patient fails medical therapy.

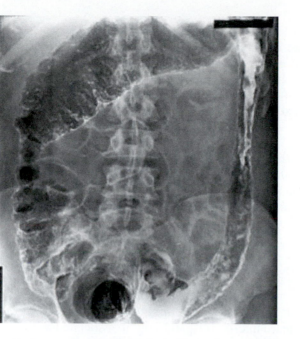

FIGURE 2.6-4.   Barium enema showing colonic dilation in ulcerative colitis.

Note the dilation of the transverse colon; the multiple irregular densities in the lumen (pseudopolyps); and the loss of haustral markings. (Reproduced, with permission, from Way LW, Doherty GM. *Current Surgical Diagnosis & Treatment*, 11th ed. New York: McGraw-Hill, 2003: 744.)

- **Follow-up: Surveillance colonoscopy with multiple biopsies** 8–10 years after diagnosis and biannually or annually thereafter.
- Some patients may elect to get a **prophylactic colectomy** given that the incidence of colon cancer is 0.5–1% per year after 10 years of disease.

IRRITABLE BOWEL SYNDROME (IBS)

A GI disorder characterized by abdominal pain and altered bowel function (diarrhea or constipation), with or without bloating. Possible etiologies include altered gut motor function, **autonomic nervous system abnormalities,** and **psychological factors.**

SYMPTOMS/EXAM

- Characterized by **abdominal pain** with complete or incomplete relief by defecation, **intermittent diarrhea or constipation,** a feeling of incomplete rectal evacuation, urgency, passage of mucus, and bloating.
- Abdominal pain is poorly localized, migratory, and variable in nature.

DIAGNOSIS

- A **diagnosis of exclusion** based primarily on the history and physical exam. Basic labs to exclude other causes should include CBC, BMP, calcium, TSH, and stool O&P.
- The **Rome III criteria** can be used to aid in diagnosis:
  - Improvement of pain with bowel movement
  - Often associated with change in frequency of bowel movement
  - Onset associated with change in form/appearance of stool

Pain unrelated to defecation or pain induced with activity, menstruation, or urination is unlikely to be IBS.

- **High-fiber diet** (20–30 g/day), **exercise,** and adequate fluid intake.
- **TCAs** are often used even in the absence of depression, especially in the setting of chronic pain and diarrhea.
- Additional treatment options depend on symptom predominance.
    - **If constipation predominates:** Use bulking agents (psyllium), lactulose, PEG, or enemas. Tegaserod, a 5-HT$_4$ receptor agonist, also can be used.
    - **If diarrhea predominates:** Give loperamide, cholestyramine, or TCAs.
    - **If bloating predominates:** Simethicone, charcoal, or *Lactobacillus* may be used.
    - **Postprandial symptoms:** Treat with anticholinergic agents, dicyclomine, or hyoscyamine.

DIARRHEA

Described as watery consistency and/or ↑ frequency of bowel movements. Stool weight is > 200–300 g/day. Small bowel pathology will show voluminous watery diarrhea; large bowel pathology is associated with more frequent but smaller-volume output. Distinguish acute from chronic diarrhea as follows:

- **Acute diarrhea:** Defined as < 2 weeks in duration; usually infectious.
- **Chronic diarrhea:** Defined as lasting > 4 weeks.

SYMPTOMS/EXAM

- The most important goal is to assess the degree of fluid loss/dehydration and nutritional depletion. If bloating predominates, it is suggestive of malabsorption. If fever is present, think of infectious causes. If guaiac ⊕, consider inflammatory processes or enteroinvasive organisms.
- Etiologies can be further distinguished as follows:
    - **Infectious:** The **leading cause of acute diarrhea.** Characterized by vomiting, pain, fever, or chills. If stools are bloody, think of enteroinvasive organisms. To characterize, check stool leukocytes, Gram stain, culture, and O&P. Treat severe disease with ciprofloxacin or metronidazole for *Clostridium difficile.*
    - **Osmotic:** Associated with lactose intolerance and with the ingestion of magnesium, sorbitol, or mannitol; ↑ stool osmotic gap. Bloating and gas are prominent with malabsorption. Treat by stopping the offending agent.
    - **Secretory:** Caused by hormonal stimulation (gastrin, VIP) or by viruses or toxins. Stool osmotic gap is normal; no change in the diarrhea occurs with fasting. Treatment is mainly supportive. Viral syndromes are common and self-limited.
    - **Exudative:** Associated with mucosal inflammation, enteritis, TB, colon cancer, and IBD. Labs reveal ↑ ESR and C-reactive protein (CRP). Characterized by tenesmus, often small volume, and frequent diarrhea. Diagnose by colonoscopy, endoscopy with small bowel biopsies (celiac disease), and imaging studies. Treatment varies depending on the etiology.
    - **Rapid transit:** Associated with laxative abuse or, rarely, hyperthyroidism. Management involves checking TSH or stopping laxative use.
    - **Slow transit:** Small bowel bacterial overgrowth syndromes, structural abnormalities (small bowel diverticulum, fistulas), radiation damage, slow motility (DM, scleroderma). Treat the underlying cause; give a short course of antibiotics to ↓ bacterial growth.

DIAGNOSIS

- **Evaluation of acute diarrhea:**
  - In the setting of high fever, bloody diarrhea, or duration > 4–5 days, obtain fecal leukocytes and bacterial cultures and test for *C. difficile* toxin for inpatients; obtain an O&P for immunocompromised patients.
  - If symptoms start within six hours of ingestion, think of a preformed toxin such as *Bacillus cereus*. If symptoms start after 12 hours, the etiology is more likely to be bacterial or viral, especially if these symptoms are accompanied by vomiting.
- **Evaluation of chronic diarrhea:**
  - Consider malabsorption syndromes, lactose intolerance, previous bowel surgery, medications, systemic disease, and IBD.
  - Tests to consider include fecal leukocytes, occult blood, flexible sigmoidoscopy with biopsy, endoscopy with small bowel biopsies, small bowel imaging, or colonoscopy.
- **Calculate the osmotic gap:** 290 − 2 (stool Na + stool K). A normal gap is < 50.
  - **Normal gap:** If the stool is of normal weight, consider IBS and factitious causes. If weight is ↑, consider a secretory cause or laxative abuse.
  - **↑ gap:** Normal stool fat points to lactose intolerance or sorbitol, lactulose, or laxative abuse. ↑ stool fat is associated with small bowel malabsorption, pancreatic insufficiency, or bacterial overgrowth.

Common bugs in acute diarrhea:

- **Bacterial:** *E. coli, Shigella, Salmonella, Campylobacter jejuni, Vibrio parahaemolyticus, Yersinia.*
- **Viral:** Rotavirus, norovirus.
- **Parasitic:** *Giardia, Cryptosporidium, Entamoeba histolytica.*

TREATMENT

Treat according to the etiology as indicated above. General treatment guidelines are as follows:

- If acute, give oral or IV fluids, electrolyte repletion, and loperamide.
- Avoid antimotility agents in the presence of a high fever, bloody diarrhea, severe abdominal pain, or systemic toxicity.
- If *C. difficile* toxin is ⊕, treat initially with oral metronidazole.

Patient on antibiotics → think C. difficile.

CELIAC SPRUE

Usually affects people of **northern European** ancestry. Can be **familial**; thought to be an **autoimmune disease** triggered by an environmental agent (wheat, rye, barley, and some oats). Associated with osteoporosis, an ↑ risk of GI malignancies (small bowel lymphoma), and **dermatitis herpetiformis.**

SYMPTOMS/EXAM

Celiac sprue → **malabsorption** with **chronic diarrhea.** Patients complain of **steatorrhea** and **weight loss.** Can also present with nonspecific symptoms (nausea, abdominal pain, weight loss), iron-deficiency anemia, or muscle wasting.

DIAGNOSIS

- Histology reveals **flattening or loss of villi** and inflammation.
- Antibody assays are often ⊕ for **antiendomysial antibody** or **anti–tissue transglutaminase.**
- A gluten-free diet improves symptoms and the histology of the small bowel.

TREATMENT

Gluten-free diet. Gluten is found in most grains in the Western world (e.g., wheat, barley, additives, many prepared foods).

PANCREATITIS

Causes of acute pancreatitis— GET SMASH'D

Gallstones
Ethanol
Trauma
Steroids
Mumps
Autoimmune
Scorpion bites
Hyperlipidemia
Drugs

Gallstones and **alcohol** account for 70–80% of acute cases. Other causes include **obstruction** (pancreatic or ampullary tumors), **metabolic** factors (severe hypertriglyceridemia, hypercalcemia), abdominal **trauma,** endoscopic retrograde cholangiopancreatography (**ERCP**), **infection** (mumps, CMV, clonorchiasis, ascariasis), and **drugs** (thiazides, azathioprine, pentamidine, sulfonamides).

SYMPTOMS

- Acute pancreatitis often presents with abdominal pain, typically in the **midepigastric** region, that **radiates to the back,** may be relieved by sitting forward, and lasts hours to days.
- Nausea, vomiting, and fever also are seen.

EXAM

- Exam reveals **midepigastric tenderness,** ↓ bowel sounds, guarding, jaundice, and fever.
- **Cullen's sign** (periumbilical ecchymoses) and **Grey Turner's sign** (flank ecchymoses) reflect hemorrhage.

DIAGNOSIS

- Typically, both **amylase and lipase** will be elevated; however, amylase may be normal, especially if the disease is due to hyperlipidemia. **Lipase** has the **greatest specificity and remains more significantly elevated than amylase in acute pancreatitis.**
- **CXR** may show a **pleural effusion and an elevated hemidiaphragm;** AXR may show **calcification of the pancreas** or a **"sentinel loop" of a small bowel ileus.**
- **Abdominal CT** is especially useful in detecting complications of pancreatitis. In **chronic pancreatitis (especially alcohol), calcifications** may be seen.
- **Elevated ALT levels suggest gallstone pancreatitis.**
- If patients are female and > 60 years of age or if patients abstain from alcohol or use it only moderately, gallstones are the more likely etiology.
- Ultrasound may allow visualization of gallstones or sludge in the gallbladder.
- In **chronic pancreatitis, a 72-hour fecal fat test** (100-g/day fat diet) is ⊕ if there are **> 7 g/day of fat in the stool.** The etiology of chronic pancreatitis includes alcohol, cystic fibrosis, and idiopathic causes but not gallstones.

TREATMENT

- **Acute:**
    - **Supportive** (NPO, IV fluids, pain management).
    - In the setting of **gallstone pancreatitis,** ERCP with papillotomy is appropriate if the common bile duct is obstructed or if there is evidence of cholangitis. If the gallstone has passed, perform a cholecystectomy once the patient is sufficiently stable for surgery.

- **Prophylactic antibiotics** are used for severe pancreatitis and consist of imipenem monotherapy or fluoroquinolone + metronidazole.
- **Chronic:**
  - Treat malabsorption with pancreatic enzyme and vitamin B_{12} replacement.
  - Treat glucose intolerance; encourage alcohol abstinence.
  - Management of chronic pain.

COMPLICATIONS

- Acute: **Pseudocyst,** peripancreatic effusions, **necrosis,** abscess, ARDS, hypotension, splenic vein thrombosis.
- Chronic: **Malabsorption,** osteoporosis, DM, **pancreatic cancer.**

APPROACH TO LIVER FUNCTION TESTS

The algorithm in Figure 2.6-5 outlines a general approach toward the interpretation of LFTs.

GALLSTONE DISEASE

In the United States, gallstone disease is most likely due to **cholesterol stones.** In trauma patients, burn patients, or those on TPN, acute cholecystitis may occur in the absence of stones (**acalculous cholecystitis**).

SYMPTOMS/EXAM

- Most patients with gallstones are **asymptomatic** (80%).
- **Biliary colic:** Characterized by **episodic RUQ** or epigastric pain that may radiate to the right shoulder; usually **postprandial** and accompanied by vomiting. **Nocturnal** pain that awakens the patient is common. Associated with **fatty food** intolerance.
- **Cholangitis:** Suggested by the presence of fever and persistent RUQ pain.
  - **Charcot's triad:** RUQ pain, jaundice, and fever/chills.
  - **Reynolds' pentad:** Charcot's triad plus shock and altered mental status may be seen in suppurative cholangitis.
- Look for RUQ tenderness and **Murphy's sign** (inspiratory arrest during deep palpation of the RUQ). Look for jaundice as a sign of common bile duct obstruction.

Symptoms of cholangitis:

- *RUQ pain*
- *Fever*
- *Jaundice*

DIAGNOSIS

- Labs reveal **leukocytosis,** $\uparrow$ amylase, and $\uparrow$ LFTs.
- **Ultrasound** is 85–90% sensitive for gallbladder gallstones and cholecystitis (**echogenic focus that casts a shadow;** pericholecystic fluid = acute cholecystitis). A thickened gallbladder wall and biliary sludge are less specific findings (see Figure 2.6-6).
- If ultrasound is equivocal and suspicion for acute cholecystitis is high, proceed to a **HIDA** scan.

Risk factors for cholecystitis—the 5 F's

Female
Fertile
Fat
Forties
Familial

TREATMENT

- **Acute cholecystitis:**
  - IV antibiotics (generally a third-generation cephalosporin plus metronidazole in severe cases), IV fluids, electrolyte repletion.

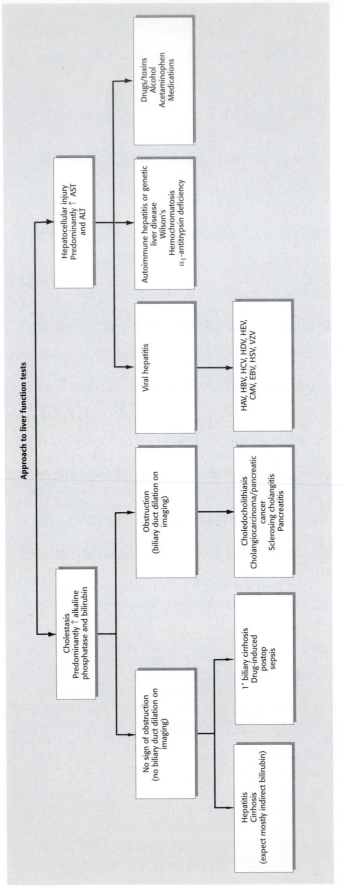

Approach to liver function tests

Cholestasis
Predominantly ↑ alkaline phosphatase and bilirubin

Hepatocellular injury
Predominantly ↑ AST and ALT

No sign of obstruction
(no biliary duct dilation on imaging)

Obstruction
(biliary duct dilation on imaging)

Viral hepatitis

Autoimmune hepatitis or genetic liver disease
Wilson's
Hemochromatosis
α₁-antitrypsin deficiency

Drugs/toxins
Alcohol
Acetaminophen
Medications

Hepatitis
Cirrhosis
(expect mostly indirect bilirubin)

1° biliary cirrhosis
Drug-induced
postop
sepsis

Choledocholithiasis
Cholangiocarcinoma/pancreatic cancer
Sclerosing cholangitis
Pancreatitis

HAV, HBV, HCV, HDV, HEV, CMV, EBV, HSV, VZV

FIGURE 2.6-5. Abnormal liver tests.

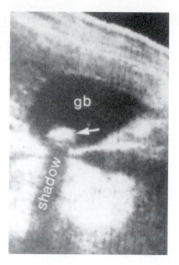

FIGURE 2.6-6.   Gallstone.

An ultrasound through the right upper quadrant showing a distended gallbladder (gb) with a single large stone (arrow) and its acoustic shadow. (Adapted, with permission, from Kasper DL et al. *Harrison's Principles of Internal Medicine,* 16th ed., www.AccessMedicine.com, ©2007 McGraw-Hill Companies.)

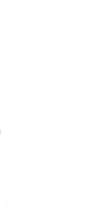

- Early cholecystectomy within 72 hours with an intraoperative cholangiogram to look for common bile duct stones. If the patient is a high-risk surgical candidate, elective surgery may be appropriate if the clinical condition allows.
- If the patient is not a candidate for surgery, consider percutaneous biliary drain.
- **Cholangitis:**
  - Admission, NPO, hydration, pressors if needed, **IV antibiotics** (ciprofloxacin is preferred).
  - **For very ill patients who are not responsive to medical treatment, urgent next-day ERCP with endoscopic sphincterotomy** may be needed. Other emergency options are ERCP with stent placement, percutaneous transhepatic drainage, and operative decompression.

VIRAL AND NONVIRAL HEPATITIS

May be acute and self-limited or chronic and symptomatic. May not be detected until years after the initial infection.

SYMPTOMS/EXAM

- In **acute** cases, patients may present with anorexia, **nausea,** vomiting, malaise, and fever but are frequently **asymptomatic.**
- Exam is often normal but may reveal an enlarged and tender liver, dark urine, and jaundice.

DIFFERENTIAL

- In the setting of a **high level of transaminase elevation (> 10–20 times the upper limit of normal),** consider acute viral infection as well as ischemia ("shock liver"), acute choledocholithiasis, or toxins (acetaminophen).

- With **moderate transaminase elevation,** consider chronic viral infection, autoimmune disorders, nonalcoholic fatty liver disease, mononucleosis, CMV, 2° syphilis, drug-induced illness, and Budd-Chiari syndrome.
- With mild transaminase elevation, also consider hemochromatosis, celiac disease, IBD, and right-sided heart failure.

DIAGNOSIS

Diagnose on the basis of the following:

- The presence of hepatitis based on clinical presentation as well as ↑ transaminases.
- Serology and/or PCR testing confirming a specific virus (see Tables 2.6-1 and 2.6-2).
- Biopsy showing hepatocellular necrosis (rarely indicated).
- An RUQ ultrasound may be performed to see if the liver is enlarged in acute hepatitis (vs. cirrhotic nodular liver in the advanced disease state).

TREATMENT

Treat according to subtype as outlined in Table 2.6-1. Additional guidelines are as follows:

- Rest during the acute phase.
- Avoid hepatotoxic agents; avoid morphine; avoid elective surgery.
- Although most symptoms resolve in 3–16 weeks, LFTs may remain elevated for much longer.

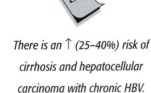

There is an ↑ (25–40%) risk of cirrhosis and hepatocellular carcinoma with chronic HBV.

TABLE 2.6-1. Viral Hepatitis and Serologic Tests

TYPE OF VIRAL HEPATITIS	⊕ SEROLOGY
Acute HAV	Anti-HAV IgM.
Previous HAV	Anti-HAV IgG.
Acute HBV	HBsAg; HBeAg; HBcAb IgM.
Acute HBV, window period	HBcAb IgM only.
Chronic active HBV	HBsAg, HBsAb IgG, HBeAg, HBcAb IgG.
Recovery HBV	HBsAb IgG, HBcAb IgG, normal ALT.
Immunized HBV	HBsAb IgG.
Acute HCV with recovery	HCV RNA early; anti-HCV Ab; recombinant immunoblot assay (RIBA); ALT elevated early.
Acute HCV with chronic infection	HCV RNA, anti-HCV Ab, RIBA, elevated/normal ALT.
Recovery HCV	Anti-HCV Ab and normal ALT.

TABLE 2.6-2. Etiologies, Diagnosis, and Treatment of Viral Hepatitis

SUBTYPE	TRANSMISSION	CLINICAL/LAB FINDINGS	TREATMENT	OTHER KEY FACTS
HAV	Transmitted via contaminated food, water, milk, and shellfish. Known day-care-center outbreaks have been identified. **Fecal-oral transmission;** has a six-day to six-weeks incubation period. Virus is shed in stool up to two weeks before symptom onset.	No chronic infection.	Supportive; generally no sequelae.	Give **immunoglobulin** to close contacts without HAV infection or vaccination.
HBV	Transmitted by **infected blood,** through **sexual contact,** or **perinatally.** Incubation is six weeks to six months. HDV can coinfect persons with HBV.	High prevalence in men who have sex with men, prostitutes, and IV drug users. Fewer than 1% of cases are fulminant. Adult acquired infection usually does not become chronic.	Interferon, **lamivudine,** and other nucleotide/ nucleoside analogs. (The goal is to ↓ viral load and improve liver histology; cure is uncommon.)	Vaccinate patients with chronic HBV against HAV. Associated with arthritis, glomerulonephritis, and **polyarteritis nodosa.** Chronic infection can result in hepatocellular carcinoma.
HCV	Transmitted through **blood transfusion or IV drug use** as well as through intranasal cocaine use or body piercing. Incubation is 6–7 weeks.	Illness is often mild or asymptomatic and is characterized by **waxing and waning aminotransferases.** HCV antibody is not protective. Antibody appears six weeks to nine months after infection. Diagnose acute infection with HCV RNA. Over 70% of infections become chronic.	Interferon + **ribavirin** combination therapy.	Vaccinate patients with HCV against HAV and HBV. Complications include **cryoglobulinemia** and membrano-proliferative glomerulonephritis, as well as hepatocellular carcinoma in patients with cirrhosis.

HIGH-YIELD FACTS

GASTROENTEROLOGY

SUBTYPE	TRANSMISSION	CLINICAL/LAB FINDINGS	TREATMENT	OTHER KEY FACTS
HDV	Requires a coexistent **HBV** infection. Percutaneous exposure. Usually found in **IV drug users** and high-risk **HBsAg carriers.**	Anti-HDV IgM is present in acute cases. Immunity to HBV implies immunity to HDV.	Similar to HBV infection.	If acquired as a superinfection in chronic HBV, there is an ↑ in the severity of the infection. Fulminant hepatitis or severe chronic hepatitis with rapid progression to cirrhosis can occur. Associated with an ↑ risk of **hepatocellular carcinoma.**
HEV	Fecal-oral transmission.	Will test ⊕ on serology for HEV.	Supportive.	Self-limited; endemic to India, Afghanistan, Mexico, and Algeria. Carries a 10–20% mortality rate in **pregnant** women.

ACETAMINOPHEN TOXICITY

SYMPTOMS/EXAM

Within 2–4 hours of an acute overdose, patients present with nausea, vomiting, diaphoresis, and pallor. Within 24–48 hours, hepatotoxicity is manifested by RUQ tenderness, hepatomegaly, and ↑ transaminases.

TREATMENT

- Supportive measures; oral administration of activated charcoal or cholestyramine within 30 minutes of ingestion to prevent absorption of residual drug.
- Begin **N-acetylcysteine** administration up to 36 hours after ingestion if the acetaminophen level is > 200 μg/mL measured at 4 hours or > 100 μg/mL at 8 hours after ingestion or if the time of ingestion is unknown and ↑ levels are seen (see Figure 2.6-7). Even late treatment can be helpful.

HEREDITARY HEMOCHROMATOSIS

- An **autosomal-recessive** disorder of **iron overload.** Usually affects **middle-aged Caucasian men** at a rate of 1 in 300.
- **Sx/Exam:** Presents with **mild transaminitis, DM, arthritis, infertility,** and heart failure.
- **Dx:** Diagnosis is made with ↑ iron saturation (> 60% in men and > 50% in women), ↑ ferritin, ↑ transferrin saturation, and the presence of the **HFE gene mutation.**
- **Tx:** Treat with **phlebotomy** to ↓ the iron burden. Genetic counseling is useful to assess the likelihood of transmission.

HIGH-YIELD FACTS

GASTROENTEROLOGY

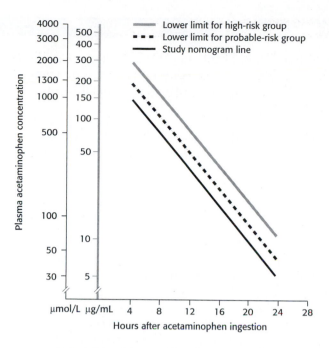

FIGURE 2.6-7. **Estimation of the severity of acetaminophen ingestion.**

(Reproduced, with permission, from Kasper DL et al. *Harrison's Principles of Internal Medicine*, 16th ed. New York: McGraw-Hill, 2005: 1841.)

WILSON'S DISEASE

- An **autosomal-recessive** disorder of **copper overload.**
- **Sx/Exam:** Exam may reveals **Kayser-Fleischer rings** and **neuropsychiatric** disorders.
- **Dx:** Labs reveal ↑ urinary copper, ↓ serum **ceruloplasmin**, and ↑ hepatic copper content on liver biopsy.
- **Tx:** Treatment is via **chelation** with penicillamine and trientine.

α_1-ANTITRYPSIN DISORDER

- Usually affects the **liver** (cirrhosis) and the **lung** (emphysema).
- **Dx:** Diagnosed by the quantitative absence of α_1-antitrypsin on serum protein electrophoresis (SPEP), as well as genotype analysis (autosomal recessive).
- **Tx:** Treatment is via **liver transplantation** and α_1-antitrypsin replacement for the lung.

AUTOIMMUNE HEPATITIS

- Primarily affects **young women;** usually suspected when transaminases are elevated.
- **Dx:** Hypergammaglobulinemia is seen on SPEP; autoantibodies are sometimes seen (**ANA**, anti–smooth muscle antibody [**ASMA**], liver/kidney microsomal antibody [**LKMA**]). Ultimately, a **liver biopsy** is needed to confirm the diagnosis.
- **Tx:** Treat with **corticosteroids and azathioprine.** A significant number of patients relapse when off therapy and thus require long-term treatment.

1° BILIARY CIRRHOSIS

- **Autoimmune** destruction of intrahepatic bile ducts. Usually occurs with other autoimmune diseases. More commonly occurs in **women.**
- **Sx/Exam:** Presents with fatigue, **pruritus,** fat **malabsorption, and osteoporosis.**
- **Dx:** Suggested by markedly ↑ alkaline phosphatase, ↑ bilirubin (late), and **antimitochondrial antibody (AMA).** Confirmed by biopsy.
- **Tx:** Ursodeoxycholic acid, fat-soluble vitamins, cholestyramine for pruritus, and transplantation.

1° SCLEROSING CHOLANGITIS

- **Idiopathic** intra- and extrahepatic fibrosis of bile ducts. Affects **men** 20–50 years of age; associated with **IBD, usually ulcerative colitis.**
- **Sx/Exam:** Can present with **RUQ pain** and pruritus but is often **asymptomatic.**
- **Dx:** Look for ↑ bilirubin and alkaline phosphatase; ⊕ **ASMA;** ⊕ **p-ANCA;** and multiple areas of beaded bile duct strictures on ERCP.
- **Tx:** Treat with ursodeoxycholic acid, cholestyramine, fat-soluble vitamins, stenting of the strictures, and ultimately liver transplantation.

CIRRHOSIS AND ASCITES

Chronic irreversible changes of the hepatic parenchyma, including fibrosis and regenerative nodules. The most common cause in the United States is alcohol abuse, followed by chronic viral hepatitis.

SYMPTOMS/EXAM

- Cirrhosis can be asymptomatic for long periods. Symptoms reflect the **severity** of hepatic damage, **not** the underlying etiology of the liver disease.
- ↓ hepatic function → jaundice, edema, coagulopathy, and metabolic abnormalities (see Figure 2.6-8).
- Fibrosis and distorted vasculature → portal hypertension → gastroesophageal varices and splenomegaly.
- ↓ hepatic function and portal hypertension → ascites and hepatic encephalopathy.

DIAGNOSIS

Cirrhosis is diagnosed as follows:

- **Labs:**
    - Laboratory abnormalities may be absent in quiescent cirrhosis.
    - ALT/AST levels are elevated during active hepatocellular injury. However, levels may not be elevated in cirrhosis because a large portion of the liver is replaced by fibrous tissue, and little new cell injury may be occurring.
    - Additional lab findings include anemia from suppressed erythropoiesis; leukopenia from hypersplenism or leukocytosis from infection; thrombocytopenia from alcoholic marrow suppression; ↓ hepatic thrombopoietin production and splenic sequestration; and prolonged PT from failure of hepatic synthesis of clotting factors.

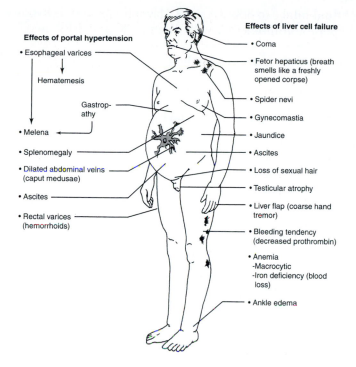

Effects of portal hypertension

- Esophageal varices
- Hematemesis
- Gastrop-athy
- Melena
- Splenomegaly
- Dilated abdominal veins (caput medusae)
- Ascites
- Rectal varices (hemorrhoids)

Effects of liver cell failure

- Coma
- Fetor hepaticus (breath smells like a freshly opened corpse)
- Spider nevi
- Gynecomastia
- Jaundice
- Ascites
- Loss of sexual hair
- Testicular atrophy
- Liver flap (coarse hand tremor)
- Bleeding tendency (decreased prothrombin)
- Anemia
  -Macrocytic
  -Iron deficiency (blood loss)
- Ankle edema

FIGURE 2.6-8. Clinical effects of cirrhosis.

(Reproduced, with permission, from Chandrasoma P, Taylor CE. *Concise Pathology*, 3rd ed. Originally published by Appleton & Lange. Copyright © 1998 by The McGraw-Hill Companies, Inc.)

- **Imaging:**
  - **Ultrasound:** Used to assess liver size and to detect ascites or hepatic nodules. Doppler ultrasound can establish the patency of the splenic, portal, and hepatic veins.
  - **CT with contrast:** Used to characterize hepatic nodules. A biopsy may be needed to rule out malignancy.
- Liver biopsy is the most accurate means of assessing disease severity.

Ascites is diagnosed in the following manner:

- **Ultrasound** and **paracentesis:** Check cell count, differential, albumin, and bacterial cultures +/− acid-fast stain and +/− cytology. The etiology of the ascites can be further characterized as follows:
  - **Related to portal hypertension (serum-ascites albumin gradient [SAAG] ≥ 1.1):** Cirrhosis, heart failure, Budd-Chiari syndrome (hepatic vein thrombosis).
  - **Unrelated to portal hypertension (SAAG < 1.1):** Peritonitis (e.g., TB), cancer, pancreatitis, trauma, nephrotic syndrome.
- If a patient with cirrhosis and established ascites presents with worsening ascites, fever, altered mental status, renal dysfunction, or abdominal pain, think of **spontaneous bacterial peritonitis (SBP)**.

Diagnose SBP with ⊕ cultures or a peritoneal fluid neutrophil count > 250.

TREATMENT

Treatment for **cirrhosis** is as follows:

- Abstain from alcohol.
- The diet should include ample protein. Dietary protein should not be restricted except occasionally in refractory hepatic encephalopathy.

- Restrict fluid intake to 800–1000 mL/day if the patient is hyponatremic.
- Treat hypoprothrombinemia with vitamin K and FFP if clinically indicated.
- Treat anemia with iron (in iron-deficiency anemia) or folic acid (in alcoholics).
- Liver transplantation is required in the setting of progressive liver disease.

Treatment for **ascites** includes the following:

- **Portal hypertension:**
    - **Sodium restriction** to < 2 g/day.
    - **Diuretics:** Furosemide and spironolactone in combination.
    - Large-volume paracentesis for painful distention.
    - Transjugular intrahepatic portosystemic shunt (TIPS) can be used in refractory cases, but this ↑ the rate of encephalopathy.
    - Ultimately, liver transplant if the patient is a candidate.
- **No portal hypertension:** Treat the underlying disorder. Therapeutic paracentesis also can be performed.
- Treat SBP with a **third-generation cephalosporin** (first-line therapy) or a **fluoroquinolone**. Often recurs.

Treat hepatic encephalopathy with lactulose and neomycin.

UPPER GI BLEED

Bleeding in the section of the GI tract extending from the upper esophagus to the duodenum at the **ligament of Treitz.** Mostly due to **PUD, gastritis, varices, or Mallory-Weiss syndrome** (see Figure 2.6-9).

SYMPTOMS

- May present with **dizziness,** lightheadedness, weakness, and nausea.
- Patients may also report vomiting of blood or dark brown contents (**hematemesis**—vomiting of fresh blood, clots, or coffee-ground material) or passing black stool (**melena**—dark, tarry stools composed of degraded blood from the upper GI tract).

EXAM

- Associated with pallor, **abdominal pain,** tachycardia, and hypotension; rectal exam reveals blood.

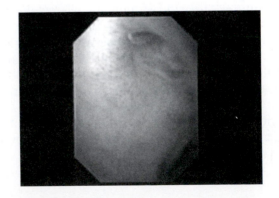

FIGURE 2.6-9. **Duodenal ulcer with oozing.**

(Courtesy of Kenneth R. McQuaid, MD.)

- Patients show signs of **cirrhosis** (telangiectasia, spider angiomata, gynecomastia, testicular atrophy, palmar erythema, caput medusae).
- **Vital signs** reveal **tachycardia** at 10% volume loss, orthostatic **hypotension** at 20% blood loss, and **shock** at 30% loss.

DIAGNOSIS

- Assess the severity of the bleed beginning with the **ABCs**.
- Check **hematocrit** (may be normal in acute blood loss), **platelet count, BUN/creatinine** (an ↑ ratio reflects volume depletion), PT/PTT, and LFTs.
- NG tube placement and lavage to assess the activity and severity of the bleed (if clear, the bleed could be intermittent or from the duodenum).
- If perforation is suspected, obtain upright and abdominal x-rays.
- Endoscopy can be both diagnostic and therapeutic in some cases.

TREATMENT

- Start with the **ABCs.** Use at least **two large-bore** peripheral IV catheters. **Transfusion** and intravascular volume replacement are indicated.
- Consult GI and surgery if bleeding does not stop or if difficulty is encountered with resuscitation 2° to a brisk bleed.
- Treat **variceal bleeds** with **octreotide**, endoscopic **sclerotherapy**, or **band ligation.** If the bleed is severe, balloon tamponade is appropriate, followed by embolization or **TIPS** if endoscopic therapy fails.
- To prevent variceal bleeds, treat with **nonselective** β-blockers (e.g., propranolol), obliterative endoscopic therapy, **shunting,** and, if the patient is an appropriate candidate, liver transplantation.
- For **PUD,** use **PPIs,** endoscopic epinephrine injection, thermal contact, and laser therapy. Begin *H. pylori* eradication measures.
- **Mallory-Weiss tears** usually stop bleeding **spontaneously.**
- Treat **esophagitis/gastritis** with PPIs or H_2 antagonists. Avoid aspirin and NSAIDs.

LOWER GI BLEED

Bleeding that is distal to the ligament of Treitz.

SYMPTOMS/EXAM

- Presents with **hematochezia** (fresh blood or clot per rectum).
- Diarrhea, tenesmus, bright red blood per rectum, or maroon-colored stools are also seen.
- As with upper GI bleeds, check vital signs to assess the severity of the bleed. Obtain orthostatics; perform a rectal exam for hemorrhoids, fissures, or a mass.

DIFFERENTIAL

Hemorrhoids, diverticulosis (see Figure 2.6-10), angiodysplasia, carcinoma, enteritis, IBD, polyps, Meckel's diverticulum.

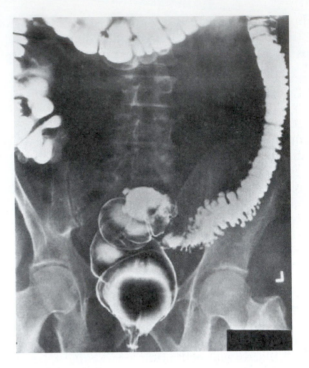

FIGURE 2.6-10. **Diverticulosis.**

Diverticulosis of the sigmoid colon on barium enema. (Reproduced, with permission, from Schwartz SI et al [eds]. *Principles of Surgery*, 5th ed. New York: McGraw-Hill, 1989: 1256.)

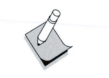

Think diverticulosis with painless lower GI bleeding.

DIAGNOSIS

- First **rule out upper GI bleed.**
- Bleeding usually **stops spontaneously.** However, colonoscopy should be performed; in the majority of cases, the diagnosis can be made at the time of visualization.
- If the bleed continues, a bleeding scan (^{99}Tc-tagged RBC scan) can be done to detect bleeding if it is > 1.0 mL/min.
- If the bleed is refractory, **arteriography** or **exploratory laparotomy** may be done.

TREATMENT

- Although bleeding generally stops spontaneously, resuscitative efforts should be initiated, as with upper GI bleeds, until the source is found and the bleeding stops.
- With diverticular disease, bleeding usually stops spontaneously, but **epinephrine injection,** catheter-directed **vasopressin,** or **embolization** can be used. In some cases, surgery may be needed.

Hematology

Anemia can be classified by the size of the red cell (mean corpuscular volume; MCV) as microcytic, normocytic, or macrocytic.

DIAGNOSIS

- Initially, order a CBC, MCV, blood smear, and reticulocyte count.
- On the basis of the initial results, order 2° tests such as iron studies (ferritin, serum iron, TIBC), serum folate, TSH, serum B_{12}, hemolysis labs (LDH, unconjugated bilirubin, haptoglobin, Coombs' test), and a DIC panel (D-dimer, fibrinogen, blood smear, soluble fibrin monomer complex).
- Look for a bleeding source, and order a cross and type if the patient is actively bleeding or symptomatic from anemia.
- Look for **pancytopenia.** Etiologies include toxins, drugs, infection, myelodysplasia, malignancy, radiation, vitamin B_{12}/folate deficiency, SLE, and congenital causes.

TREATMENT

Patients with severe anemia and those who are symptomatic initially require fluid resuscitation and RBC transfusion. Transfuse to keep serum hemoglobin > 7 g/dL, or > 8 g/dL for CAD patients. Identify the cause of the anemia and treat the underlying disorder.

Microcytic Anemia

Anemia with an MCV < 80 fL. Anemia with an **MCV < 70 fL** is due to either **iron-deficiency anemia or thalassemia.** Other causes include anemia of chronic disease and sideroblastic anemia (see the mnemonic **TICS**).

SYMPTOMS/EXAM

Iron-deficient patients may have **pica.** Ask about melena and blood in the stools; check for fecal occult blood. For females, ask about heavy menstrual periods. A family history of anemia should raise suspicion for thalassemia.

DIAGNOSIS

Examine iron studies, a blood smear, and a CBC to identify the cause of the microcytic anemia (see Table 2.7-1). Suspect **colorectal cancer** in elderly patients with microcytic anemia, and refer these patients for a colonoscopy.

TREATMENT

- If iron-deficiency anemia is the cause, identify the site of blood loss and initiate oral iron supplementation (patients intolerant of oral therapy and those with GI disease may need parenteral therapy). **Treatment should be continued 3–6 months after lab values are normal to help replenish stores.**
- Erythropoietin (**Epogen**) should be administered to patients with anemia of chronic disease, particularly chronic renal disease.
- The treatment of thalassemia is detailed separately in the discussion below.

HIGH-YIELD FACTS

HEMATOLOGY

Causes of microcytic anemia—TICS

Thalassemia
Iron deficiency
Chronic disease
Sideroblastic anemia

Serum ferritin, a measure of iron stores, is ↓ in iron-deficiency anemia but is ↑ in infection and inflammation (anemia of chronic disease).

TABLE 2.7-1.   Causes of Microcytic Anemia

	IRON-DEFICIENCY ANEMIA	THALASSEMIA	ANEMIA OF CHRONIC DISEASE (LATE)	SIDEROBLASTIC ANEMIA
Serum ferritin	↓ (may be normal in inflammatory states, including cancer)	Normal to ↑	↑ (may be normal in early stages)	↑
Serum iron	↓	Normal to ↑	Slightly ↓	↓
Iron-binding capacity	↑	Normal to ↑	**Normal to ↓**	Normal
Other tests	**Wide RDW.**	**Normal RDW.** **Order hemoglobin electrophoresis to confirm the diagnosis.**		**Smear shows normal and dimorphic RBCs with basophilic stippling.** Confirm the diagnosis with bone marrow biopsy (shows erythroid hyperplasia and ringed sideroblasts).
Comments	Etiologies include malabsorption, chronic blood loss, and malnutrition. Thrombocytosis is common.	Characterized by ↓ or absent production of one or more globin chains in the hemoglobin. Also marked by an elevated MCHC and an MCV/RBC < 13.	Etiologies include chronic inflammation, infection, and malignancy.	Etiologies include chronic alcohol use, drugs (antitubercular, chloramphenicol), and lead poisoning. Has ↑ transferrin levels. Order lead levels if lead toxicity is suspected.

THALASSEMIA

A group of disorders resulting from ↓ synthesis of α- or β-globin protein subunits. α-thalassemia is most common among **Asians** and African-Americans; β-thalassemia is most frequently found in people of **Mediterranean** origin as well as in Asians and African-Americans.

SYMPTOMS/EXAM

Clinical presentation varies according to subtype:

- α-thalassemia: If **all four** α alleles are affected, babies are stillborn with **hydrops fetalis** or die shortly after birth. **HbH** disease with **three** affected alleles → **chronic hemolytic microcytic anemia** and **splenomegaly.** Carriers of one or two affected alleles are usually asymptomatic.
- β-thalassemia: β-thalassemia **major** (homozygous; no β-globin production and hence no HbA) presents in the first year of life as the fraction of HbF declines. Manifestations include growth retardation, **bony deformities,** hepatosplenomegaly, and jaundice. β-thalassemia **minor** (heterozygous) is usually less severe and is diagnosed by an ↑ HbA$_2$ on electrophoresis.

DIAGNOSIS

CBC reveals severe microcytic anemia with normal RDW and an ↑ RBC count (unlike iron deficiency). Hemoglobin electrophoresis is the definitive diagnostic test.

TREATMENT

- Although the treatment of choice for patients with thalassemia is allogeneic bone marrow transplantation, blood transfusions should be given as necessary for symptomatic control, and patients must receive folate supplementation.
- To prevent 2° hemosiderosis due to iron overload, deferoxamine, an iron chelator, is usually given concomitantly.
- Prenatal diagnosis is now available, and genetic counseling should be offered to high-risk families.

Treat iron overload and 2° hemosiderosis—a common complication of repeated blood transfusions for thalassemia—with an iron chelator such as deferoxamine.

Macrocytic Anemia

Anemia with an MCV > 100 fL. Causes include the following:

- **Folate deficiency:** Common causes include poor dietary intake (including that which occurs with **alcoholism**) and **drugs** (e.g., phenytoin, zidovudine, TMP-SMX, methotrexate, and other chemotherapeutic agents).
- **B_{12} deficiency:** Commonly caused by a strict vegetarian diet, **pernicious anemia,** gastrectomy, and ileal dysfunction (Crohn's disease, surgical resection). B_{12} deficiency can cause **neurologic deficits** (paresthesias, gait disturbance, and mental status changes).
- **Other:** Liver disease, hypothyroidism, alcohol abuse, myelodysplasia.

An MCV > 110 fL is usually due to vitamin B_{12} or folate deficiency.

DIAGNOSIS

- Emphasis should be placed on obtaining a serum B_{12} level, an RBC folate level, and a **blood smear** to look for megaloblastic anemia, which shows **oval macrocytes** and hypersegmented neutrophils (see Figure 2.7-1).
- If B_{12} deficiency is suspected, check intrinsic factor antibody and anti–parietal cell antibody for pernicious anemia. A Schilling test may be used to confirm the cause.
- Methylmalonic acid levels will confirm the diagnosis in patients with borderline levels.

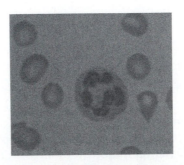

FIGURE 2.7-1. **Hypersegmented neutrophil seen in megaloblastic anemia.**

(Courtesy of Peter McPhedran, MD, Yale University.)

TREATMENT

- Treat B_{12} deficiency with monthly B_{12} shots; treat folate deficiency with oral replacement.
- Discontinue any medications that could be contributing to megaloblastic anemia; minimize alcohol use.

Normocytic Normochromic Anemia

Anemia with an MCV of 80–100 fL. May be due to **blood loss (hemorrhage)**, **hemolysis**, or $\downarrow$ **production**.

SYMPTOMS/EXAM

Look for evidence of acute bleeding on history and exam. Patients with **hemolytic anemia** may present with jaundice and dark urine from unconjugated hyperbilirubinemia as well as with pigment gallstones and splenomegaly.

DIAGNOSIS

The initial workup should focus on reticulocyte count, creatinine, hemolysis labs, and blood smear.

- **Normal reticulocyte count:** Anemia of chronic disease or chronic renal failure.
- $\uparrow$ **reticulocyte count with normal hemolysis labs:** Hemorrhage.
- $\uparrow$ **reticulocyte count,** $\uparrow$ **LDH,** $\uparrow$ **unconjugated bilirubin,** and $\downarrow$ **haptoglobin:** Hemolysis. Causes include the following:
  - **Microangiopathic hemolytic anemia:** Schistocytes or helmet cells are seen on blood smear; see below.
  - **Hereditary spherocytosis:** Characterized by spherocytes, a $\oplus$ family history, and a $\ominus$ Coombs' test.
  - **Autoimmune hemolytic anemia:** Marked by spherocytes with a $\oplus$ **Coombs' test.**
  - **Cold agglutinin disease:** Acrocyanosis in cold exposure. The cold agglutinin test is $\oplus$. Seen with mycoplasmal infection and mononucleosis.
  - **Sickle cell anemia:** See below.
  - **G6PD deficiency:** Hemolysis in the presence of infection or drugs (primarily sulfa drugs). Peripheral blood smear may show characteristic bite cells (has the appearance of a bite taken out from the periphery). G6PD levels may be normal during hemolytic episodes but are $\downarrow$ thereafter.
  - **Paroxysmal nocturnal hemoglobinuria (PNH):** Intravascular hemolysis (with ensuing hemoglobinuria) and **recurrent thrombosis.** May involve pancytopenia. Diagnosed by **flow cytometry.**

TREATMENT

- Patients who are hemorrhaging must be resuscitated with fluids and RBC transfusions. The cause of the bleeding must be identified and treated.
- **Hereditary spherocytosis** usually responds to **splenectomy.**
- Treatment for **autoimmune hemolytic anemia** includes **steroids,** immunosuppressive agents, IVIG, and, if necessary, splenectomy.

MICROANGIOPATHIC HEMOLYTIC ANEMIA

Defined as the presence of **intravascular hemolysis with fragmented RBCs (schistocytes and helmet cells** on blood smear). Constitutes a **medical emergency.** Distinguished as follows (see also Table 2.7-2):

- **DIC:** Overwhelming systemic activation of the coagulation system stimulated by serious illness. Causes include sepsis, shock, malignancy, obstetric complications, and trauma.
- **HUS:** The triad of hemolytic anemia, thrombocytopenia, and ARF. Causes include viral illness and *E. coli* O157:H7.
- **TTP:** Presents as a **pentad** of the HUS triad plus fever and fluctuating neurologic signs, although patients may not have all five. Causes include HIV, pregnancy, and OCP use.

TREATMENT

- **DIC:** Treat the underlying condition; transfuse platelets; give cryoprecipitate (to replace fibrinogen) and FFP (to replace coagulation factors).
- **HUS:** Treat with dialysis for ARF.
- **TTP:** The treatment of choice is **plasmapheresis.** In urgent situations, give FFP until plasmapheresis becomes available. Do not give platelets, as this may exacerbate the TTP.

SICKLE CELL ANEMIA

An autosomal-recessive disease resulting from the substitution of valine for glutamic acid at the sixth position in the globin chain.

SYMPTOMS/EXAM

Seen predominantly among African-Americans, who often have a ⊕ family history. Clinical features include stigmata of chronic hemolysis such as gallstones, poorly healing ulcers, jaundice, splenomegaly (usually during childhood), and CHF.

TABLE 2.7-2. Differential of Microangiopathic Hemolytic Anemia

	PLATELETS	PT/PTT	D-DIMER	OTHER FINDINGS
TTP or HUS	↓↓↓	Normal	Normal	ARF, CNS dysfunction.
DIC	↓↓	↑	↑↑	↑ fibrin split products, ↓ fibrinogen.
Mechanical valve	Normal	Normal	Normal	Heart murmur.
Severe vasculitis, severe hypertension, HELLP	↓	Normal	Normal	Elevated liver enzymes in HELLP.

DIAGNOSIS

Blood smear reveals sickled cells, Howell-Jolly bodies, and evidence of hemolysis. Hemoglobin electrophoresis is the definitive diagnostic test.

TREATMENT

- Vaccinate all patients for *Streptococcus pneumoniae*, *Haemophilus influenzae*, and HBV.
- Give folic acid supplementation.
- Consider transfusions for severe anemia, sickle cell crisis, and priapism.
- Instruct patients to avoid dehydration, hypoxia, intense exercise, and high altitudes.
- In patients with frequent pain crisis, hydroxyurea or bone marrow transplantation should be considered.

COMPLICATIONS

- **Pain crisis:**
  - Sickled cells cause occlusion of arterioles → tissue infarction. Characterized by pain in the back, limbs, abdomen, and ribs.
  - Precipitated by dehydration, acidosis, infection, fever, or hypoxia.
  - Treat with hydration, analgesia, and supplemental O_2.
- **Aplastic crisis:** A sudden ↓ in hemoglobin and reticulocyte count caused by parvovirus B19. Support with transfusions.
- **Acute chest crisis:**
  - Sickled cells cause occlusion of pulmonary blood supply and lung infarctions.
  - Clinical findings include fever, chest pain, cough, wheezing, tachypnea, and new pulmonary infiltrate on CXR.
  - Treat with O_2, analgesia, transfusions, and antibiotics (a second-generation cephalosporin with erythromycin).
- **Lungs:** Pulmonary infarcts can cause pulmonary hypertension.
- **Heart:** Sickle cell cardiomyopathy → heart failure.
- **GI tract:** Cholecystitis, splenic infarcts.
- **Kidneys:** Sickling of cells can cause infarcts → papillary necrosis and ARF (particularly in sickle cell trait).
- **Genital:** Priapism, impotence in males.
- **Infections:** The absence of a functional spleen predisposes patients to encapsulated organisms, including *S. pneumoniae*, *H. influenzae*, *Neisseria meningitidis*, and gram-⊖ bacterial infections.
- **Bones:** Avascular necrosis, *Salmonella* osteomyelitis.
- **Pregnancy:** Patients are at ↑ risk of spontaneous abortions.

POLYCYTHEMIA VERA (PCV)

A myeloproliferative syndrome in which the predominant abnormality is ↑ RBCs. Classically affects males > 60 years of age. The most common cause of erythrocytosis is **chronic hypoxia** 2° to lung disease rather than 1° PCV.

SYMPTOMS/EXAM

- Patients present with malaise, fever, pruritus (especially after a warm shower), and signs of vascular sludging (e.g., **stroke**, angina, MI, claudication, hepatic vein thrombosis, headache, and blurred vision).
- Exam may reveal **plethora,** large retinal veins on funduscopy, and **splenomegaly.**

DIAGNOSIS

- Labs show ↑ **hematocrit** (≥ 50%), ↑ RBC mass, and a normal **erythropoietin** level (↑ in chronic hypoxia-induced polycythemia). Basophilia suggests proliferative myelopoiesis. JAK-2 ⊕.
- Establish the diagnosis by bone marrow biopsy, which shows a hypercellular marrow.
- Table 2.7-3 outlines the laboratory features of PCV in contrast to those of other myeloproliferative disorders.

Distinguish polycythemia vera from other causes of 2° polycythemia through an erythropoietin level.

TREATMENT

Treatment includes **serial phlebotomy** until hematocrit is < 45 (men) and < 42 (women) along with **daily ASA**. Hydroxyurea is appropriate for those at high risk of thrombosis (age over 70, prior thrombosis, platelet count > 1,500,000/μL, presence of cardiovascular risk factors). Anagrelide can be used to ↓ platelets in refractory patients.

COMPLICATIONS

PCV, like other myeloproliferative syndromes, is associated with an ↑ **risk of conversion** to other myeloproliferative syndromes or AML.

BLEEDING DISORDERS

Disorders in **coagulation or platelets** that predispose patients to bleed (see Table 2.7-4).

DIAGNOSIS

- Initial tests to order include PT/PTT, CBC, platelet count, and DIC panel (D-dimer, fibrinogen, blood smear). Use these laboratory data to determine if the cause of the bleeding is 2° to a coagulopathy or a platelet problem.
  - Think **thrombocytopenia** when the platelet count is < 90,000 cells/μL (see the discussion of platelet pathology below).
  - Think **coagulopathy** if the PT or PTT is ↑ (see the discussion of coagulopathies).
- If platelet count and PT/PTT are normal, check bleeding time (PFA-100 test) and thrombin time. An ↑ bleeding time suggests a **platelet dysfunction**. An ↑ thrombin time suggests a **defect in the cross-linking of fibrin** such as that in **dysfibrinogenemia or DIC**.

Petechiae = **P**latelet deficiency.
Cavity/joint bleeding = **C**lotting factor deficiency.

TABLE 2.7-3. Laboratory Features of Myeloproliferative Disorders

	WBC COUNT	HEMATOCRIT	PLATELET COUNT	RBC MORPHOLOGY
CML	↑↑	Normal	Normal or ↑	Normal
Myelofibrosis	Normal or ↓/↑	Normal or ↓	Normal or ↓/↑	**Abnormal**
PCV	Normal or ↑	↑	Normal or ↑	Normal
Essential thrombocytosis	Normal or ↑	Normal	↑↑	Normal

Reproduced, with permission, from Tierney LM et al (eds). *Current Medical Diagnosis & Treatment: 2004.* New York: McGraw-Hill, 2004: 481.

CLINICAL FEATURE	PLATELET DISORDER	COAGULOPATHY
Amount of bleeding after surface cuts	Excessive, prolonged.	Normal to slightly ↑.
Onset of bleeding after injury	Immediate bleeding.	Delayed bleeding after surgery or trauma. Spontaneous bleeding into joints or hematoma.
Clinical presentation	Superficial and mucosal bleeding (GI tract, gingival, nasal). Petechiae, ecchymosis.	Deep and excessive bleeding into joints, muscles, GI tract, and GU tract.

TREATMENT

- Patients who are hemodynamically unstable need immediate resuscitation with IV fluids. The source of hemorrhage should be identified and stopped.
- Blood transfusions should be given to maintain a hemoglobin > 8 g/dL. FFP should be given to normalize PTT and PT. Platelets should be given as needed.

Platelet Disorders

Disorders associated with a ↓ in the number of platelets (**thrombocytopenia**) or a ↓ in the functioning of platelets that predisposes patients to bleed (**platelet dysfunction**). Look for petechiae and easy bruising. In addition to TTP and HUS, common platelet disorders include the following:

- **Thrombocytopenia:**
  - **Drug-induced thrombocytopenia:** One of the most common causes of mild asymptomatic thrombocytopenia. Common drugs include quinine, antibiotics, sulfa drugs, and glycoprotein IIb/IIIa inhibitors. Usually resolves within one week of stopping the implicated drug.
  - **ITP:** Severe thrombocytopenia due to **platelet-associated IgG** antibodies. A diagnosis of exclusion. DIC panel is ⊖. Treatment involves **prednisone** and, if the patient is unresponsive to steroids, splenectomy.
  - **Heparin-induced: Immune-mediated** thrombocytopenia occurring 4–14 days after the initiation of heparin. Platelet factor-4 (PF-4) antibodies are used for diagnosis. Treat by stopping heparin immediately and are starting an alternative anticoagulant such as lepirudin, argatroban, or danaparoid sodium (**not** warfarin).
- **Platelet dysfunction:** Normal platelet count.
  - **Acquired:** Severe liver disease, severe renal disease, DIC, aspirin use, multiple myeloma. Treat with desmopressin, OCPs for menorrhagia, and FFP or cryoprecipitate for major bleeding. Do not use ASA.
  - **Inherited:** Includes Bernard-Soulier syndrome, Glanzmann's thrombasthenia, and storage pool disease. Treatment is the same as that for acquired disease.

Lymphoma

Lymphomas result from monoclonal proliferation of cells of lymphocyte lineage. Approximately 90% are derived from B cells, 9% from T cells, and 1% from monocytes or natural killer (NK) cells.

Hodgkin's Lymphoma

Malignancy of neoplastic Reed-Sternberg (RS) cells, which are of B-cell origin. EBV infections play a role in the pathogenesis of this disease. Usually affects young adults.

EBV is a common cause of aggressive lymphoma in patients with immune deficiencies.

Symptoms/Exam

- Usually presents with cervical lymphadenopathy and spreads in a predictable manner along the lymph nodes. The spleen is the most commonly involved intra-abdominal site.
- **"B symptoms"** may be present and include **10% weight loss in six months, night sweats requiring a change of clothes, and fever > 38.5°C.** These symptoms indicate bulky disease and a worse prognosis.

Diagnosis

- Diagnosis is usually based on biopsy of an enlarged lymph node that demonstrates the presence of RS cells.
- Staging is predicated on the anatomically based **Ann Arbor system** and on the presence of prognostic factors. Chest and abdominal/pelvic CT as well as bilateral bone marrow biopsies and aspirates are routine.

Reed-Sternberg cells ("owl's eye" nuclei) are pathognomonic for Hodgkin's lymphoma.

Treatment

Treat with chemotherapy consisting of doxorubicin, bleomycin, vinblastine, and dacarbazine (**ABVD cocktail**) with or without radiation of the involved field.

Non-Hodgkin's Lymphoma (NHL)

- Classified as low, intermediate, or high grade on the basis of histologic type.
- Associated with infections—EBV with Burkitt's lymphoma; HIV with CNS lymphoma; HTLV with T-cell lymphoma; and *H. pylori* with gastric MALToma.
- **Dx:** Diagnosis is similar to that of other lymphomas. LDH is a prognostic marker.
- **Tx:**
  - The addition of **rituximab** (monoclonal anti-CD20) to the chemotherapeutic regimen appears to improve outcomes.
  - The treatment of **high-grade NHL** may be complicated by **tumor lysis syndrome,** which consists of **hyperkalemia, hyperphosphatemia, hyperuricemia,** and **hypocalcemia. Treat with aggressive hydration and allopurinol.**
  - Gastric MALTomas can be treated with antibiotics for *H. pylori* as initial therapy.
  - All HIV-related NHL requires immediate institution of antiretroviral therapy (HAART).

Multiple Myeloma

A malignancy of **plasma cells** within bone marrow, often with unbalanced, excessive production of immunoglobulin heavy/light chains. Typically seen in **older adults**.

SYMPTOMS/EXAM

- Symptoms include **back pain** (the presenting symptom in 80% of patients), **hypercalcemic symptoms** ("stones, bones, abdominal moans, and psychiatric overtones"), **pathologic fractures**, fatigue, and frequent infections (2° to dysregulation of antibody production).
- Exam may reveal pallor, fever, bone tenderness, and lethargy.

DIFFERENTIAL

Waldenström's macroglobulinemia is a plasma cell disorder that is similar to multiple myeloma but has a predominance of IgM as well as a higher incidence of cold agglutinins and hyperviscosity syndrome (visual disturbance, dizziness, headache). The latter is treated with urgent plasmapheresis.

DIAGNOSIS

Plain radiographs of the axial skeleton show the characteristic lytic lesions of multiple myeloma. Bone scans are not helpful, since they show blastic activity.

- Critical tests to evaluate for the presence of multiple myeloma (and to distinguish it from MGUS) include **UPEP** (to examine for **Bence Jones protein**) **and SPEP** (to look for monoclonal immunoglobulin, most commonly **IgG, > 3 g/dL**).
- **Bone marrow aspirate** can enumerate **plasma cells (> 10%)**, and a full-body skeletal survey can demonstrate **punched-out osteolytic lesions** of the skull and long bones.
- LAP levels are normal (lesions are osteolytic, not osteoblastic).

TREATMENT

- Treatment is aimed at reducing tumor burden, relieving symptoms, and preventing complications. β-microglobulin is a prognostic marker.
- **Chemotherapy involves use of melphalan and steroids +/− thalidomide. Stem cell transplantation** is used for patients who are < 60 years of age and in advanced stages of disease.
- Treatment measures aimed at alleviating symptoms or preventing complications include the following:
  - **Hypercalcemia:** Treat with hydration, glucocorticoids, and diuresis.
  - **Bone pain/destruction/fractures:** Treat with bisphosphonates and local radiation.
  - **Renal failure:** Give hydration to aid in the excretion of light-chain immunoglobulins.
  - **Infections:** Vaccinate against preventable infections; diagnose early and treat aggressively.
  - **Anemia:** Administer erythropoietin.

BREAST CANCER

The most common cancer and the second most common cause of cancer death in women in the United States (after lung cancer). Routine annual mammography is universally recommended after age 50 (or earlier for high-risk cases and patients with a family history of breast cancer). Routine mammography for those who are 40–50 years of age and are not at high risk is controversial. Risk factors include the following:

- Female gender
- Older age
- Breast cancer in first-degree relatives
- A prior history of breast cancer
- A history of atypical ductal or lobular hyperplasia or carcinoma in situ
- Early menarche, early menopause, or late first full-term pregnancy (before age 35)
- HRT use for > 5 years
- Obesity
- Prior radiation (e.g., for treatment of Hodgkin's lymphoma)

SYMPTOMS/EXAM

- Most masses are discovered by the patient and present as a **hard, irregular, immobile, painless breast lump,** possibly with nipple discharge.
- **Skin changes** (dimpling, erythema, ulceration) and **axillary adenopathy** indicate more advanced disease.
- Any breast mass in postmenopausal women is breast cancer until proven otherwise. The most common location is the **upper outer quadrant.**

DIAGNOSIS

- Diagnosis is suggested by a palpable mass or by **mammographic abnormalities** (e.g., microcalcifications, hyperdense regions, irregular borders) and is confirmed by biopsy.
- In clinically suspicious cases—e.g., those involving patients > 35 years of age with any breast lump—a ⊖ mammogram should be followed by **ultrasound** (to look for cysts vs. solid masses), **FNA** (for palpable lumps), **stereotactic** core biopsy (for nonpalpable lesions), or **excisional** biopsy until convincing evidence has been gathered to support the absence of cancer.
- Biopsied specimens should be tested for prognostic factors such as estrogen/progesterone receptors **(ER/PR)** and **HER2.**
- Special forms of breast cancer include the following:
  - **Inflammatory breast cancer:** A highly aggressive, rapidly growing cancer that invades the lymphatics and causes skin inflammation (i.e., mastitis). Has a poor prognosis.
  - **Paget's disease:** Ductal carcinoma in situ (DCIS) of the nipple with unilateral itching, burning, and nipple erosion. May be mistaken for infection; associated with a focus of invasive carcinoma.

TREATMENT

- **Intraductal carcinoma (DCIS,** or pure ductal carcinoma in situ) warrants **only local therapy** (either mastectomy or wide excision plus radiation therapy).
- Lobular carcinoma in situ (LCIS) is associated with a high risk (up to 20%) of developing a subsequent infiltrating breast cancer, including cancer in the contralateral breast. Therapy options include close monitoring, mastectomy, or the use of tamoxifen for prophylaxis.
- **The choice of treatment for invasive breast cancer is based on lymph node status, tumor size, and hormone receptor status.**
  - Those with **node-⊖ disease** (stage I) can be treated with **breast conservation therapy** (wide tumor excision) or **modified radical mastectomy with radiation therapy.**

Women should be tested for BRCA-1 and BRCA-2 mutations if they have a "genetic" risk: i.e., a strong family history of breast and/or ovarian cancer.

The sensitivity of mammography for breast cancer is 75–80%, so do not stop workup with a ⊖ mammogram in clinically suspicious cases.

ER/PR-⊕ status is a good prognostic indicator in breast cancer, and such patients should be treated with hormonal therapy.

Breast conservation therapy is generally as effective as modified radical mastectomy in patients with a unifocal tumor size of < 4 cm.

- **Adjuvant chemotherapy** (two or more agents such as 5-FU, methotrexate, doxorubicin, cyclophosphamide, or epirubicin for 3–6 months) is usually given for **tumors > 2 cm or those with axillary lymph node involvement (stages II–III)**.
- **Endocrine** therapy such as tamoxifen or raloxifene is beneficial only for patients with **ER-⊕ or PR-⊕ tumors**.
- Trastuzumab (Herceptin) is beneficial for those with HER2-⊕ tumors.

LUNG CANCER

The **leading cause of cancer death**. The major risk factor is **tobacco** use. Other risk factors include radon and asbestos exposure. Subtypes include the following:

- **Adenocarcinoma:** The most common lung cancer; has a **peripheral** location. More common in women.
- **Bronchoalveolar type of adenocarcinoma:** Associated with multiple nodules, bilateral lung infiltrates, and metastases late in the disease course.
- **Squamous cell carcinoma:** Presents **centrally** and is **usually cavitary**.
- **Large cell/neuroendocrine carcinomas:** Least common.
- **Small cell lung cancer (SCLC):** Highly related to **cigarette exposure**. Usually **centrally** located and always presumed to be **disseminated** at the time of diagnosis.

> **The 3 C's of squamous cell carcinoma:**
>
> **C**entral
> **C**avitary
> hyper**C**alcemia

SYMPTOMS/EXAM

- In some cases, an asymptomatic lesion is discovered incidentally on either x-ray or chest CT.
- Most patients, however, develop signs that herald a problem—e.g., chronic **cough, hemoptysis, weight loss,** or **postobstructive pneumonia.**
- **Less frequently, patients may present late with complications of a large tumor burden:**
  - **Pancoast's syndrome:** Presents with shoulder pain, Horner's syndrome (miosis, ptosis, anhidrosis), and lower brachial plexopathy.
  - **Superior vena cava syndrome:** Characterized by swelling of the face and arm, most often on the right side, and elevated JVP. Treated with radiation therapy.
  - **Hoarseness:** Vocal cord paralysis from entrapment of the recurrent laryngeal nerve, most often on the left.
  - **Hypercalcemia:** Most often seen with squamous cell carcinoma. Treat with bisphosphonates.
  - **Trousseau's syndrome:** A hypercoagulable state seen with adenocarcinoma.
  - **Hyponatremia/SIADH:** Small cell carcinoma.
  - **Eaton-Lambert syndrome: Similar to myasthenia gravis, except that muscle fatigue improves with repeated stimulation** (vs. myasthenia gravis, in which such measures yield no improvement).

DIFFERENTIAL

- Other common causes of lung mass include TB/other granulomatous diseases, fungal disease (aspergillosis, histoplasmosis), lung abscess, metastasis, benign tumors (bronchial adenoma), and hamartoma.
- Serial CXRs are useful for distinguishing benign lesions from malignant ones. Lesions that remain stable over > 2 years are generally not cancer-

ous. Other features suggestive of benign lesions include young age, smooth margins, small size (< 2 cm), and the presence of satellite lesions. However, any lung nodule in a smoker or ex-smoker should be evaluated for the presence of cancer.

DIAGNOSIS

- If there is a palpable lymph node (axillary, supraclavicular), consider biopsy of the node first. If not, order a CXR initially, and in doubtful/suspicious cases, obtain a **chest CT and, if needed, bronchoscopy.**
- If mediastinal lymph nodes are enlarged, consider a PET scan and mediastinoscopy for proper staging.
- **Centrally** located cancers can be diagnosed by **bronchoscopy** or **sputum cytology.**
- **Staging** includes chest and abdominal CT, bone scan, and CT or MRI of the head.

TREATMENT

- Non–small cell lung cancer (**NSCLC**) **is potentially curable with resection of localized disease** but is **only modestly responsive to chemotherapy.** Patients are classified into one of three clinical groups at the time of diagnosis:
  - **Stages I and II:** Early-stage disease. Represents candidacy for surgical resection.
  - **Locally or regionally advanced disease** (supraclavicular or mediastinal lymphadenopathy or chest wall/pleural/pericardial invasion): Treated with combination chemotherapy and radiation; surgery is not indicated.
  - **Distant metastases:** The goal of any chemotherapy or radiation is **palliation only.**
- For **SCLC, chemotherapy** is the treatment of choice.

GI TUMORS

Pancreatic Cancer

Typically seen in patients > 50 years of age. **Ductal adenocarcinoma** accounts for 90% of 1° tumors; > 50% arise in the head of the pancreas. Risk factors include smoking, chronic pancreatitis, and diabetes mellitus (DM).

SYMPTOMS/EXAM

Common symptoms include **nausea, anorexia, lumbar back pain, new-onset DM, venous thromboembolism,** and **painless obstructive jaundice** (associated with adenocarcinoma in the **head** of the pancreas).

DIAGNOSIS

- Characterized by ↑ bilirubin, ↑ aminotransferases, and normocytic normochromic anemia.
- **Ultrasound** is useful as an initial diagnostic test. Abdominal/pelvic CT can evaluate the extent of disease; a **thin-section helical CT** through the pancreas can determine if the mass is resectable.
- **Endoscopic ultrasonography** yields excellent anatomic detail and can help confirm if the tumor is resectable.

Painless jaundice and/or palpable gallbladder–think pancreatic cancer.

TREATMENT

- **Pancreaticoduodenectomy** (Whipple procedure) is appropriate for patients with resectable tumors.
- **Chemotherapy** or **radiation** is used for **palliative care** in patients with advanced or unresectable disease.

Hepatocellular Cancer (Hepatoma)

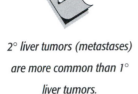

Risk factors for hepatocellular cancer (HCC) include viral hepatitis (HBV, HCV), alcoholic cirrhosis, aflatoxin, hemochromatosis, and α_1-antitrypsin deficiency. OCPs are associated with benign hepatic adenoma (vs. HCC).

2° liver tumors (metastases) are more common than 1° liver tumors.

SYMPTOMS/EXAM

Presents with abdominal discomfort together with laboratory abnormalities (↑ aminotransferases, ↑ bilirubin, coagulopathy) that warrant abdominal imaging.

TREATMENT

- Surgical resection and liver transplantation can yield long-term survival.
- Alternatives for unresectable tumors include percutaneous alcohol injections, arterial chemoembolization, and radiofrequency ablation.

Colorectal Cancer

Most cases occur after age 50. Suspect hereditary nonpolyposis colorectal cancer (HNPCC) in a younger person with colon cancer and a family history of colon, ovarian, and endometrial cancer. Table 2.8-1 discusses risk factors. Screen all asymptomatic individuals > 50 years of age with annual fecal occult blood testing (FOBT) and flexible sigmoidoscopy every 5 years, or with colonoscopy every 10 years.

If there is a family history of polyps or colorectal cancer, start screening when the patient is 10 years younger than the age of the affected relative at the time of diagnosis.

SYMPTOMS/EXAM

Symptoms depend on the site of the 1° tumor and may include a change in bowel habits, melena, bright red blood per rectum, weight loss, fatigue, vomiting, and abdominal discomfort.

TABLE 2.8-1. Risk Factors for Colorectal Cancer

PATIENT AGE	PERSONAL HISTORY	FAMILY HISTORY	
		COLORECTAL CANCER OR ADENOMATOUS POLYPS	HEREDITARY COLORECTAL CANCER SYNDROMES
> 50 years	Previous colorectal cancer Adenomatous polyps IBD, particularly ulcerative colitis	One first-degree relative < 60 years of age or two first-degree relatives of any age	Familial adenomatous polyposis (FAP) HNPCC Hamartomatous polyposis syndromes

DIAGNOSIS

- Diagnosed by a mass palpated by DRE or by a ⊕ FOBT.
- Iron-deficiency anemia or ↑ transaminases may be seen.
- Confirm the diagnosis via colonoscopy and biopsy in suspected cases.

TREATMENT

- Treatment decisions are influenced by tumor stage at diagnosis. 1° surgical resection involves resection of the bowel segment with adjacent mesentery and regional lymph nodes. Solitary liver/lung metastases can be resected.
- Stage I patients have an excellent prognosis with surgery alone (90% survival at five years).
- **Adjuvant chemotherapy (5-FU based)** is warranted for patients at stage III and above.

Miscellaneous GI Tumors

ESOPHAGEAL TUMORS

- **Sx/Exam:** The classic symptom is **dysphagia in the elderly,** especially in smokers, and tumors are usually squamous in nature. Esophageal adenocarcinoma can arise from long-standing esophageal reflux with Barrett's disease.
- **Dx:** Confirm the diagnosis by EGD with biopsy.
- **Tx:** Treatment involves resection for localized disease and radiation therapy with chemotherapy for advanced disease.

GASTRIC TUMORS

- More common among those of Asian ethnicity.
- **Sx/Exam:** Classically presents as **iron-deficiency anemia with vague abdominal pain in the elderly.**
- **Dx:** Confirm the diagnosis via EGD with biopsy.
- **Tx:** Treatment involves resection for localized disease and radiation therapy with chemotherapy for advanced disease.

CARCINOID TUMORS

- Usually occur in the appendix or small bowel.
- **Sx/Exam:** Clinical features include flushing, abdominal pain, diarrhea, and tricuspid regurgitation (carcinoid syndrome).
- **Dx:** Diagnosed by **elevated levels of 5-HIAA** or chromogranin A.
- **Tx:** Surgical resection is curative in localized disease. Consider **octreotide for symptomatic control.**

ISLET CELL TUMORS

- **Sx/Exam:** Presentation depends on tumor type.
  - **Insulinoma (elevated proinsulin, C-peptide, and insulin levels):** Should be suspected with a triad consisting of hypoglycemic symptoms, fasting blood sugar < 40, and immediate relief with glucose administration.
  - **VIPoma (elevated VIP levels):** Suspect in the setting of profuse watery diarrhea that causes hypokalemia.

- **Glucagonoma (elevated glucagon levels):** Characterized by persistent hyperglycemia with necrolytic erythema.
- **Dx:** Islet cell tumors and their metastases can be localized by somatostatin receptor scintigraphy (SRS).

Bladder Cancer

The **most common** malignant tumor of the urinary tract; usually **transitional cell carcinoma.** Risk factors include **smoking,** exposure to aniline (rubber) dyes, and chronic bladder infections (e.g., **schistosomiasis**).

Symptoms/Exam

Gross hematuria is the most common presenting symptom. Other urinary symptoms, such as frequency, urgency, and dysuria, may also be seen.

Diagnosis

- **UA** is the most basic diagnostic modality and often shows hematuria (macro- or microscopic). Lack of dysmorphic RBCs helps distinguish this from glomerular bleeding. Cytology may show dysplastic cells (first morning specimen is best).
- **IVP** can examine the upper urinary tract as well as defects in bladder filling.
- **Cystoscopy with biopsy is diagnostic.**

Treatment

Treatment depends on the extent of spread beyond the bladder mucosa.

- **Carcinoma in situ (CIS):** Intravesicular chemotherapy.
- **Invasive cancers without metastases:** Aggressive surgery, radiation therapy, or both.
- **Patients with distant metastases:** Chemotherapy alone.

Prostate Cancer

The most common cancer in men. Ninety-five percent are adenocarcinomas. Risk ↑ linearly with age.

Incidental asymptomatic prostate cancer is especially common among those > 80 years of age and does not always need treatment.

Symptoms/Exam

- Many patients are asymptomatic and are incidentally diagnosed either by **DRE** or by a **PSA** level that is obtained for screening purposes.
- If symptomatic, patients may present with **urinary urgency/frequency/hesitancy** and, in late or aggressive disease, with anemia, hematuria, or low back pain.
- Screening with **DRE** or **PSA** should be done in patients > 50 years of age with > 10 years of life expectancy.

Diagnosis

- Ultrasound-guided needle biopsy of the prostate allows for both diagnosis and staging.

- The **Gleason score (2–10)** remains the best predictor of tumor biology. It sums the scores of the two most dysplastic biopsy samples on a scale of 1–5 (well differentiated to poorly differentiated).

TREATMENT

Treatment choice is based on the aggressiveness of the tumor and on the patient's risk of dying from the disease.

- **Watchful waiting** may be the best approach for elderly patients with low Gleason scores.
- **Consider radical prostatectomy** or **radiation therapy** (e.g., brachytherapy or external beam) for node-$\ominus$ disease. Treatment is associated with an ↑ risk of incontinence and/or impotence.
- Treat node-$\oplus$ and metastatic disease with **androgen ablation** (e.g., GnRH agonists, orchiectomy, flutamide) and chemotherapy.

Testicular Cancer

The most common solid malignant tumor in men 20–35 years of age. It is highly treatable and often curable. Risk factors include **cryptorchid testis** and Klinefelter's syndrome. Ninety-five percent are germ cell tumors.

SYMPTOMS/EXAM

- A **unilateral scrotal mass is testicular cancer until proven otherwise.**
- Other presentations include testicular discomfort or swelling suggestive of orchitis or epididymitis.

DIAGNOSIS

- Serum levels of α-fetoprotein (**AFP**), **LDH,** and β-**hCG** should be measured.
- Definitive diagnosis is made by radical inguinal orchiectomy.
- Staging evaluation (TNM is widely used) should include serum LDH, AFP, β-hCG, and CT of the chest/abdomen and pelvis.

TREATMENT

Radical inguinal orchiectomy +/– chemotherapy/radiation therapy is the treatment of choice.

Ovarian Cancer

More than 90% are adenocarcinomas. Risk factors include age, use of infertility drugs, and familial cancer syndromes (e.g., BRCA-1, BRCA-2). Risk is ↓ with sustained use of OCPs, having children, breast-feeding, bilateral tubal ligation, and TAH-BSO.

SYMPTOMS/EXAM

- Usually **asymptomatic** until the disease has reached an advanced stage.
- Patients may have abdominal pain, bloating, pelvic pressure, urinary frequency, early satiety, constipation, vaginal bleeding, and systemic symptoms (fatigue, malaise, weight loss).
- Exam findings may include a palpable solid, fixed, nodular pelvic mass; ascites; and pleural effusion (Meigs syndrome). **An ovarian mass in postmenopausal women is ovarian cancer until proven otherwise.**

Do not do a scrotal biopsy to diagnose testicular cancer, as this may result in seeding of the biopsy tract.

DIAGNOSIS/TREATMENT

- Evaluate adnexal masses with **pelvic ultrasound** and possibly CT or MRI; obtain serum **CA-125** and a **CXR.**
- Staging is surgical and includes **TAH-BSO, omentectomy,** and **tumor debulking.**

Cervical Cancer

Infection with HPV types 16, 18, and 31 ↑ the risk of cervical cancer. An HPV vaccine has been approved for the prevention of cervical cancer.

Despite the **screening Pap smear,** cervical cancer remains the third most common gynecologic malignancy. Risk factors include **HPV infection, tobacco use,** early onset of sexual activity, multiple sexual partners, immunocompromised status (e.g., HIV), and STDs. An **HPV vaccine** has recently been approved by the FDA for the prevention of cervical cancer.

SYMPTOMS/EXAM

- Patients are usually asymptomatic and are diagnosed on routine **Pap smear.**
- If symptomatic, patients may present with menorrhagia and/or metrorrhagia, **postcoital bleeding,** pelvic pain, and vaginal discharge.

DIAGNOSIS

In suspicious cases, the Pap smear should be followed by colposcopy and biopsy.

- **Colposcopy** and biopsy in patients with an abnormal Pap smear or visible cervical lesions.
- Cancers are categorized as **invasive cervical carcinoma** (depth > 3 mm, width > 7 mm) or **cervical intraepithelial neoplasia (CIN).**

TREATMENT

- **CIN I (mild dysplasia or low-grade squamous intraepithelial lesion; LGSIL):** Most regress spontaneously. Reliable patients can be observed via Pap smears and colposcopy every three months for one year.
- **CIN II/III:** Treat with **cryosurgery,** laser surgery, or **LEEP.**
- **Invasive cancer:** Early-stage disease can be treated with **radical hysterectomy and lymph node dissection.** Advanced disease requires **radiation and chemotherapy.**

SKIN TUMORS

Melanoma

> **The ABCDEs of melanoma:**
>
> **A**symmetric shape
> **B**orders irregular
> **C**olor variegated
> **D**iameter > 6 mm
> **E**nlargement of any lesion

An aggressive malignancy of melanocytes and the **leading cause of death** from skin disease. Risk factors include **sun exposure,** fair skin, a family history, a large number of nevi, and the presence of dysplastic nevi.

SYMPTOMS/EXAM

- **A pigmented skin lesion that has recently changed in size or appearance should raise concern.**
- Lesions are characterized by the **ABCDEs** of melanoma (see mnemonic) and may occur **anywhere** on the body. They are most commonly found on the **trunk for men** and on the **legs for women.**

Skin biopsy shows **melanocytes with marked cellular atypia** and melanocytic invasion into the dermis.

TREATMENT

- **Surgical excision** is the treatment of choice. **The thickness of the melanoma (depth of invasion)** is the most important prognostic factor.
- Depending on depth, lymph node dissection may be necessary. Systemic **chemotherapy** is used for metastatic disease.

Basal Cell Carcinoma

The **most common skin cancer;** associated with excessive sun exposure.

SYMPTOMS/EXAM

- Exam reveals a **pearl-colored papule** of variable size. The external surface is frequently covered with fine **telangiectasias** and appears **translucent.**
- Lesions may be located anywhere on the body but are most commonly found on **sun-exposed** areas, **particularly the face.** Large ulcers are described as "**rodent ulcers.**"

DIAGNOSIS

Skin biopsy shows characteristic basophilic **palisading cells with retraction.**

TREATMENT

- Therapy depends on the size and location of the tumor, the histologic type, the history of prior treatment, the underlying health of the patient, and cosmetic considerations.
- Options include curettage, surgical excision, cryosurgery, and radiation.

Squamous Cell Carcinoma

Risk factors include exposure to **sun** or ionizing radiation, prior **actinic keratosis, immunosuppression,** arsenic exposure, and exposure to industrial carcinogens.

SYMPTOMS/EXAM

- Lesions are usually slowly evolving and **asymptomatic;** occasionally, bleeding or pain may develop.
- Exam reveals small, red, **exophytic nodules** with varying degrees of scaling or crusting. Lesions are commonly found in **sun-exposed areas, particularly the lower lip.**

DIAGNOSIS

Biopsy shows irregular masses of anaplastic epidermal cells proliferating down to the dermis.

TREATMENT

- **Surgical excision** is necessary for larger lesions and for those involving the periorbital, periauricular, perilabial, genital, and perigenital areas.

- **Mohs' micrographic surgery** may be performed for recurrent lesions and on areas of the face that are difficult to reconstruct.
- **Radiation** may be necessary in cases in which surgery is not a viable option.

CNS TUMORS

1° brain tumors make up < 2% of all tumors diagnosed. Meningioma, glioma, vestibular schwannoma, pituitary adenoma, and 1° CNS lymphoma are the most common CNS tumors in adults and can occur in association with AIDS.

Meningioma

- The **most common** tumor of the brain; **usually benign.**
- **Sx/Exam:** Most tumors are small, asymptomatic, and discovered incidentally. When symptoms are present, they usually consist of **progressive headache** or a **focal neurologic deficit** reflecting the location of the tumor.
- **Dx:** CT of the head typically demonstrates a partially **calcified, homogeneously enhancing extra-axial mass adherent to the dura.** Craniopharyngioma is another highly calcified tumor in children but is present **around the pineal gland** and can cause bitemporal hemianopia.
- **Tx:** Surgical resection is appropriate for large or symptomatic tumors; **observation with serial scans** is the preferred approach for **small or asymptomatic lesions.**

MRI is superior to CT for viewing skull-base/cerebellar lesions but is less reliable for detecting calcifications.

Glial Tumors

- Include astrocytomas, oligodendrogliomas, mixed gliomas, and ependymomas.
- **Sx/Exam:**
  - Headache is the most common symptom; it may be generalized or unilateral, often **awakens** the patient from sleep and induces **vomiting,** and is **worse with the Valsalva maneuver.**
  - Tumors appear as a **diffusely infiltrating area** of low attenuation on CT or an ↑ T2 signal on MRI.
  - **Glioblastoma multiforme** is usually a **unifocal and centrally necrotic** enhancing lesion with surrounding edema and mass effect.
- **Dx:** Biopsy is required for definitive diagnosis.
- **Tx: Surgical resection** followed by **external beam radiation** is used for high-grade tumors. Chemotherapy is reserved for high-grade gliomas in patients < 60 years of age.

TUMOR MARKERS

Usually sensitive but not specific. Thus, they are most useful for monitoring of recurrence and disease activity following resection. However, tumor markers can also be useful in diagnosis if they are supported by clinical evidence. Common tumor markers and associated malignancies include the following:

- **CA 125:** Ovarian cancer.
- **CA 15-3:** Breast cancer.

- **CA 19-9:** Pancreatic cancer.
- **CEA:** GI cancer, particularly of the colon.
- **AFP:** Liver, yolk sac (testicular) cancer.
- **hCG:** Choriocarcinoma (testicular/ovarian).
- **PSA:** Prostate cancer.
- **LDH:** Lymphoma.
- **Calcitonin:** Medullary thyroid carcinoma.
- **Chromogranin A:** Carcinoid tumor.

Common tumor markers:

CEA = **C**olon cancer
hCG =
    Choriocarcinoma
PSA= **P**ro**S**tate
LDH = **L**ymp**H**oma

TABLE 2.9-4. Antibiotic Regimens for Bacterial Meningitis

PATHOGEN	THERAPY OF CHOICE
S. pneumoniae	Vancomycin + third-generation cephalosporin +/– dexamethasone.
N. meningitidis	Ampicillin or third-generation cephalosporin.
L. monocytogenes	Ampicillin **(not cephalosporins).**
Streptococcus agalactiae	Ampicillin.
H. influenzae type b	Third-generation cephalosporin.

- **Dx:** Diagnosis is based on clinical findings. Radiographic imaging or CT may help (air-fluid level, inflammation of tissues).
- **Tx:** If symptoms persist after seven days or are suggestive of bacterial sinusitis, empiric therapy consists of a 10-day course of amoxicillin +/– clavulanate or cefpodoxime.

Chronic Sinusitis

- Defined as sinus symptoms lasting > 4 weeks.
- **Dx:** Sinus CT with bone windows is the imaging modality of choice.
- **Tx:**
  - Amoxicillin +/– clavulanate for 21 days.
  - Intranasal steroid sprays are beneficial.
  - Refractory cases require endoscopic surgery.

Otitis Media

- Causative agents are similar to those of acute sinusitis.
- **Sx/Exam:**
  - Typical features include **fever** and unilateral **ear pain.**
  - There may also be hearing loss, and children may be irritable or may tug at their ears.
  - The tympanic membrane is typically erythematous, lacks a normal light reflex, and may be bulging. Look for perforation of the tympanic membrane along with pus in the ear canal.
- **Tx:**
  - First-line treatment is with amoxicillin or TMP-SMX for 10 days. However, many recent studies suggest that a five- to seven-day course may be adequate if the patient is > 2 years of age and has no history of recurrent otitis media.
  - Patients who do not respond to antimicrobial therapy and develop hearing loss should have tympanostomy tubes placed.

Otitis Externa

- Predisposing factors include **swimming,** eczema, hearing aid use, and mechanical trauma (e.g., cotton swab insertion). In most patients, the causative organism is *Pseudomonas*. *S. aureus* is implicated in acute otitis externa.

- **Sx/Exam:**
    - Patients have a painful ear along with foul-smelling drainage. The **external ear canal** will be swollen and erythematous. There may also be pus.
    - Patients have tenderness upon **movement of the pinna** or tragus.
- **Tx:** Remove any foreign material from the ear canal and start a topical antimicrobial (typically **ofloxacin**) with **steroids.**

Pharyngitis

Typically due to **viral causes** such as rhinovirus or adenovirus. **Group A streptococcus** is implicated in up to 25% of cases. Untreated group A streptococcal infection can → acute pyogenic complications and **rheumatic fever.**

SYMPTOMS/EXAM

Symptoms include sore throat and fever +/− cough. Look for tonsillar exudates and tender anterior cervical adenopathy.

DIAGNOSIS

- Think about infectious mononucleosis in patients with lymphadenopathy and malaise.
- In adults with pharyngitis, always consider HIV infection and acute retroviral syndrome.
- In children, think about epiglottitis (febrile patients with complaints of severe sore throat and dysphagia with minimal findings on exam).
- For streptococcal infection, check a rapid antigen test (good sensitivity and specificity) as well as a throat swab for culture.

TREATMENT

- Treat group A streptococcal infections with penicillin. Use a macrolide for patients with penicillin allergy.
- Chronic carriers (i.e., those who have a ⊕ throat culture or are asymptomatic) should be treated with clindamycin for eradication.

PNEUMONIA

Community-Acquired Pneumonia (CAP)

Pneumonia still ranks as the sixth leading cause of death overall and is the leading cause of death from infection. Etiologies are as follows:

- **Typical pathogens:** *S. pneumoniae, H. influenzae, S. aureus* (in the setting of influenza virus).
- **Atypical pathogens:** *Mycoplasma, Chlamydia, Moraxella.*

SYMPTOMS/EXAM

- Think of pneumonia in any patient with acute onset of fever, **chills, productive cough,** and **pleuritic chest pain.**
- **Atypical organisms** present with low-grade fever, nonproductive cough, and myalgias ("walking pneumonia").
- Look for evidence of consolidation (dullness to percussion, crackles, bronchial breath sounds) on lung exam.

DIAGNOSIS

- There should be radiographic evidence of an infiltrate in all immunocompetent patients as well as recovery of a pathogenic organism from blood, sputum, or pleural fluid.
- **Urine _Legionella_ antigen** should be sent in patients with risk factors.
- Remember to check an ABG to determine the acid-base status of patients who appear to be in distress.
- If the patient is hospitalized, check blood cultures.

TREATMENT

- Decide whether the patient needs to be hospitalized based on clinical risk factors. Admit patients who are > 50 years of age or those who have chronic underlying disease (e.g., COPD, CHF, cancer), unstable vital signs, or a high fever.
- Initiate empiric antimicrobial therapy based on the patient's risk factors (e.g., community-dwelling and healthy vs. diabetic). **Think about MRSA** in patients with a history of colonization or in those who have been hospitalized (see Table 2.9-5).

Ventilator-Associated Pneumonia

- **Dx:** Typical agents in this setting include methicillin-sensitive _S. aureus_, MRSA, _Pseudomonas_, _Legionella_, _Acinetobacter_, and other gram-⊖ rods.

Think of Legionella infection in a smoker with pneumonia, diarrhea, and elevated LDH.

The sputum sample should have < 10 epithelial cells.

TABLE 2.9-5. Empiric Antibiotic Treatment Strategies for CAP

PATIENT PROFILE	INCLUDE COVERAGE FOR	EMPIRIC ANTIBIOTIC CHOICE
Community-dwelling outpatients	S. pneumoniae H. influenzae Atypicals	Azithromycin PO
Patients with comorbidities (age > 60, DM, EtOH use, COPD)	S. pneumoniae Klebsiella Legionella	Fluoroquinolone or azithromycin PO
Inpatient (severe or multilobar pneumonia)	As above	Ceftriaxone IV + azithromycin IV
Nursing home–acquired CAP	Gram-negative rods Pseudomonas MRSA	Ceftriaxone IV + azithromycin IV +/– vancomycin
Patients with cystic fibrosis	Pseudomonas	Ceftazidime IV + levofloxacin IV + aminoglycoside
Aspiration	Anaerobes Gram-negative rods S. aureus	Ceftriaxone IV + azithromycin IV + clindamycin IV

- **Tx: Always obtain sputum cultures before starting or changing antimicrobials.** Tailor empiric therapy as soon as culture data become available. Treatment should be for eight days.

Pneumocystis jiroveci Pneumonia (PCP)

Can be present in HIV-⊕ patients (CD4 < 200) as well as in anyone on immunosuppressive therapies.

SYMPTOMS/EXAM

- Presents with fever, nonproductive cough, and dyspnea on minimal exertion that resolves quickly on rest.
- Patients may have findings consistent with atypical pneumonia, or there may be few physical exam findings. Look for pneumothorax.

DIAGNOSIS

- CXR ranges from normal to bilateral interstitial or alveolar infiltrates. The classic appearance is that of "ground-glass" infiltrates.
- Other findings include ↑ LDH.
- Obtain a silver stain of sputum or bronchoalveolar lavage to look for PCP.

TREATMENT

- First-line therapy is with IV TMP-SMX. Alternatives include IV pentamidine.
- Use **concomitant prednisone if PaO$_2$ is < 70 mmHg** or if the patient has an alveolar-arterial (A-a) oxygen gradient of > 35 mmHg on room air.

BRONCHITIS

Infection of the upper airways (bronchi), with risk factors including cigarette smoking and COPD.

SYMPTOMS/EXAM

Presents with cough with or without sputum production, dyspnea, fever, and chills. Lungs are clear with possible upper airway noise.

DIFFERENTIAL

URI, pneumonia, allergic rhinitis.

DIAGNOSIS

CBC, CXR, sputum Gram stain and culture.

TREATMENT

- Depending on comorbidities and severity, patients may need hospitalization.
- If a bacterial etiology is suspected, give antimicrobials to cover S. *pneumoniae* and atypicals.

May be 1°, latent, or extrapulmonary.

SYMPTOMS/EXAM

- **1° TB:** Usually involves the middle or lower lung zones and is associated with hilar adenopathy (Ghon complex).
- **Latent TB infection (LTBI):** Characterized by the presence of acid-fast bacilli but the absence of active infection. Reactivation occurs in about 10% of patients and typically involves the upper lungs and cavitation.
- **Extrapulmonary TB:** Usually associated with HIV-⊕ persons; may involve any organ.

DIAGNOSIS

- Screening should be conducted for LTBI in **high-risk groups** — e.g., immigrants from endemic areas, HIV-⊕ patients, homeless persons, health care workers, IV drug users, and patients with chronic medical conditions (COPD, chronic renal failure, DM, post-transplant, cancer).
- BCG vaccination status should be disregarded in the interpretation of test results (see Table 2.9-6).

TREATMENT

- The most commonly used regimen includes four drugs described by the mnemonic **RIPE** — **R**ifampin, **I**soniazid (INH), **P**yrazinamide, and **E**thambutol — given daily for eight weeks, followed by INH and rifampin for an additional 16 weeks. Table 2.9-7 outlines the common side effects of these drugs.
- Treatment of LTBI requires nine months of INH.
- Patients coinfected with TB and HIV should be treated with rifabutin instead of rifampin, since the latter can interact with anti-HIV medications.

Give vitamin B₆ to prevent INH-associated neuropathy.

Cystitis

- Some 10% of U.S. women have at least one uncomplicated UTI each year. The most common pathogen is *E. coli*.
- **Sx/Exam:** Dysuria, urgency, and frequency of urination are the most common complaints.

TABLE 2.9-6.   PPD Interpretation

POPULATION	⊕ TB SKIN TEST
Low risk of disease	≥ 15 mm
Patients with exposure risk (health care workers, immigrants, diabetics)	≥ 10 mm
HIV-⊕, immunocompromised, recent contact with TB, CXR c/w previous TB infection	≥ 5 mm

TABLE 2.9-7.   Common Side Effects of Tuberculosis Drugs

TUBERCULOSIS DRUGS	SIDE EFFECTS
Rifampin	Red-orange body fluids, hepatitis.
Isoniazid	Peripheral neuropathy (consider giving pyridoxine, or vitamin B_6, with medication), hepatitis, lupus-like syndrome.
Pyrazinamide	Hyperuricemia, hepatitis.
Ethambutol	Optic neuritis.

- **Dx:**
  - Think about urethritis/cervicitis in sexually active patients. Renal stones may also present with colicky pain and dysuria.
  - Check a UA for the presence of bacteria, WBCs, leukocyte esterase, and nitrite.
- **Tx:** Give a three-day course of either TMP-SMX or a fluoroquinolone. Cultures are not necessary. A seven-day course is recommended for diabetics, patients with symptoms of > 7 days' duration, and men.

Pyelonephritis

- **Sx/Exam:**
  - Findings are similar to those of UTI except that patients are more acutely ill.
  - Be sure to check for **CVA tenderness.** Also look for signs of bacteremia such as fever, tachycardia, and hypotension.
- **Dx:** Urine specimens usually demonstrate significant bacteriuria, pyuria, and occasional WBC casts. A urine culture should be sent on all patients. **Always obtain blood cultures on admission, as 15–20% of patients will be bacteremic.**
- **Tx:** Begin a fluoroquinolone IV. If there is no clinical response, look for an intrarenal abscess or foreign bodies such as **renal calculi** with CT or ultrasound.

Prostatitis

- **Sx/Exam:**
  - Presenting symptoms include spiking fevers, chills, dysuria, cloudy urine, and even obstructive symptoms if prostate swelling is significant.
  - In patients with chronic infection, low back pain or perineal/testicular discomfort may be present.
  - The gland is exquisitely tender on prostate DRE.
- **Dx:** Obtain urine cultures before and after a prostatic massage to look for gram-⊖ rods.
- **Tx:** Treat with TMP-SMX or a fluoroquinolone for 14 days. For those with chronic prostatitis, treatment should be extended to one month with a fluoroquinolone or to three months with TMP-SMX.

HIGH-YIELD FACTS

INFECTIOUS DISEASE

Syphilis

Caused by *Treponema pallidum*. Transmissible during early disease (1° and 2° syphilis) through exposure to open lesions (loaded with spirochetes!).

SYMPTOMS

- **1° syphilis:** Develops within several weeks of exposure; involves one or more painless, indurated, superficial ulcerations (chancre).
- **2° syphilis:** After the chancre has resolved, patients may develop malaise, anorexia, headache, diffuse lymphadenopathy, or rash (involves the mucosal surfaces, palms, and soles).
- **3° syphilis:** Includes cardiovascular, neurologic, and gummatous disease (e.g., general paresis, tabes dorsalis, aortitis, meningovascular syphilis).

EXAM

Findings depend on the stage of syphilis—the painless chancre for 1° disease; maculopapular rash or diffuse lymphadenopathy for 2° disease; and multiple neurologic and/or cardiovascular signs for 3° disease (see above).

DIAGNOSIS

- **1°:** Do a nontreponemal serologic test (RPR or VDRL). Darkfield microscopy of the lesion's exudate will show the spirochetes. Direct antigen tests (MHA-TP or FTA-ABS) are used for confirmation.
- **2°:** Diagnosed by the presence of clinical illness and ⊕ serologic tests.
- **3°:** Perform an LP when neurologic or ophthalmic signs and symptoms are present, in the setting of treatment failure, or with a VDRL of ≥ 1:32. Correlate with cardiovascular, neurologic, and systemic symptoms.

TREATMENT

- **1°/2°:** Penicillin G 2.4 MU in a single IM dose. Alternatives include doxycycline or erythromycin for 14 days. If the disease duration is > 1 year, give three doses of penicillin G IM a week apart.
- **Neurosyphilis:** Penicillin G IV for 14 days.

Patients who have had HIV or syphilis longer than a year should always undergo LP.

Genital Herpes

- Painful grouped vesicles in the anogenital region. Caused by human herpes simplex virus, usually type 2.
- **Sx/Exam:** Frequently associated symptoms include tender inguinal lymphadenopathy, fever, myalgias, headaches, and aseptic meningitis. Symptoms are usually more pronounced during the initial episode and grow less frequent with recurrences.
- **Dx:** Diagnosis can be confirmed by viral PCR of the vesicle fluid.
- **Tx:**
  - Use acyclovir for 7–10 days for 1° infections. Treatment should begin within one week of symptoms.
  - Severe recurrences may necessitate repeat treatment with either acyclovir or valacyclovir for five days. Daily suppressive therapy for frequent recurrences can be used.

Counsel patients regarding safe-sex practices. HSV transmission can occur even in the absence of visible vesicles.

Cervicitis/Urethritis

- Chlamydial and gonococcal infections often present as cervicitis or urethritis. *Mycoplasma genitalium* is an emerging pathogen in this syndrome.
- **Sx/Exam:** Dysuria, dyspareunia, and mucopurulent vaginal discharge are frequent complaints in women. In men, dysuria and purulent penile discharge predominate.
- **Dx:** A ⊕ endocervical or urethral culture or a ⊕ urine PCR for chlamydia/gonorrhea is diagnostic.
- **Tx:**
  - Always **treat for both infections simultaneously, and treat sexual partners.**
  - Treat chlamydia with a single PO dose of azithromycin.
  - Treat gonorrhea with a single PO dose of ofloxacin or ciprofloxacin or with a single IM dose of ceftriaxone.

Pelvic Inflammatory Disease (PID)

IUDs greatly ↑ the risk of PID and should be removed in women who have been diagnosed with an STD.

- An upper genital tract infection in women that is usually a complication of chlamydia and/or gonorrhea infection.
- **Sx/Exam:** Presents with pelvic pain, dyspareunia, vaginal discharge, fever, and menstrual irregularities as well as with lower abdominal tenderness, adnexal tenderness, and cervical motion tenderness.
- **Dx:** A finding of > 10 WBCs/low-power field on Gram stain and endocervical smear is consistent with a diagnosis of PID.
- **Tx:** Treat with a second-generation cephalosporin IV and doxycycline IV.

ACUTE HIV INFECTION

Acute retroviral syndrome occurs in 50–90% of cases. The incubation period is usually 2–6 weeks. Acute symptoms last 1–4 weeks, with an average of two weeks.

SYMPTOMS/EXAM

Patients have a typical viral prodrome (e.g., malaise, low-grade fever) followed by the development of adenopathy. Unusual presentations include Bell's palsy, peripheral neuropathy, radiculopathy, cognitive impairment, and psychosis.

DIAGNOSIS

- HIV serology (ELISA) detects antibody to HIV. Serology becomes ⊕ 2–3 months after exposure, with > 95% seroconversion at six months. Send a confirmatory Western blot in patients with a ⊕ ELISA screen.
- For patients with suspected acute retroviral syndrome, check a viral load, since the ELISA may not have had time to turn ⊕.

TREATMENT

- Begin highly active antiretroviral therapy (HAART) in any of the following situations:
  - In symptomatic patients (any CD4 or viral load).
  - In asymptomatic patients with a CD4 < 350 and any viral load.
  - In pregnant women.
  - In the setting of a needle stick involving blood from an HIV-⊕ patient.
- Regimens should include three drugs, **preferably from different categories** (see Table 2.9-8).

TABLE 2.9-8. **Categories of Antiretroviral Drugs**

MAJOR ANTIRETROVIRAL CLASSES	EXAMPLES	COMMON SIDE EFFECTS
Nucleoside reverse transcriptase inhibitors (NRTIs)	Zidovudine (AZT)	Myopathy and bone marrow suppression.
	Didanosine (ddl)	Pancreatitis.
	Abacavir	Hypersensitivity reaction (e.g., fever, chills, dyspnea).
	Emtricitabine (FTC) and lamivudine (3TC)	Diarrhea, nausea, and headache.
	Tenofovir (TNV)	Renal toxicity.
Non-nucleotide reverse transcriptase inhibitors (NNRTIs)	Efavirenz	CNS toxicity and teratogenicity.
	Nevirapine	Rash and hepatic failure.
Protease inhibitors (PIs)	Atazanavir	Benign indirect hyperbilirubinemia.
	Indinavir	Kidney stones.
	Nelfinavir	Diarrhea.
	Ritonavir	Potent P-450 inhibitor.
	Saquinavir	Rare side effects.
		All PIs can ↑ lipids, redistribute fat, and cause DM.
Fusion inhibitor	Enfuvirtide (T20)	Injection site reactions.

COMPLICATIONS

Complications are numerous and typically involve opportunistic infections and side effects from drugs. See Table 2.9-9 for prophylaxis indications.

TABLE 2.9-9. **Prophylaxis in HIV**

DISEASE	INDICATION	TREATMENT
PCP	CD4 < 200 or previous PCP or thrush.	TMP-SMX, dapsone, or atavaquone.
Mycobacterium avium-intracellulare (MAI)	CD4 < 50.	Azithromycin weekly.
Toxoplasma gondii	CD4 < 100 and Toxo IgG ⊕.	TMP-SMX or dapsone + leucovorin + pyrimethamine.
TB	Recent contact or PPD > 5 mm.	INH for nine months.
Pneumococcal pneumonia	All HIV-⊕.	Vaccine every five years.
Influenza	All HIV-⊕.	Yearly vaccine.
Hepatitis B	Surface antigen/core antibody ⊕.	Hepatitis B vaccine.

Malaria Prophylaxis

- Prophylaxis must be tailored to reflect the prevalence of resistant *Plasmodium falciparum* (high mortality) in the area of proposed travel. Most regimens start a week or two prior to travel and continue for a month after return.
- Weekly chloroquine is the mainstay of therapy in chloroquine-sensitive areas.
- Mefloquine is active against chloroquine-resistant *P. falciparum* and is also given weekly. Mefloquine resistance is emerging in Southeast Asia.
- Daily doxycycline or daily Malarone (atovaquone and proguanil) can be used in those people who are unable to take mefloquine or who are traveling to chloroquine-resistant areas. Malarone can be used for short trips.
- **Precautions:**
  - Mefloquine has the potential for neuropsychiatric side effects. Caution should thus be exercised in prescribing it to people with recent or active depression, psychosis, schizophrenia, or anxiety disorders.
  - Other effects include sinus bradycardia and QT-interval prolongation; avoid in patients on β-blockers or in those with known conduction disorders.

Traveler's Diarrhea (TD)

- Roughly 40–60% of people traveling to developing countries develop TD (see Table 2.9-10).
- **Sx/Exam:** Patients with uncomplicated TD have watery, unformed stools without systemic symptoms. Those with complicated TD can have bloody diarrhea along with systemic symptoms such as nausea, vomiting, abdominal pain, and fever.
- **Dx:** Since uncomplicated TD is self-limited (48–72 hours), studies are usually not warranted, and treatment is symptomatic. Exceptions are as follows:
  - A stool culture should be considered in those with blood in the stool, fever, and symptoms of colitis.
  - Viral studies should be considered if symptoms persist for 10–14 days.
  - Stool examination for *Giardia* should be done in patients with predominantly upper GI symptoms—e.g., nausea, bloating, gas, and persistent nonbloody diarrhea.

TABLE 2.9-10.   Common Pathogens Causing Traveler's Diarrhea

BACTERIA	VIRUSES	PARASITES
ETEC (enterotoxic *E. coli*)	Rotavirus	*Giardia*
Campylobacter	Enteric adenovirus	*Cryptosporidium*
Salmonella		*Cyclospora*
Shigella		Microsporidia
Vibrio		*Isospora belli*
Yersinia		*Entamoeba histolytica*

- **Tx:**
  - Fluid replacement should be initiated in all cases; oral rehydration should be started in children with cholera. Antimicrobials are indicated for moderate to severe disease.
  - **Fluoroquinolone or azithromycin** is the first choice. Antimotility agents should not be used in severe TD.

Lyme Disease

A systemic disease caused by *Borrelia burgdorferi*, a spirochete carried by the deer tick (*Ixodes* genus). Patients may reside in the Northeast or Midwest.

SYMPTOMS/EXAM

- **Stage 1:** Presents with erythema migrans (target or bull's-eye lesion), fever, arthralgias, myalgias, and lymphadenopathy.
- **Stage 2:** Characterized by myocarditis, possibly accompanied by varying degrees of AV block, Bell's palsy (unilateral or bilateral), peripheral neuropathy, and meningitis.
- **Stage 3:** Marked by arthritis and possibly chronic neurologic symptoms.

DIFFERENTIAL

Erythema migrans is pathognomonic for Lyme disease. The differential for other nonspecific symptoms is broad.

DIAGNOSIS

A Western blot or PCR can be used to confirm the diagnosis.

TREATMENT

Treat with doxycycline or amoxicillin. **If cardiac or neurologic symptoms are present, treat with ceftriaxone.**

Ehrlichiosis

- A systemic disease with nonspecific symptoms that include fever, chills, malaise, myalgias, and headache in the absence of physical exam findings. Caused by *Ehrlichia* and *Anaplasma* bacteria, which are transmitted by several different ticks, typically during the summer.
- **Sx/Exam:** Patients may have **thrombocytopenia, leukopenia,** and **elevated transaminases.**
- **Dx:** Diagnose with serology or PCR.
- **Tx:** Treat with doxycycline.

Babesiosis

- A systemic disease caused by *Babesia* organisms that infect RBCs → a hemolytic anemia.
- **Sx/Exam:**
  - Presents with nonspecific symptoms that include fever, chills, fatigue, and myalgias.
  - Patients have typically visited the northeast, particularly Cape Cod, Martha's Vineyard, or Nantucket.

- **Dx:** Diagnose with a peripheral blood smear or PCR.
- **Tx:** Treat with clindamycin and quinine.

NEUTROPENIC FEVER

Most often occurs after chemotherapy. Defined as a single temperature of > 38.3°C (101.3°F), or a sustained temperature > 38°C (100.4°F) for > 1 hour in a neutropenic patient (ANC = PMNs + bands < 500).

SYMPTOMS/EXAM

- The skin should be examined for signs of erythema, rash, cellulitis, ulcers, or line infection.
- All indwelling lines should be carefully examined for subtle signs of infection, as erythema, tenderness, fluctuance, or exudate may be the only evidence of a serious "tunnel infection."
- Do not conduct a DRE unless perirectal abscess is suspected.

DIAGNOSIS

- Obtain a CBC with differential, a complete metabolic panel, amylase, lipase, and a CXR.
- Cultures of urine, blood, sputum, and stool should be sent. LP is warranted only if CNS symptoms are present.

TREATMENT

Elderly patients or those on corticosteroids may not be able to mount a fever that meets diagnostic criteria for neutropenic fever.

- Empiric antimicrobials should cover *Pseudomonas*. Use **cefepime** IV or carbapenem IV.
- Consider vancomycin in patients with a history of MRSA infections, hypotension, persistent fever on empiric therapy, or skin or catheter site infections.
- Think about fungal infections (especially *Candida* and *Aspergillus*) in patients with 5–7 days of persistent fever, and begin amphotericin B or voriconazole.

SEPSIS

Defined as two systemic inflammatory response syndrome (SIRS) criteria **with evidence of infection.** Divided into three levels of severity (see Table 2.9-11). SIRS criteria are as follows:

- **Temperature:** < 36°C or > 38°C.
- **Heart rate:** > 90 bpm.
- **Respiratory rate:** > 24 breaths/min, or a P_{CO_2} < 32.
- **Leukocytes:** > 12,000 cells/mm^3, < 4000 cells/mm^3, or > 10% bands on peripheral blood smear.

SYMPTOMS/EXAM

- Presents with nonspecific infectious symptoms such as fever, chills, and fatigue.
- Symptoms and signs suggestive of cellulitis, necrotizing fasciitis, meningitis, sinusitis, pneumonia, endocarditis, UTI, or GI infection are seen.
- Vital signs are abnormal (see the SIRS criteria above).
- Evidence of hypoperfusion → cool, pale extremities, ↓ pulses, altered mental status, and ↓ urine output.

TABLE 2.9-11.   Severity of Sepsis

SEVERITY	CRITERIA
Sepsis	Meets at least two of the SIRS criteria with evidence of infection.
Severe sepsis	Meets the criteria for sepsis with evidence of end-organ damage.
Septic shock	Meets the criteria for sepsis with BP not responding to fluid resuscitation and necessitating the initiation of pressors and/or inotropes.

DIFFERENTIAL

MI, PE, cardiac tamponade, acute pancreatitis, acute hemorrhage, transfusion reactions, drug reactions, anaphylaxis, acute adrenal insufficiency, myxedema coma.

DIAGNOSIS

- Find the focus of infection.
- If no clear infectious focus can be found, obtain a CXR, a UA, and urine Gram stain and culture. Consider obtaining sputum, CSF, pleural fluid, and peritoneal fluid samples; a transesophageal echocardiogram (TEE); and an ultrasound of preexisting catheters or other foreign bodies (e.g., pacemakers).
- Always obtain blood cultures and sensitivities.
- Obtain a CBC, electrolytes, glucose, lactate, AST, ALT, aPTT, and PT, and consider an ABG if respiratory failure is a concern.

Early initiation of appropriate antimicrobials is critical in the management of sepsis.

TREATMENT

- Treat hypotension with **rapid fluid resuscitation.**
- Consider central line access for cardiovascular and pulmonary monitoring as well as administration of high-volume fluid resuscitation, blood products, and/or pressors/inotropes.
- Consider an arterial line for continuous monitoring of BP.
- If an infectious focus is identified, **appropriately tailor antimicrobial treatment.** If the source cannot be identified, start broad-spectrum antimicrobials in accordance with patient risk factors (e.g., immune compromise, nursing home residency, recent hospitalization).
- Use an insulin drip to **maintain glucose between 80 and 110.**
- If the patient does not respond to fluid resuscitation, consider relative adrenal insufficiency, administer IV corticosteroids, and obtain an ACTH stimulation test.
- If the patient meets the criteria for severe sepsis or septic shock and has multiorgan failure or ARDS, consider starting activated protein C.

COMPLICATIONS

Can → ARDS, DIC, multiorgan failure, and death.

DIVERTICULITIS

Inflammation and microperforation of diverticula.

SYMPTOMS/EXAM

Presents with fever, chills, nausea, vomiting, and abdominal pain, classically in the LLQ. Occasionally there may be a palpable mass in the LLQ.

DIFFERENTIAL

Ulcerative colitis, Crohn's disease, perforating colon cancer.

DIAGNOSIS

A clinical diagnosis, but often made with CT scan. Do not scope patients, as they are at high risk for perforation. Obtain a CBC and blood cultures.

TREATMENT

Bowel rest and antimicrobial coverage of gram-$\ominus$ and anaerobic organisms (e.g., ciprofloxacin and metronidazole). If diverticular abscess is present, manage surgically with a drain or resection.

COMPLICATIONS

Abscess, sepsis, death.

*If diverticulitis is suspected, do **not** perform lower endoscopy until the acute process resolves, since patients are at high risk for perforation.*

FUNGAL INFECTIONS

Typically affect immunocompromised patients and should always be considered in this population.

Cryptococcosis

- Affects patients with **depressed T-cell immunity.**
- **Sx/Exam:** Presents as a disseminated infection, frequently causing meningoencephalitis. In healthy patients, it typically causes pneumonia that is often self-limited.
- **Dx:**
    - Diagnose with fungal culture and antigen testing (e.g., CSF, blood, sputum). Silver stains of biopsies can aid in diagnosis.
    - Although largely replaced by the antigen test, an India ink test may show a halo 2° to the capsule.
- **Tx:**
    - Treat mild to moderate disease with fluconazole for 6–12 months.
    - Patients with severe disease, immunocompromised hosts, and those with CNS infections should be treated with amphotericin (+/– flucytosine) followed by long-term fluconazole.

Histoplasmosis

- Affects both healthy and immunocompromised patients.
- **Sx/Exam:**
    - Usually manifests as a respiratory illness, but can present as a disseminated disease in the immunocompromised.

- Disseminated disease can present with palate ulcerations, fever, weight loss, splenomegaly, anemia, and an elevated ESR.
- Patients have commonly visited the **Ohio/Mississippi river valleys** or have a **history of exposure to bird excrement, bat guano, or construction sites.**
- **Dx:** Diagnosis is best made with silver staining and culture of biopsied infected tissue, but *Histoplasma* antigen tests of urine and serum are available.
- **Tx:** Mild cases in healthy patients do not require treatment. Amphotericin should be used in severe cases, and itraconazole can be given if there is no CNS involvement.

Coccidioidomycosis

- Typically affects immunocompromised individuals, but not exclusively.
- **Sx/Exam:**
  - 1° disease is usually a self-limited pneumonitis with dry cough and fever; however, disseminated disease affects the CNS (meningitis), skin (erythema nodosum), bones, and joints.
  - Patients have **commonly visited the southwestern United States, particularly Arizona or the San Joaquin Valley in California.**
- **Dx:** Diagnose with silver stains of culture or biopsy, serologic studies, or antibody detection in CSF if meningitis is present.
- **Tx:** Treat with fluconazole and amphotericin if the disease is progressive or disseminated or if the patient is immunocompromised.

SECTION II

Musculoskeletal

Joint aspiration aids in the preliminary diagnosis of arthritis by helping distinguish inflammatory from noninflammatory disease as well as infectious and hemorrhagic processes (see Table 2.10-1).

SYSTEMIC LUPUS ERYTHEMATOSUS (SLE)

A multisystem, chronic inflammatory disease that is 2° to ANA complex formation and deposition. Patients may experience acute flare-ups of their symptoms. SLE is generally 1° but sometimes occurs 2° to drug use (hydralazine, penicillamine, and procainamide). 2° SLE is reversible.

SYMPTOMS/EXAM

Patients tend to be young African-American females. Findings by organ system are as follows:

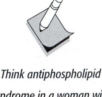

Think antiphospholipid syndrome in a woman with recurrent spontaneous abortion or premature delivery.

- **Constitutional:** Fatigue, weight loss, fever.
- **Arthritis:** Usually migratory and asymmetric; involves the hands.
- **Skin: Malar rash** (butterfly rash over the cheeks and nose), **discoid rash** (scaling papules that can leave residual scarring), alopecia, painless **oral ulcers,** Raynaud's phenomenon, **photosensitive rash.**
- **Renal failure.**
- **Pulmonary: Pleuritis,** pleural effusion, interstitial lung disease, pulmonary hypertension.
- **Cardiovascular: Pericarditis,** pericardial effusion.
- **CNS:** Seizures, neuropathies, headache.
- **Psychological:** Anxiety, depression, psychosis.
- **Hematologic:** Thrombocytopenia, hemolytic anemia, leukopenia.
- **GI:** Peritonitis.

TABLE 2.10-1. Interpretation of Joint Aspiration

	NORMAL	**NONINFLAMMATORY**	**INFLAMMATORY**	**INFECTIOUS**	**HEMORRHAGIC**
Color	Clear	Xanthochromic	Yellow	Opaque	Bloody
Viscosity	High	High	Low	Low	Variable
WBCs/mm^3	< 200	200–3000	3000–50,000	> 50,000	Variable
% PMNs	< 25	< 25	> 50	> 75	Variable
Crystals	None	None	May be present	None	None
Differential	None	Osteoarthritis, SLE, trauma, aseptic necrosis, scleroderma, Charcot's joint	Gout, pseudogout, rheumatoid arthritis, SLE, TB, scleroderma, ankylosing spondylitis, psoriatic arthritis	Bacterial, TB	Coagulopathy, trauma

DIAGNOSIS

- The diagnostic criteria for SLE are summarized in the mnemonic **DOPAMINE RASH.** Diagnosis requires at least four of the 11 criteria.
- ANA is highly sensitive but nonspecific, whereas anti-dsDNA and anti-Sm antibodies are highly specific.
- Obtain anticardiolipin antibody and lupus anticoagulant assays to screen for antiphospholipid antibody syndrome in patients with SLE.
- Active SLE flare-ups are characterized by ↓ C3 and C4 but ↑ CRP and ESR.

TREATMENT

- Arthritis and mild serositis are treated with NSAIDs. Hydroxychloroquine is used for rashes and for arthritis that is unresponsive to NSAIDs. Steroids and immunosuppressants are used in the presence of significant organ involvement.
- Patients undergoing active SLE flare-ups are treated with steroids, which are tapered once remission has been induced. Those with antiphospholipid antibody syndrome need lifelong anticoagulation with warfarin.

COMPLICATIONS

SLE patients who become pregnant have a higher incidence of spontaneous abortion. Neonates can get congenital complete heart block. Patients can have antiphospholipid antibody syndrome, which predisposes them to arterial and venous thrombosis.

> **SLE criteria—DOPAMINE RASH**
>
> **D**iscoid rash
> **O**ral ulcers
> **P**hotosensitive rash
> **A**rthritis
> **M**alar rash
> **I**mmunologic criteria
>   (⊕ anti-dsDNA or
>   ⊕ anti-Sm)
> **NE**urologic or
>   psychiatric symptoms
> **R**enal disease
> **A**NA ⊕
> **S**erositis (pleural,
>   peritoneal, or
>   pericardial)
> **H**ematologic disorders
>   (thrombocytopenia,
>   anemia, or
>   leukopenia)

RHEUMATOID ARTHRITIS (RA)

A chronic, symmetrical, and erosive synovitis.

SYMPTOMS/EXAM

Insidious onset of a symmetrical arthritis. **Nonspecific** complaints include fever, fatigue, anorexia, and weight loss. Affected joints are swollen and tender. Other findings include joint deformities (see Figure 2.10-1), atlantoaxial joint subluxation, carpal tunnel syndrome, and Baker's cyst rupture. **Extra-**

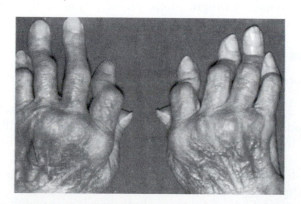

FIGURE 2.10-1.   Rheumatoid arthritis.

The swan-neck deformities of the digits and severe involvement of the PIP joints are characteristic. (Reproduced, with permission, from Chandrasoma P. *Concise Pathology*, 3rd ed. Stamford, CT: Appleton & Lange, 1998: 978.)

articular features may include neuropathy, episcleritis, Sjögren's syndrome (dry eyes and mouth), pulmonary fibrosis, hepatosplenomegaly, Hashimoto's thyroiditis, pleuritis, lung nodules, pericarditis, and myocarditis.

Typical RA hands:

- *MCP and PIP involvement*
- *Sparing of the DIP joint*
- *Ulnar deviation*
- *Symmetric*
- *Swan-neck deformities*

Methotrexate for RA is contraindicated in pregnant patients and in those with HIV, liver disease, renal failure, or bone marrow suppression.

Monoarthritis? Think:

- *Gout*
- *Septic arthritis*
- *Lyme disease*
- *Traumas*

Avoid allopurinol during acute gout attacks.

DIAGNOSIS

- Diagnosed in the presence of four or more of the following criteria for six weeks:
    - Morning stiffness (> 1 hour).
    - Arthritis of three or more joint areas (most commonly the PIP, MCP, wrist, elbow, knee, or ankle).
    - Arthritis of the hand joints (MCP, PIP, or wrists).
    - Symmetric arthritis.
    - Rheumatoid nodules (most commonly found at the elbow).
    - ↑ serum RF.
    - Radiographic changes (obtain plain films of affected joints in all RA patients).
- RF is nonspecific but is ⊕ in 75% of RA cases. Joint aspiration is inflammatory (see Table 2.10-1). Look for periarticular osteoporosis with erosions around the affected MCP and PIP joints on x-rays (see Figure 2.10-1).

TREATMENT

- Mild cases are treated with NSAIDs; add hydroxychloroquine if NSAIDs are inadequate.
- Moderate to severe cases are treated with NSAIDs and methotrexate.
- If methotrexate fails or is contraindicated, give anti-TNF treatment (etanercept, infliximab, adalimumab).
- Immunosuppressants are used in patients who fail methotrexate and etanercept therapy.
- Acute exacerbations of RA (i.e., patients who are febrile, toxic, or experiencing a rapid decline in function) are treated with a short course of prednisone.
- Other measures include weight loss, rest, and physiotherapy.

GOUT

A metabolic condition resulting from the intra-articular deposition of monosodium urate crystals. Complications include nephrolithiasis and chronic urate nephropathy.

SYMPTOMS/EXAM

- Typically presents in **middle-aged, obese men** (90%) from the Pacific Islands.
- Acute gout attacks often occur at night between periods of remission.
- Patients initially present with severe pain, redness, and swelling in a single, unilateral, lower extremity joint (typically the first MTP joint); subsequent attacks may present in additive fashion with multiple joints.
- Differentiate from pseudogout, in which symptoms are less severe and often affect the knee (> 50%).
- Common precipitants of attacks include a high-purine diet (e.g., meats, alcohol), dehydration (2° to diuretic use), trauma, or tumor lysis syndrome.
- Patients with long-standing disease may develop tophi that → joint deformation.

DIAGNOSIS

- Joint aspiration is inflammatory with needle-shaped, negatively birefringent (**yeLLow** when **paraLLel** to the condenser) crystals (see Figure 2.10-2 and Table 2.10-2). Radiographs are normal in early gout. Characteristic punched-out erosions with overhanging cortical bone ("rat bites") are seen in more advanced disease.
- Most patients have ↑ serum uric acid (which is neither sensitive nor specific). Roughly 90% are underexcreters of uric acid, while the remainder are overproducers.
- A 24-hour urine collection for uric acid while patients are off hyperuricemia-inducing medications (diuretics, alcohol, cyclosporine) helps differentiate between the two (see Table 2.10-3).

TREATMENT

- For acute attacks, administer high-dose NSAIDs (e.g., indomethacin) or colchicine. Use steroids when first-line therapy fails.
- Once the acute attack resolves, begin maintenance therapy to ↓ serum uric acid levels. Overproducers are treated with allopurinol; undersecreters are treated with probenecid.
- Avoid precipitants of acute attacks; consume a low-purine diet (eggs, cheese, fruit, and vegetables).

OSTEOARTHRITIS (OA)

A chronic, noninflammatory joint disease marked by degeneration of the articular cartilage, **hypertrophy** of the bone margins, and changes in the synovial membrane. OA can be 1° or 2° to trauma, chronic arthritis, congenital joint disease, or a systemic metabolic disorder (hemochromatosis, Wilson's disease).

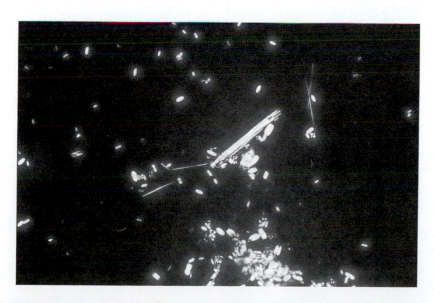

FIGURE 2.10-2.   Gout crystals.

Note the needle-shaped, negatively birefringent crystals. (Reproduced, with permission, from Milikowski C. *Color Atlas of Basic Histopathology*, 1st ed. Stamford, CT: Appleton & Lange, 1997: 546.)

DIAGNOSIS

Obtain an **ESR** (often > 100), a prompt ophthalmologic evaluation, and a **temporal artery biopsy.** Biopsy will reveal thrombosis, necrosis of the media, and lymphocytes, plasma cells, and giant cells.

TREATMENT

Treat immediately with **high-dose prednisone** (40–60 mg/day) and continue for 1–2 months before tapering. Do not delay treatment, as blindness is permanent. Conduct serial eye exams for improvements or changes.

POLYMYALGIA RHEUMATICA

- Sx/Exam:
  - Typical symptoms include **pain and stiffness of the shoulder and pelvic girdle** areas with **fever,** malaise, weight loss, and minimal joint swelling.
  - Patients classically have difficulty getting out of a chair or lifting their arms above their heads but have **no objective weakness.**
- Dx: Look for concurrent **anemia** and a ↑↑ **ESR.**
- Tx: Treat with **low-dose prednisone** (5–20 mg/day).

FIBROMYALGIA

- Sx/Exam:
  - Presents as a syndrome of myalgias, weakness, and fatigue in the absence of inflammation; laboratory testing is $\ominus$.
  - Associated with depression, anxiety, and irritable bowel syndrome (IBS); most commonly affects **women > 50 years of age.**
  - Suspect with 11 of 18 **trigger points** (see Figure 2.10-3) that reproduce pain with palpation. Otherwise, consider myofascial pain syndrome.
- Tx:
  - Treat with supportive measures such as stretching and heat application.
  - Consider hydrotherapy, transcutaneous electrical nerve stimulation (TENS), stress reduction, psychotherapy, or low-dose antidepressants.

POLYMYOSITIS

A progressive, systemic connective tissue disease characterized by striated muscle inflammation. One-third of patients have **dermatomyositis** with coexisting cutaneous involvement. Patients may also develop myocarditis, cardiac conduction deficits, or malignancy. More commonly seen in **older women** (50–70 years of age).

SYMPTOMS/EXAM

- **Symmetric,** progressive proximal muscle weakness and pain → the classic complaint of difficulty rising from a chair. Patients may eventually have difficulty breathing or swallowing.
- Dermatomyositis may present with a **heliotrope rash** (violaceous periorbital rash) and **Gottron's papules** (papules located on the dorsum of the hands over bony prominences).

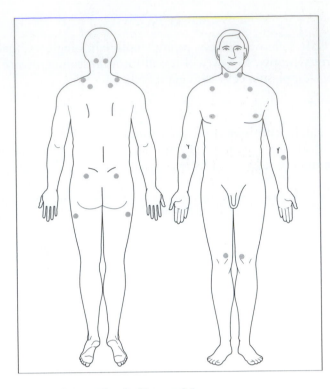

FIGURE 2.10-3. Trigger points in fibromyalgia.

(Reproduced, with permission, from Le T et al. *First Aid for the USMLE Step 2 CK*, 6th ed. New York: McGraw-Hill, 2007: 255.)

DIAGNOSIS

Look for ↑ **serum creatinine, aldolase, and CK.** EMG demonstrates fibrillations. Muscle biopsy shows inflammatory cells and muscle degeneration.

TREATMENT

High-dose **corticosteroids** generally → improved muscle strength in 4–6 weeks and can be tapered to a lower dose for maintenance therapy. If patients are unresponsive to initial treatment, immunosuppressive medication may be used. Monitor for malignancy.

> ### CREST SYNDROME
>
> **C**alcinosis
> **R**aynaud's
>   phenomenon
> **E**sophageal dysmotility
> **S**clerodactyly
> **T**elangiectasias

SCLERODERMA

- A multisystem disease with **symmetric thickening** of the skin on the face and extremities.
- Typically affects **women** 30–65 years of age.
- **Dx:** There are two subtypes: limited and systemic (see Table 2.10-8).

TABLE 2.10-8. **Limited vs. Diffuse Scleroderma**

	LIMITED (CREST)	DIFFUSE
Skin involvement	Distal, face only	Generalized
Progression	Slow	Rapid
Diagnosis	Anticentromere antibody	Anti-Scl-70 antibody
Prognosis	Fair	Poor
Calcinosis	+++	+
Telangiectasia	+++	+
Renal failure	0	++

SECTION II

Nephrology

Glomerular Filtration Rate (GFR) and Surrogates

■ GFR, which is literally defined as the amount of fluid entering Bowman's space from the glomeruli per minute, is a marker of renal function. It cannot be directly measured but is approximated using creatinine clearance (CrCl).

■ Normal values are 97–137 mL/min in males and 88–128 mL/min in females.

■ Oliguria is generally defined as urine < 500 cc/day, or approximately 20 cc/hr.

Interpreting a Urinalysis (UA)

Tables 2.11-1 and 2.11-2 are guidelines for interpreting a UA.

TABLE 2.11-1. Interpretation of UAs

TEST	INTERPRETATION
Proteinuria	A urine dip generally requires 100–150 mg/dL of protein to be ⊕; many dip tests can detect only albumin (not globulins or Bence Jones proteins). UA can detect both albumin and non-albumin proteins, but there must be at least 1–10 mg of protein/dL for the UA to be ⊕.
Glucosuria	Indicates the possibility of hyperglycemia; consider diabetes.
Ketonuria	Occurs with starvation, poorly controlled diabetes (e.g., DKA), and alcohol intoxication. Urine ketones can also be elevated following recent exercise and during pregnancy.
Hematuria/blood	A ⊕ value indicates myoglobin, hemoglobin, or RBCs in the urine.
Nitrite	Can become ⊕ with gram-⊖ bacteriuria.
Leukocyte esterase	Produced by WBCs, which are not normal in urine; suggestive of a UTI.
pH	Alkalosis is most common with *Proteus* UTI but may also be seen with some strains of *Klebsiella, Pseudomonas, Providencia,* and *Staphylococcus.* Acidosis with nephrolithiasis suggests uric acid or cystine stones. A pH of > 5.5 in the setting of metabolic acidosis suggests distal renal tubular acidosis (RTA). A low-sensitivity test (see the section on statistics for a detailed definition of sensitivity).
Specific gravity	A rough estimate of urine osmolarity (U_{osm}).
Urobilinogen	Low sensitivity. ↑ urobilinogen occurs in hemolysis or hepatocellular disease. ↓ urobilinogen may suggest biliary obstruction.
Bilirubin	Bilirubin in the urine suggests a conjugated hyperbilirubinemia.
Epithelial cells	An excessive number of epithelial cells in the urine suggests a contaminated urine sample.

TABLE 2.11-2.   Urine Sediment Analysis

FINDING	ASSOCIATION
Hyaline casts	Normal finding, but an ↑ amount suggests a prerenal condition, although it is nonspecific.
RBC casts	Glomerulonephritis.
WBC casts	Pyelonephritis.
Eosinophils	Allergic interstitial nephritis.
Glomerular, "muddy brown" casts	Acute tubular necrosis (ATN).
RBCs	Indicates hematuria. The absence of RBCs when the dipstick is ⊕ for blood suggests hemoglobinuria from hemolysis or myoglobinuria from rhabdomyolysis.
WBCs	More than a few is always abnormal, except when contaminated (e.g., epithelial cells). Causes include infection, nephrolithiasis, neoplasm, acute interstitial cystitis, prostatitis, acute interstitial nephritis, strictures, and glomerulonephropathy.
Crystals	See the discussion of nephrolithiasis.
Yeast, bacteria	Indicate infection if the sample is not contaminated (e.g., epithelial cells).

Fractional Excretion of Sodium (Fe$_{Na}$)

- Fe$_{Na}$ is calculated using measured plasma and urine levels of sodium and creatinine:

$$Fe_{Na} = (U_{Na} \times P_{Cr}) / (P_{Na} \times U_{Cr})$$

- An Fe$_{Na}$ of < 1% suggests a **prerenal** state such as CHF, dehydration, hepatorenal syndrome, or drug effects (e.g., NSAIDs, ACEIs).
- An Fe$_{Na}$ of > 2% suggests **intrinsic** renal disease such as ATN, acute interstitial nephritis, vasculitis, or anything causing renal ischemia.
- Note that Fe$_{Na}$ can be unreliable under any conditions, but particularly in the setting of sepsis or recent diuretic use. It is best used in the oliguric patient.

ELECTROLYTES

Hyponatremia

Serum sodium < 135 mEq/L.

SYMPTOMS/EXAM

- Often asymptomatic, but may present with **confusion, lethargy,** muscle cramps, and nausea.
- When serum sodium is low enough or in the setting of rapid changes, hyponatremia may → cerebral edema that in turn → seizures, status epilepticus, coma, or even death.

DIAGNOSIS

Hyponatremia is classified by serum osmolarity (P$_{osm}$), as listed below. To make the differential, order a P$_{Na}$, osmolarity, total protein, glucose, and lipid panel.

In pseudohyponatremia, measured serum sodium may be falsely ↓ by hyperlipidemia or hyperproteinemia.

- **Hypertonic ($P_{osm} > 295$ mOsm/kg):** Hyperglycemia; hypertonic infusion (e.g., mannitol, radiocontrast).
- **Isotonic ($P_{osm} = 280–295$ mOsm/kg):** Hyperlipidemia (triglycerides, chylomicrons), hyperproteinemia.
- **Hypotonic ($P_{osm} < 280$ mOsm/kg):** Hypotonic hyponatremia is further categorized according to volume status (see Table 2.11-3). Useful tests to aid in evaluation include serum BUN, creatinine, sodium, and Fe_{Na} (U_{Na}, U_{Cr}).

TREATMENT

- **Hypertonic and isotonic hyponatremia** are best addressed through the correction of their underlying causes.
- **Hypotonic hyponatremia** can cause problems independent of its etiology, requiring specific treatment (see Table 2.11-4). The most important factor in treatment is volume status; however, acuity is also relevant.
- Correcting too rapidly can → **central pontine myelinolysis** (flaccid paralysis, dysarthria, dysphagia), so correction should generally be done gradually through use of normal saline (NS). However, with symptomatic hyponatremia (altered mental status or seizures), correction should initially be more rapid, using 3% **hypertonic saline** to ↑ P_{Na} by 5–6 mEq/L over the first 2–3 hours. Concurrent furosemide may be necessary to prevent volume overload. Maximum target correction should not exceed **8–10 mEq/L/day.** A patient whose volume status has been normalized and is correcting too rapidly can, paradoxically, be treated with free water to slow down the sodium correction.

Hypernatremia

Serum sodium > 147 mEq/L.

SYMPTOMS/EXAM

May present with lethargy, mental status changes, focal neurologic deficits (e.g., hyperreflexia, tremors, rigidity), and seizures. Abrupt, severe hypernatremia can → intracranial hemorrhage.

DIAGNOSIS

- Take a thorough history and assess the patient's volume status to determine the etiology of the hypernatremia. Check U_{osm}, P_{osm}, potassium, BUN/creatinine, calcium, and glucose.

TABLE 2.11-3. Classification of Hypotonic Hyponatremia by Volume Status

HYPOVOLEMIC		EUVOLEMIC	HYPERVOLEMIC
EXTRARENAL SALT LOSS **($Fe_{Na} < 1\%$)**	**RENAL SALT LOSS** **($Fe_{Na} > 2\%$)**		**EDEMATOUS** **STATES**
Dehydration	Diuretic use	SIADH	CHF
Diarrhea	Nephropathies	Hypothyroidism	Liver disease
Vomiting	Mineralocorticoid deficiency	Psychogenic polydipsia	Nephrotic syndrome
		Beer potomania	Advanced renal failure

TABLE 2.11-4. Treatment of Hypotonic Hyponatremia

Volume Status	Treatment
Hypovolemic	Replace fluids with NS.
Euvolemic	Fluid restriction (free water < 1 L/day).
Hypervolemic	Restrict salt and fluid; diuresis if necessary.

- Etiologies can be distinguished as follows:
  - Hypernatremia from **hypovolemia** usually presents in the setting of dehydration, **when the patient has limited access to free water.** U_{osm} is usually > 700 mOsm/kg. Causes include ↑ insensible losses (burns, sweating, endotracheal intubation) and diarrhea.
  - Hypernatremia from ↑ **total body sodium** generally does **not** present with hypovolemia. Causes include excessive hydration with hypertonic fluids, dysfunction of central regulation, and mineralocorticoid excess (consider if the patient has hypokalemia and hypertension).
  - Hypernatremia from **renal losses** (see Table 2.11-5) usually occurs in the setting of hypovolemia and a U_{osm} < 700 mOsm/kg. Consider the clinical context in the setting of the U_{osm}/P_{osm} ratio to help determine the cause.

Hypernatremia often occurs with dehydration when a patient has no access to free water.

TREATMENT

- Always treat underlying causes (e.g., DDAVP for central diabetes insipidus).
- Correct the free-water deficit with hypotonic saline, D_5W, or oral water depending on volume status.
- To prevent cerebral swelling, correction of hypernatremia should not occur at a rate of > 12 mEq/L per day.

Hypokalemia

Serum potassium < 3.5 mEq/L.

TABLE 2.11-5. Causes of Hypernatremia 2° to Renal Losses

	Etiology	Comments
Osmotic diuresis	**Causes:** Mannitol, hyperglycemia, high protein feeds, postobstructive diuresis.	U_{osm}/P_{osm} > 0.7.
Central diabetes insipidus	The pituitary does not make ADH. **Causes:** Tumor, trauma, neurosurgery, infection.	U_{osm}/P_{osm} < 0.7. U_{osm} should ↑ by 50% in response to DDAVP.
Nephrogenic diabetes insipidus	The kidneys are unresponsive to ADH. **Causes:** Renal failure, hypercalcemia, demeclocycline, lithium, sickle cell anemia.	U_{osm}/P_{osm} < 0.7. U_{osm} should not respond to DDAVP challenge.

SYMPTOMS/EXAM

May present with fatigue, **muscle weakness or cramps, ileus,** hyporeflexia, paresthesias, and flaccid paralysis if severe. ECG may show **T-wave flattening, U waves** (an additional wave after the T wave), ST depression, and QT prolongation followed by AV block and subsequent cardiac arrest.

DIAGNOSIS

- Order an ECG and check urine potassium.
- Diagnose as follows:
  - **Urine potassium > 20 mEq/L:** Usually indicates that the kidneys are wasting potassium. Acid-base status must be examined to further stratify the etiology.
    - **Metabolic acidosis:** Type 1 RTA (e.g., amphotericin), lactic acidosis, or ketoacidosis.
    - **Metabolic alkalosis:** 1° or 2° hyperaldosteronism (check plasma renin activity and plasma aldosterone concentration), Cushing's syndrome (check 24-hour urine cortisol), diuretics (e.g., loop or thiazide), vomiting, NG suction.
    - **Variable pH:** Gentamicin, platinum-containing chemotherapeutics, hypomagnesemia.
  - **Urine potassium < 20 mEq/L:** Usually indicates a nonrenal source of hypokalemia. This could be from **transcellular shift** (e.g., insulin, β_2-agonists, alkalosis, periodic paralysis) or from **GI losses** (e.g., diarrhea, chronic laxative abuse).

The greatest determinant of urinary potassium wasting is the urinary flow rate. The greater the urine volume production, the more potassium is wasted.

TREATMENT

- Treat the underlying disorder.
- Provide oral and/or IV **potassium repletion.** Oral administration is preferred, as a burning sensation may result when potassium is given through a peripheral IV.
- Replace **magnesium,** as this deficiency makes potassium repletion more difficult. Monitor ECG and plasma potassium levels frequently during replacement.

Hyperkalemia

Serum potassium > 5 mEq/L.

SYMPTOMS/EXAM

May be asymptomatic or may present with nausea, vomiting, **intestinal colic, areflexia, weakness,** flaccid paralysis, and paresthesias. ECG findings follow a pattern consisting of **tall, peaked T waves,** PR prolongation, a wide QRS, and loss of P waves that together progress to **sine waves,** ventricular fibrillation, and cardiac arrest (see Figure 2.11-1).

DIAGNOSIS

- Begin by confirming the hyperkalemia with a **repeat blood draw** unless the suspicion is already high.
- Then exclude **spurious** causes of hyperkalemia, which include hemolysis (e.g., from fist clenching during blood draws), extreme leukocytosis, severe thrombocytosis, or rhabdomyolysis. Order an ECG and use urine potassium levels as a guide to help determine the etiology of the hyperkalemia.
  - **Urine potassium < 40 mEq/L:** Usually indicates that the hyperkalemia is caused by ↓ potassium excretion by the kidneys. Causes include re-

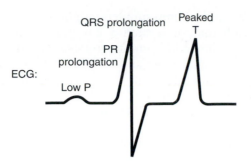

FIGURE 2.11-1. **Effects of hyperkalemia as seen on ECG.**

(Reproduced, with permission, from Cogan MF. *Fluid and Electrolytes.* Stamford, CT: Appleton & Lange, 1991: 170.)

nal insufficiency, drugs (e.g., spironolactone, triamterene, amiloride, ACEIs, trimethoprim, NSAIDs) and mineralocorticoid deficiency (type 4 RTA). A plasma renin activity and plasma aldosterone concentration should be ordered if a mineralocorticoid deficiency is suspected.

- **Urine potassium > 40 mEq/L:** Usually indicates a nonrenal etiology. Causes include **cellular shifts** resulting from tissue injury, tumor lysis, insulin deficiency, drugs (e.g., succinylcholine, digitalis, arginine, α-blockers), and **iatrogenic** factors.

TREATMENT

- Values > 6.5 mEq/L or ECG changes (especially PR prolongation or wide QRS) require emergent treatment.
- **Calcium gluconate** for cardiac cell membrane stabilization should be given immediately to prevent arrhythmias, followed by **bicarbonate** and/or **insulin and glucose** to temporarily shift potassium into the cells.
- Patients can be given **Kayexalate** and/or **furosemide** with hydration to promote potassium excretion.
- **Restrict potassium** in the diet and discontinue any medications that may be contributing to the hyperkalemia.
- Severe or symptomatic hyperkalemia, hyperkalemia refractory to the above management, or patients on **chronic** hemodialysis may require acute **hemodialysis.**

Hypercalcemia

Serum calcium > 10.6 mg/dL. The most common causes are **hyperparathyroidism and malignancy** (e.g., squamous cell carcinomas, myelomas).

SYMPTOMS/EXAM

May present with **bones** (fractures), **stones** (kidney stones), abdominal **groans** (anorexia, nausea, constipation), and **psychiatric overtones** (weakness, fatigue, altered mental status). Consider in patients with pancreatitis, refractory PUD, a personal or family history of kidney stones, or bone pain.

DIAGNOSIS

- Confirm hypercalcemia with a repeat calcium; if measuring total serum calcium rather than ionized calcium, check a serum albumin and correct by 0.8 mg/dL for each 1-g/dL deviation in albumin.

> *Causes of hypercalcemia—*
> ***CHIMPANZEES***
>
> **C**alcium
>   supplementation
> **H**yperparathyroidism
> **I**atrogenic/**I**mmobility
> **M**ilk-alkali syndrome
> **P**aget's disease
> **A**ddison's
>   disease/**A**cromegaly
> **N**eoplasm
> **Z**ollinger-Ellison
>   syndrome
> **E**xcess vitamin A
> **E**xcess vitamin D
> **S**arcoidosis

Stones most commonly occur in males in the third and fourth decades of life. Risk factors include a ⊕ family history, **low fluid intake**, gout, postcolectomy/ileostomy, chronic diarrhea, sarcoid, specific enzyme disorders, RTA, and hyperparathyroidism. Stones are most commonly calcium oxalate but may also be calcium phosphate, struvite, uric acid, or cystine (see Table 2.11-9).

SYMPTOMS/EXAM

Presents with **acute onset of severe, colicky flank pain** that may **radiate to the testes or vulva** and may be associated with nausea and vomiting. Patients are unable to get comfortable and shift position frequently (vs. those with peritonitis, who remain still).

DIAGNOSIS

Labs, examination, and imaging together make the diagnosis.

- Gross or **microscopic hematuria** and an **altered urine pH** may be noted on UA. Check serum calcium, a CBC, and serum creatinine, and look for signs of UTI (which may be the cause of infection leading to struvite stones or 2° to obstruction from other stones).
- Tenderness may be present in the costovertebral areas or in either abdominal lower quadrant. It may be difficult to distinguish pain associated with nephrolithiasis from that originating in the ovaries, fallopian tubes, intestines, or gallbladder.
- Imaging is critical. A **KUB** can detect any radiopaque stones, and **IVP** can be used to detect stones that are radiolucent on KUB. **Noncontrast abdominal CT scans (CT-KUB)** are now the 1° means of diagnosis; they can identify not only stones but also other causes of flank pain.

TABLE 2.11-9. Types of Nephrolithiasis

TYPE	FREQUENCY	ETIOLOGY AND CHARACTERISTICS	TREATMENT
Calcium oxalate/ calcium phosphate	83%	The most common causes are **idiopathic hypercalciuria,** elevated urine uric acid 2° to diet, and 1° hyperparathyroidism. Alkaline urine. Radiopaque.	Hydration, thiazide diuretic.
Struvite (Mg-NH$_4$-PO$_4$)	9%	"Triple phosphate stones." Associated with urease-producing organisms (e.g., *Proteus*). Form staghorn calculi. Alkaline urine. Radiopaque.	Hydration; treat UTI if present.
Uric acid	7%	Associated with gout and high purine turnover states. Acidic urine (pH < 5.5). **Radiolucent.**	Hydration; alkalinize urine with citrate, which is converted to HCO$_3^-$ in the liver.
Cystine	1%	Due to a defect in renal transport of certain amino acids (**COLA**—**C**ystine, **O**rnithine, **L**ysine, and **A**rginine). **Hexagonal crystals.** Radiopaque.	Hydration, alkalinize urine, penicillamine.

Reproduced, with permission, from Le T et al. *First Aid for the USMLE Step 2 CK*, 6th ed. New York: McGraw-Hill, 2007: 443.

- All urine should be strained, and if a stone is passed, it should be recovered and sent to the lab for analysis.

TREATMENT

- **Hydration and analgesia** are the initial treatment; additional treatment is based on the size of the stone.
  - Stones < 5 mm in diameter can pass through the urethra.
  - Stones up to 3 cm in diameter can be treated with **extracorporeal shock-wave lithotripsy** (ESWL) or percutaneous nephrolithotomy.
- Preventive measures include hydration and prophylactic measures that depend on stone composition.

RENAL TUBULAR ACIDOSIS (RTA)

May occur 2° to renal or adrenal disease, or may be a 1° disease. Due to a net ↓ in either tubular hydrogen (H^+) secretion or bicarbonate reabsorption that → a **non-anion-gap metabolic acidosis**. There are four types of RTA (see Table 2.11-10), but only three are clinically important. **Type IV (distal)** is the most common; type III is uncommon and is seen only in children.

DIAGNOSIS

Usually asymptomatic. There are fewer urinary anions (mostly Cl^-) than cations (Na^+, K^+) in distal RTA; in proximal RTA, there is high urinary bicarbonate despite low serum bicarbonate.

TABLE 2.11-10. Types of RTA

	TYPE I (DISTAL)	TYPE II (PROXIMAL)	TYPE IV (DISTAL)
Defect	H^+ secretion.	HCO_3^- reabsorption.	Aldosterone deficiency or resistance → defects in Na^+ reabsorption, H^+ and K^+ excretion, ↓ ammoniagenesis.
Serum K^+	High or low.	Low.	High.
Urinary pH	> 5.3.	> 5.3 initially; < 5.3 once serum is acidic.	< 5.3.
Etiologies (most common)	Hereditary, amphotericin, collagen vascular disease, cirrhosis, nephrocalcinosis.	Hereditary, carbonic anhydrase inhibitors, Fanconi's syndrome.	Hyporeninemic hypoaldosternism with DM; HTN, chronic interstitial nephritis.
Treatment	Potassium citrate.	Potassium citrate.	Furosemide, Kayexalate.
Complications	Nephrolithiasis.	Rickets, osteomalacia.	Hyperkalemia.

Reproduced, with permission, from Le T et al. *First Aid for the USMLE Step 2 CK,* 6th ed. New York: McGraw-Hill, 2007: 435.

SECTION II

Neurology

Table 2.12-1 distinguishes the pathophysiology and clinical presentation of UMN lesions from that of LMN lesions.

Bell's palsy involves damage to the facial nerve → diminished taste, hyperacusis, ↑ tearing, and variable hyperesthesia of the face.

STROKES

Acute onset of focal neurologic deficits that result from ↓ blood flow. Strokes persist for **at least 24 hours.** In **transient ischemic attacks (TIAs),** the neurologic deficit resolves in < 24 hours, often lasting only 5–15 minutes. Risk factors include untreated hypertension, atrial fibrillation (AF), diabetes, cigarette smoking, recent myocardial infarction, valvular heart disease, carotid artery disease, TIA, OCP use, illicit drugs use (e.g. cocaine, amphetamines), and hyperlipidemia. **Ischemic strokes** account for 85% of strokes; 1° intracranial hemorrhage accounts for 15%. Etiologies are as follows:

- **Ischemic strokes** are usually due to an occlusion of a large cerebral vessel by a **thrombosis** that extends within an atherosclerotic extracranial or intracerebral artery; or an **embolus** from the heart, aortic arch, or proximal arterial vessels.
- **Intracranial hemorrhage** usually results from rupture of an aneurysm or a small vessel.

SYMPTOMS/EXAM

- **Ischemic strokes** have an abrupt, dramatic onset of focal neurologic symptoms. Small, deep ischemic lesions are seen in lacunar strokes.
- By contrast, **intracranial hemorrhagic strokes** may evolve over a 5- to 30-minute period.
- Specific symptoms are as follows:
    - **Superior division MCA stroke:** Contralateral hemiparesis that affects the face, hand, and arm; contralateral hemisensory deficit in the same distribution; ipsilateral gaze preference; facial droop. If the dominant hemisphere is affected, **Broca's aphasia** results.
    - **Inferior division MCA stroke:** Contralateral homonymous hemianopia; neglect of the contralateral limbs; apraxia. If the nondominant hemisphere is affected, **Wernicke's aphasia** results.
    - **Anterior cerebral artery stroke:** Leg paresis.
    - **Posterior cerebral artery stroke:** Homonymous hemianopia with macular sparing; prosopagnosia (inability to recognize familiar faces).
    - **Basilar artery stroke:** Coma, cranial nerve palsies, locked-in syndrome.
    - **Lacunar stroke:** Pure motor or sensory deficit; dysarthria–clumsy hand syndrome; hemiparesis; facial droop.

Broca's (expressive) aphasia involves nonfluent speech; good auditory comprehension; and poor repetition and naming.

DIFFERENTIAL

Seizure, brain tumor or abscess, subdural or epidural hematoma, hypo- or hyperglycemia, MS, TIA.

DIAGNOSIS

- **Head CT without contrast** to rule out bleed.
- **MRI with diffusion-weighted imaging (DWI) and perfusion-weighted imaging (PWI):** DWI shows dying tissue; PWI shows penumbra, or tissue at risk of dying.
- **MRA:** To evaluate vessels, including the carotids and circle of Willis.

Wernicke's (receptive) aphasia involves fluent speech and poor auditory comprehension, repetition, and naming.

HIGH-YIELD FACTS

NEUROLOGY

TABLE 2.12-1. UMN vs. LMN Lesions

	UMN LESIONS	LMN LESIONS
Anatomy	The corticospinal tract path extends from the brain **down to but not including** the anterior horn cells of the spinal cord ("CNS lesions").	Extends from the anterior horn cells to the peripheral nerve ("PNS lesions").
Paresis (muscle weakness)	Affect the upper extremity extensors more than the flexors, and the lower extremity flexors more than the extensors.	Distribution of motor neurons, dermatome, and root. Affect the trunk, cord, or nerves.
Tone	Spasticity.	Flaccidity.
Wasting	Absent.	Present.
DTRs	Hyperactive.	Hypoactive or absent.
Plantar reflexes	Upgoing ($\oplus$ Babinski's).	Downgoing (normal).
Fasciculations	Absent.	Present.
Examples	Lesions in the cerebrum, basal ganglia, brain stem, cerebellum, or spinal cord: strokes, TIA, brain tumors, head trauma, AIDS, MS.	Guillain-Barré syndrome, neuropathies, myopathies, myasthenia gravis, **Bell's palsy**, herpes zoster, Lyme disease, acoustic neuroma.

- **Transesophageal echocardiography (TEE):** To evaluate for cardiac emboli and patent foramen ovale.
- **Labs:** CBC, electrolytes, coagulation studies, HbA_{1c}, fasting lipids.

TREATMENT

- Check airway, breathing, and circulation (**ABCs**); order STAT glucose. **Keep NPO** until intracranial hemorrhage has been ruled out and the patient has been assessed for dysphagia (aspiration risk).
- Admit to the ICU or to a telemetry-monitored bed.
- Maintain adequate BP (e.g., > 160/> 80) to optimize intracranial perfusion. **Do not precipitously lower BP.**
- In the setting of a 1° intracranial bleed, **obtain an urgent neurosurgical evaluation** for possible evacuation.
- If the head CT shows a normal or hypodense area consistent with **acute ischemic stroke,** consider the following:
  - **Antiplatelet agents:** Aspirin ↓ the incidence of a second event. Patients already on aspirin may be given clopidogrel, ticlopidine, or dipyridamole.
  - **Thrombolytics:** IV recombinant tPA has strict inclusion and exclusion criteria.
    - **Inclusion criteria** include symptom duration of < **3 hours** and a measurable neurologic deficit.
    - **Exclusion criteria** include stroke or head trauma within the prior three months; a history of intracranial hemorrhage; major surgery within two weeks; acute myocardial infarction within the prior three months; lumbar puncture within seven days; uncontrolled hyper-

Causes of peripheral neuropathy—

"DANG THE PAPIST"

Diabetes
Alcohol
Nutrition (B_1, B_{12} deficiency)
Guillain-Barré syndrome
Trauma
Hereditary
Environmental (lead, drugs)
Paraneoplastic
Amyloid
Porphyria
Inflammatory
Syphilis
Tumor of nerves

HIGH-YIELD FACTS

NEUROLOGY

tension requiring aggressive threrapy; pregnancy or lactation; and evidence of cerebral hemorrhage.

- Patients with **basilar artery thrombosis** may receive intra-arterial tPA up to **six hours after symptom onset.**
- If there is > 70% carotid stenosis on angiogram, consider carotid end-arterectomy.
- Give warfarin for anticoagulation in the presence of AF or if the LVEF is ≤ 15%.

PREVENTION

1° and 2° stroke prevention involves smoking cessation, antiplatelet agents, lipid-lowering agents, and antihypertensives.

Seizures are paroxysmal events due to abnormal, excessive, hypersynchronous discharges from a group of CNS neurons.

SYMPTOMS

- **Partial seizures:** Involve only part of the brain. There are two subtypes, both of which can progress to a **generalized tonic-clonic (GTC) seizure.**
  - **Simple partial seizures:** Characterized by **normal consciousness;** arise from a discrete region in one of the cerebral hemispheres. Manifestations may be motor (e.g., jacksonian march), sensory, or autonomic.
  - **Complex partial seizures:** Marked by **abnormal** consciousness; usually involve the **temporal lobes.**
- **Generalized seizures:** Involve the entire brain. There are four major subtypes:
  - **GTC ("grand mal") seizures:** Present with sudden loss of consciousness, loss of postural control, and tonic extension of the back and extremities followed by clonic movements (rhythmic muscular jerking). There may also be cyanosis, incontinence, or tongue biting. Some seizure patients experience a preictal aura, a sensory prodrome such as automatisms (e.g., lip smacking, chewing, picking at clothes), blushing, cognitive sensations (e.g., déjà vu), or an affective state (e.g., fear). GTC is usually accompanied by postictal acidosis with a low HCO_3, elevated serum **CK,** and elevated serum **prolactin.**
  - **Status epilepticus:** > 30-minute or repetitive seizures that develop spontaneously or when antiepileptic drugs (AEDs) are withdrawn too rapidly. A medical emergency with a 20% mortality rate. Treat with IV lorazepam or diazepam and phenytoin.
  - **Absence ("petit mal") seizures:** Seen in **children;** resolve by adulthood. Involve brief, subtle episodes of impaired consciousness without loss of postural control. Episodes last a few seconds and occur up to hundreds of times per day. EEG shows generalized **spike-and-wave discharges at 3 Hz.**
  - **Myoclonic seizures:** Shocklike jerks of muscle groups.

EXAM

- **Fever** suggests CNS infection or status epilepticus.
- Look for **tongue biting, urinary incontinence,** and **meningeal signs** (nuchal rigidity, ⊕ Brudzinski's, ⊕ Kernig's).

Jacksonian march presents as progressive jerking that spreads from one limb to the next.

Postictally, seizure patients may have a focal neurologic deficit that mimics a stroke (e.g., Todd's paralysis) and resolves within minutes to days.

HIGH-YIELD FACTS

NEUROLOGY

DIFFERENTIAL

- Intracranial hemorrhage, acute or **old stroke (particularly cortical), SAH,** meningitis, head injury, subdural hematoma, migraines.
- **Hyponatremia, EtOH withdrawal,** cocaine or amphetamine intoxication.
- Medications associated with seizures include imipramine, meperidine, INH, metronidazole, bupropion, and **fluoroquinolones.**
- 1° **CNS tumor** or brain metastases.

DIAGNOSIS

- **Labs:** Order a CBC, electrolytes, glucose, magnesium, calcium, ammonia, EtOH level, a toxicology screen, and an AED level if appropriate.
- **EEG:** To establish a baseline, localize the focus and confirm the diagnosis. If a focal deficit is present, get a **CT** or **MRI** of the brain.
- If CNS infection is suspected, get an LP—but only if there is **no evidence of ↑ ICP.**

TREATMENT

- **Acute:**
  - Check **ABCs; intubation may be required to protect the airway.**
  - Gently turn the patient onto his left side to prevent aspiration. Unless the patient is being intubated, do not put anything into his mouth (e.g., tongue blade, fingers)!
  - Always check a **glucose level,** as hypoglycemia is a common cause of convulsions. If the patient is hypoglycemic, give IV thiamine and then glucose. If the glucose level is normal, give lorazepam 0.1 mg/kg in 2-mg increments each over 2–3 minutes up to 8 mg.
  - If the seizure continues, give phenytoin 15–20 mg/kg at a rate no faster than 50 mg/min. If the seizure persists, consider phenobarbital coma.
- **Chronic:** Table 2.12-2 outlines pharmacotherapeutic options for the long-term prevention of seizures.

Most antiepileptic drugs are teratogenic. Rule out pregnancy before starting treatment.

Signs and symptoms of elevated ICP: headache on awakening, nausea/vomiting, drowsiness, diplopia, blurry vision, papilledema, CN VI palsies.

BRAIN DEATH

A coma suggests a life-threatening event affecting the brain hemispheres and/or the brain stem. Clinical criteria for the determination of brain death are as follows:

- The patient is comatose (unresponsive to verbal, tactile, or painful stimuli).
- The following are absent:
  - Motor responses.
  - Pupillary light reflex, with pupils fixed at midposition (4–6 mm).

TABLE 2.12-2. First-Line Drugs for the Prevention of Seizure

PARTIAL	TONIC-CLONIC	ABSENCE	MYOCLONIC
Carbamazepine	Valproate	Ethosuximide	Valproate
Phenytoin	Lamotrigine	Valproate	Lamotrigine
Lamotrigine	Phenytoin		Topiramate
Valproate	Carbamazepine		

- Corneal, gag, oculocephalic (doll's-head maneuver), and oculovestibular reflexes.
- Respiratory drive is at a $PaCO_2$ of 60 mmHg, or 20 mmHg above normal values.

DIFFERENTIAL

- **Locked-in syndrome:** A basilar pontine lesion in which the patient is quadriplegic but fully conscious.
- **Other:** Nonconvulsive status epilepticus; psychogenic coma (hysterical coma).

DIAGNOSIS

- EEG to evaluate for nonconvulsive status epilepticus; LP to rule out infection or SAH.
- **Labs:** Urine and serum toxicology screen; CBC, electrolytes, and blood cultures.
- **Imaging:** MRI of the brain; angiography; transcranial Doppler ultrasound.

TREATMENT

Manage medical causes of coma; control body temperature; treat seizures as indicated.

EPIDURAL HEMATOMA

- Typically results from head trauma associated with a lateral skull fracture and tearing of the **middle meningeal artery.** A true **neurologic emergency.**
- **Sx/Exam:** Patients may have a **lucid interval** before the onset of coma. Initial symptoms may include headache, nausea, vomiting, drowsiness, and seizures. Look for hemiparesis and a **blown pupil** (a fixed, dilated pupil due to herniation).
- **Dx:** Head CT without contrast shows **biconvex lens-shaped hyperdensity** compressing the cerebral hemisphere (see Figure 2.12-1).
- **Tx: Prompt surgical evacuation** of blood.

SUBDURAL HEMATOMA

- Typically results from blunt head trauma (commonly a fall) → rupture of the **bridging veins** (common in the **elderly** and in **alcoholics**).
- **Sx/Exam:** Presents with headache, altered mental status, and hemiparesis.
- **Dx:** Head CT shows a **crescent-shaped,** concave hyperdensity that follows the contour of the cerebral hemisphere (see Figure 2.12-2).
- **Tx: Surgical evacuation** of blood if symptoms are present or if the lesion is increasing in size.

SPINAL CORD COMPRESSION

A neurologic emergency! If trauma is suspected, **immobilize the neck.** Localize the lesion, image the spine, and **call neurosurgery.** Causes include the following:

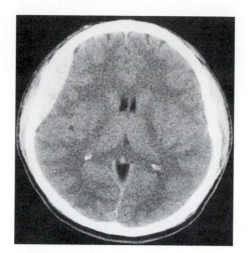

FIGURE 2.12-1.   Acute epidural hematoma.

The typical lenticular shape is due to the dura, which is tightly adherent to the skull. Epidural hematomas are usually caused by disruption of the middle meningeal artery following fracture of the temporal bone. (Reproduced, with permission, from Kasper DL et al. *Harrison's Principles of Internal Medicine*, 16th ed. New York: McGraw-Hill, 2005: 2450.)

- **Trauma:** Motor vehicle accidents; sports-related injuries.
- **Infection:** Epidural abscess in IV drug users; spinal TB (Pott's disease) in immunocompromised patients; vertebral osteomyelitis.
- **Neoplasms:** Metastases are most common.
- **Degenerative disease:** Cervical and lumbar disk herniations.
- **Vascular:** Infarction, epidural and subdural hematomas, and AVMs are rare.

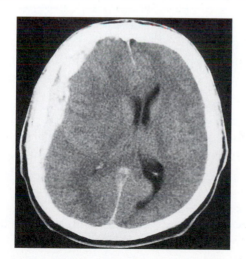

FIGURE 2.12-2.   Acute subdural hematoma in a noncontrast CT scan.

The hyperdense clot has an irregular border with the brain and typically causes more horizontal displacement (mass effect) than might be expected from its thickness. (Reproduced, with permission, from Kasper DL et al. *Harrison's Principles of Internal Medicine*, 16th ed. New York: McGraw-Hill, 2005: 2450.)

Loss of anal reflex ("anal wink") indicates a lesion in S2–S4.

Always look for a sensory level when considering a spinal cord process. The pinprick test is precise and reproducible.

SYMPTOMS/EXAM

- Presents with pain, paresthesias, and weakness. Trauma to the neck should be suspected if there is trauma to the face and body. Signs of skull fracture include the following:
  - **Battle's sign** (ecchymosis over the mastoid process).
  - **Raccoon eyes** (periorbital ecchymosis).
  - Hemotympanum and CSF rhinorrhea/otorrhea.
- Conduct a **pinprick test** to establish a sensory level. If present, a spinal sensory level is usually **one to five levels below** the level of cord compression.
  - **Conus medullaris involvement** is characterized by perineal sensory loss (**saddle anesthesia**) and loss of **anal reflex.**
  - **Cauda equina involvement** is marked by saddle anesthesia.
  - Radicular pain helps localize and confirm extramedullary spinal involvement.
  - Abrupt onset of radicular pain, flaccid weakness, sphincter dysfunction, and a sensory level indicate **cord infarction.**
  - **Hyporeflexia** is often present at the level of spinal cord injury with **hyperreflexia** below.

DIAGNOSIS

Spinal CT scan with contrast, **MRI/MRA** with gadolinium, or myelography.

TREATMENT

- **Acute spinal cord injury:** Methylprednisolone 30 mg/kg IV bolus. Wait 45 minutes; then give methylprednisolone in a 5.4-mg/kg/hr continuous infusion over the next 24 hours.
- **Spinal tumor:** Dexamethasone 100 mg IV bolus.
- **Fractures, subluxations, and dislocations:** Surgical reduction.
- **Epidural abscess:** Neurosurgical decompressive laminectomy.

HEADACHE

Headache danger signs include a change in frequency or severity, fever, neurologic signs, and new-onset headaches.

Severe, sudden-onset headache should raise concern for a subarachnoid/aneurysm rupture.

Tension Headache

A chronic disorder that begins after age 20.

SYMPTOMS/EXAM

Presents with nonthrobbing, bilateral occipital head pain that is generally not associated with nausea, vomiting, or prodromal visual disturbances. The pain is described as a **tight band around the head.**

DIFFERENTIAL

- **Sinus tenderness:** May point to sinusitis.
- **Temporal artery tenderness:** Associated with temporal arteritis.
- **Cranial bruit:** Rule out AVM.

DIAGNOSIS

Obtain a CT scan:
- If the headache is acute and extremely severe ("**thunderclap headache**").
- If the headache is progressive over days to weeks, particularly if it is not similar to previous headaches.

- In the presence of focal neurologic signs.
- In the setting of papilledema.
- If the headache has a morning onset or awakens the patient from sleep.

TREATMENT

Treat with **NSAIDs** or acetaminophen. Relaxation techniques may be helpful.

Migraine

Prevalence in the United States 18% in women and 6% in men. Has a familial predisposition, with > 50% of patients having an affected family member.

SYMPTOMS/EXAM

- **Migraine without aura ("common migraine")**: Recurrent headaches of 4–72 hours' duration characterized by at least two of the following—unilateral, pulsating, severe enough in intensity to limit daily activity, and aggravated by physical activity—plus nausea, vomiting, photophobia, or phonophobia.
- **Migraine with aura ("classic migraine")**: Common migraine that also includes a homonymous visual disturbance (e.g., scintillations, blind spots) as well as unilateral paresthesias and, rarely, weakness.

TREATMENT

- Identify and **eliminate triggers.**
- Treat according to severity:
    - **Mild:** NSAIDs plus an antiemetic such as metoclopramide.
    - **Moderate:** Abortive (**triptans** as soon as headache begins).
    - **Severe:** IV hydration, metoclopramide, dexamethasone, prochlorperazine, or ergotamine.
- **Preventive therapy:** TCAs, α-blockers, valproate, β-blockers.

Cluster Headache

- A brief, severe, **unilateral, periorbital, stabbing** headache.
- Affects men more than women; onset is at 20–30 years of age. Attacks occur in clusters over time.
- **Sx/Exam:** Exam reveals ipsilateral lacrimation, **conjunctival injection,** Horner's syndrome, and nasal congestion.
- **Tx:** Responds to 100% O_2 or low-dose prednisone.

GUILLAIN-BARRÉ SYNDROME (GBS)

Numbness, paresthesias, and **ascending weakness** from the lower extremities to the face. Classically presents with a recent history of respiratory or GI infection (particularly *Campylobacter jejuni*).

SYMPTOMS/EXAM

Presents with **absent reflexes,** ↓ sensation, cranial nerve weakness (facial nerve palsy), proximal muscle weakness, and respiratory failure.

Even if the head CT is ⊖, get an LP if there is a high suspicion for SAH. Fifteen percent of patients with an aneurysmal SAH have a ⊖ CT scan. LP will show high RBCs in all tubes and xanthochromia (yellow CSF).

Horner's syndrome presents with ipsilateral miosis (pupillary constriction), ipsilateral ptosis (eyelid droop), and ipsilateral anhidrosis (lack of sweating) of the face.

Absence of reflexes, ascending weakness, and recent infection–think GBS.

LP and EMG/NCS are crucial in diagnosing GBS.

Neuromuscular blocking agents used during anesthesia can unmask or worsen MG → prolonged postoperative weakness and ventilator dependence.

DIAGNOSIS

- **CBC:** Shows an ↑ WBC count. Obtain an ESR and a Lyme titer.
- **LP:** Typically shows ↑ protein with normal WBC levels (**"albuminocytologic dissociation"**).
- **Nerve conduction study (NCS):** Look for **denervation** and **conduction block.**

TREATMENT

- **IV immunoglobulin (IVIG),** plasmapheresis, physical therapy.
- **PFTs** to monitor for **respiratory compromise.**
- Watch for **autonomic instability,** including temperature dysregulation and cardiac **arrhythmias.**

MYASTHENIA GRAVIS (MG)

Although relatively rare, myasthenia gravis (MG) is the most common disorder of neuromuscular transmission. There is a bimodal distribution, with an earlier peak in the 30s–40s (women), and a late peak in the 70s–90s (men). MG is an autoimmune disorder in which antibodies attack the acetylcholine receptor proteins at the neuromuscular junction.

SYMPTOMS/EXAM

Characterized by **fluctuating skeletal muscle weakness,** with true fatigue in specific muscle groups (not just tiredness). Weakness fluctuates during the day but is usually worse at the end of the day or after exercise.

- **Ocular MG:** Muscle weakness limited to the eyelids and extraocular muscles, with ptosis and/or diplopia. Fifty percent go on to develop generalized MG.
- **Generalized MG:** Weakness may be seen in ocular, bulbar (dysarthria, dysphagia, fatigable chewing), facial (expressionless), limb, and respiratory muscles. Worsening respiratory muscle strength can lead to respiratory failure, or a "**myasthenic crisis.**"

DIFFERENTIAL

Generalized fatigue, motor neuron diseases (e.g., ALS), botulism, Lambert-Eaton myasthenic syndrome.

DIAGNOSIS

- **Bedside tests:**
  - **Edrophonium chloride (Tensilon)** is an acetylcholinesterase inhibitor that prolongs the presence of ACh at the neuromuscular junction. A ⊕ test results in an immediate ↑ in the strength of affected muscles.
  - The **ice pack test** can be used in patients with ptosis.
- Immunologic assays for **acetylcholine receptor antibody;** if seronegative, **MuSK antibodies.**
- **Repetitive nerve stimulation:** The most common electrodiagnostic test for MG.
- **Single-fiber electromyography:** The most sensitive diagnostic test for MG.

TREATMENT

- **Symptomatic treatment:** First-line treatment is an **acetylcholinesterase inhibitor** (pyridostigmine).
- **Chronic immunomodulating agents:** Corticosteroids, azathioprine, cyclosporine, mycophenolate mofetil.
- **For myasthenic crisis:** Plasmapheresis and/or **IVIG**.
- **Surgery:** Thymectomy.

VERTIGO

Must be distinguished from lightheadedness or presyncopal sensation. Categorized as peripheral or central:

- **Peripheral:** Lesions of the labyrinth of the inner ear or the vestibular division of the acoustic nerve (CN VIII). Tends to occur intermittently and to last for brief periods; nystagmus is fatigable and causes more distress.
- **Central:**
  - Spontaneous nystagmus that cannot be suppressed with visual fixation; nystagmus that changes direction with gaze; purely vertical, horizontal, or torsional nystagmus; saccade dysmetria (overshoot and undershoot of gaze).
  - Lesions affect the brain stem vestibular nuclei or their connections. Usually acute onset, with symptoms independent of head positioning.
  - Cranial nerve signs such as facial droop, dysarthria, and loss of corneal reflexes are also seen.

EXAM

- Examine the external auditory canal for vesicles (herpes zoster or **Ramsay Hunt** syndrome).
- Identify the type of nystagmus:
  - **Horizontal:** Rhythmic oscillation of the eyes; seen in both peripheral and central vertigo.
  - **Rotational:** Seen with peripheral vertigo.
  - **Vertical:** Seen with **central vertigo only.**
- Look for hearing loss (peripheral vertigo), diplopia (central only), and limb ataxia (central only).

DIFFERENTIAL

Distinguish vertigo-like conditions from true vertigo:

- **Mimickers of vertigo:** Orthostatic hypotension, cardiac arrhythmia, presyncope/syncope.
- **True vertigo:**
  - Medication side effects (**furosemide, aminoglycosides**).
  - **Benign paroxysmal positional vertigo (BPPV):** Episodic attacks of severe vertigo. Self-limited; probably caused by crystals floating inside the semicircular canals brushing against the sensory cilia.
  - **Labyrinthitis/neuronitis:** Viral inflammation of CN VIII or the labyrinth; usually self-limited.
  - **Ménière's disease:** Overproduction of endolymph in the vestibular canals. **Triad** of vertigo, tinnitus, and hearing loss.
  - **Brain stem stroke:** Associated neurologic deficits are seen, including weakness, ataxia, and cranial nerve dysfunction.
  - **Schwannoma:** A mass compressing CN VIII, causing hearing loss and vertigo.

If there are episodic attacks of severe vertigo associated with head position, think of BPPV.

DIAGNOSIS

- Neurologic exam.
- **Imaging:** Head CT without contrast; MRI of the brain with DWI.
- **Bárány** or **Dix-Hallpike maneuver:** The physician moves the patient from a sitting to a supine position, with the head rotated to one side. The test is ⊕ for BPPV if vertigo is recreated.

TREATMENT

- BPPV may respond to the **Epley maneuver** and **meclizine** 25 mg PO TID for 3–4 days along with desensitization exercises.
- In the setting of a posterior circulation stroke, careful monitoring is necessary for 24–48 hours followed by stroke workup.

MULTIPLE SCLEROSIS (MS)

A CNS demyelinating disease that is autoimmune mediated. **Young females** are at higher risk, as are those who reside in **northern latitudes.**

SYMPTOMS

- Visual or oculomotor symptoms commonly include blurring of vision, loss of vision, or **diplopia.**
- Also presents with weakness or **paresthesias** in a limb; uncoordinated gait; heat sensitivity; and worsening of symptoms in a **hot shower.**

EXAM

Exam reveals the following:

- Hyperreflexia, **weakness,** and ataxia.
- **Lhermitte's sign:** Radiating/shooting pain up or down the neck on flexion or extension.
- **Optic neuritis:** A swollen optic disk.
- **Afferent pupillary defect (Marcus Gunn pupil):** The pupil paradoxically dilates to a light stimulus owing to delayed conduction.
- **Internuclear ophthalmoplegia (MLF syndrome):** The classic finding is bilateral weakness on adduction of the ipsilateral eye with nystagmus on abduction of the contralateral eye, together with incomplete or slow abduction of the ipsilateral eye on lateral gaze with complete preservation of convergence.

DIAGNOSIS

- **Brain MRI with gadolinium:** Reveals multiple focal **periventricular areas of ↑ signal,** called **Dawson's fingers** (see Figure 2.12-3).
- **CSF:** Shows ↑ protein (myelin basic protein, **oligoclonal bands**).
- **Visual evoked potentials:** Show delayed conduction.

TREATMENT

- Treat acute exacerbations with corticosteroids.
- Manage relapsing-remitting disease with **interferon-α**1a or 1b.
- Glatiramer acetate, a synthetic polymer of amino acids, may reduce relapses.
- Baclofen may be given for spasticity.

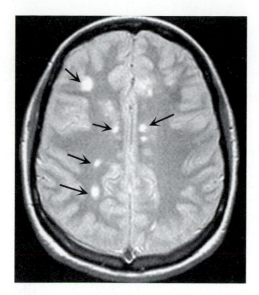

FIGURE 2.12-3. **MRI findings in multiple sclerosis.**

The multiple bright signal abnormalities in white matter are typical of multiple sclerosis. (Reproduced, with permission, from Kasper DL et al. *Harrison's Principles of Internal Medicine,* 16th ed. New York: McGraw-Hill, 2005: 2465.)

MUSCULAR DYSTROPHY

The most common form is **Duchenne's muscular dystrophy,** which is **X-linked** and presents by age six. Patients progress to being wheelchair-bound in childhood and to death in adolescence.

SYMPTOMS/EXAM

- Presents with **toe walking,** waddling gait, and inability to run or climb stairs.
- Proximal muscle **weakness** is also seen.
- In attempting to rise to standing from a supine position, patients use their arms to climb up their bodies (**Gowers' sign**).
- **Pseudohypertrophy** of the calves.

DIAGNOSIS

- Serum CK levels are ↑.
- Muscle biopsy with immunohistochemistry; genetic testing for the **dystrophin gene mutation.**

TREATMENT

There is no definitive treatment. Prednisone is used to improve muscle strength but is limited in its duration.

PARKINSON'S DISEASE

Characterized by **bradykinesia**. Due to the striatal deficiency of **dopamine** resulting from neuronal degeneration within the **substantia nigra**.

SYMPTOMS

Clinical manifestations include the following:

- **Progressive slowness** in dressing, walking, feeding, or writing.
- Difficulty rising from a chair; hesitancy in initiating gait.
- **Frequent falls** and loss of balance.
- **Loss of facial expression (masked facies).**
- **Depressed mood.**
- Patients have smaller handwriting compared to their previous pattern (**micrographia**).

EXAM

Exam reveals the following:

- **Resting tremor.**
- **Bradykinesia:** Movements are slow and diminished in amplitude. Patients have a slow blink rate and few facial expressions (masked facies).
- **Rigidity:** ↑ muscle tone that is present in all directions of movement may be **cogwheel rigidity** (ratchet-like rigidity).
- **Loss of postural reflexes:** Patients cannot remain balanced if pushed from the front or from behind.

TREATMENT

- **Levodopa (dihydroxyphenylalanine):** A precursor amino acid to dopamine that crosses the blood-brain barrier and replenishes dopamine. The gold standard of treatment.
- **Bromocriptine, pergolide, and ropinirole:** Ergot derivatives with potent dopamine receptor agonist activity.
- **Surgical pallidotomy.**

> **Key Parkinson's signs—**
>
> **PARKINSON'S**
>
> **P**ill rolling
> **A**kinesia/bradykinesia
> **R**igidity
> **K**yphosis
> **I**nstability
> **N**eck titubation
> **S**huffling gait
> **O**culogyric crisis
> **N**ose tap (e.g., glabellar tap)
> **S**mall writing

AMYOTROPHIC LATERAL SCLEROSIS (ALS)

- A chronic degenerative condition involving motor neurons in the spinal cord. Sensations and cognition are completely intact. Some 5–10% of cases are familial. Usually presents in **older males**.
- Sx/Exam:
  - Patients have progressive muscular weakness, spasticity, and respiratory insufficiency.
  - Look for generalized **muscle atrophy, dysarthria, tongue fasciculations,** proximal muscle weakness, and hyperreflexia. Eye movements are spared.
- **Dx:** EMG shows widespread denervation. Muscle biopsy shows neurogenic atrophy.
- **Tx:** ALS is an incurable, progressive disease. Treatment with **riluzole**, which inhibits glutamate release, has been associated with modest improvement.

*Look for UMN **and** LMN signs with ALS.*

Chronic, progressive cognitive decline that interferes with daily performance in occupational and social activities. Roughly 10% of dementias are reversible; 40–60% are due to Alzheimer's disease.

SYMPTOMS

- **Impairment of recent memory** is typically the first sign.
- Subsequent manifestations include the following:
    - Difficulty completing recently performed tasks (e.g., balancing the checkbook).
    - Disorientation first to time and then to place.
    - Depressed mood.

EXAM

- **Primitive reflexes** are present in advanced disease (e.g., palmar grasp, glabellar, rooting, palmomental).
- Other exam findings are as follows:
    - **Apraxia:** Inability to execute or carry out learned movements.
    - **Anomia:** Inability to remember the names of things, people, or places.
    - **Acalculia:** Inability to perform mathematical computations.

DIFFERENTIAL

- **Delirium** (see the relevant discussion in the Psychiatry chapter).
- **Alzheimer's disease.**
- **Pick's disease (frontotemporal dementia):** Involves personality changes.
- **Vascular/multi-infarct dementia:** Follows a stepwise progression. Typically presents after multiple strokelike episodes. **Focal neurologic deficits are common.**
- **Normal pressure hydrocephalus:** A treatable cause of dementia. A disorder of CSF drainage in which patients often present with a triad of **dementia, gait disturbance,** and **urinary incontinence.** Treated with a ventricular shunt.
- **Alcoholism.**
- Hypothyroidism.
- **Vitamin B$_{12}$ deficiency:** Involves loss of proprioception.
- **Depression:** "Pseudodementia."
- Subdural hematoma.

DIAGNOSIS

- Conduct a complete neurologic exam and a mini-mental status exam.
- Check a CBC, electrolytes, B$_{12}$, TSH, and a VDRL.
- Obtain an MRI of the brain.
- Conduct **neuropsychological testing.**

TREATMENT

- Current therapies are aimed at increasing CNS ACh levels. Some treatment strategies may delay admission to a nursing home by roughly six months.
- **Acetylcholinesterase inhibitors** include donepezil (Aricept), rivastigmine (Exelon), and galantamine (Reminyl). Memantine (Namenda) works as a glutamate receptor antagonist.
- Offer social support and supervision (i.e., a nursing home) if severe.

- The classic names for alcohol-induced persistent amnesia are **Wernicke's encephalopathy,** an acute set of symptoms, and **Korsakoff's syndrome,** a chronic condition. Both are due to **thiamine** (vitamin B$_1$) deficiency.
- Sx/Exam:
  - **Wernicke's encephalopathy** is usually completely reversible after treatment and presents with the classic **triad of ataxia, ophthalmoplegia, and confusion.**
  - **Korsakoff's syndrome** is characterized by **impaired short-term memory** in an alert and responsive patient. There may or may not be **confabulation,** which is the unconscious filling of gaps in memory by imagined or untrue experiences. Only 20% of patients recover completely.
- **Dx:** MRI may show mammillary body lesions.
- **Tx:** For **Wernicke's,** treat with **IV thiamine.** Ocular deficits improve within hours. Give thiamine **before** glucose, as administering glucose in the absence of thiamine may precipitate neuronal death. Treatment for Korsakoff's is PO thiamine.

SECTION II

Obstetrics

All prenatal visits should document weight, BP, extremity edema, protein and glucose (urine dipstick), fundal height (> 20 weeks), and fetal heart rate. Further recommendations are as follows:

- **Weight gain:** Average-size women should gain 25–35 lbs; obese women should gain less (15–25 lbs) and thin women more.
- The average caloric requirement is roughly 2300 kcal/day.
- An additional 300 kcal/day is needed during pregnancy and 500 kcal/day during breast-feeding.
- **Nutrition:** ↑ requirements for protein, iron, folate, calcium, and zinc. All patients should take prenatal vitamins.
- **Folate:** Supplement with 400 μg/day to ↓ the risk of neural tube defects. **Women with a prior history of a fetus with neural tube defects should have 4 mg/day of folate.**
- **Iron:** Supplement with 30–60 mg/day of elemental iron in the latter half of pregnancy to prevent anemia.
- **Calcium:** Supplement with 1500 mg/day in the later months of pregnancy and during breast-feeding.
- **Smoking cessation.**
- **Prenatal labs:** See Table 2.13-1 for scheduled lab work during pregnancy.

TABLE 2.13-1. Prenatal Labs During Pregnancy

GESTATIONAL AGE (GA)	LABS TO BE OBTAINED
Initial visit	CBC, blood type, **Rh antibody screen,** UA with culture, **Pap smear,** cervical gonorrhea and chlamydia cultures, **rubella antibody titer,** hepatitis B surface antigen, syphilis screen, PPD, HIV. Toxoplasmosis and sickle cell screening for at-risk patients. Women with prior gestational diabetes or a family history (in a first-degree relative) should get early glucose testing.
6–11 weeks	**Ultrasound** to determine GA (more accurate than later scans).
15–19 weeks	**Triple-marker screen/quadruple test** quad screen. Offer amniocentesis for those of advanced maternal age (≥ 35 years of age at delivery).
18–21 weeks	**Screening ultrasound** to survey fetal anatomy, placental location, and amniotic fluid.
26–28 weeks	**One-hour glucose challenge test.** If ≥ 140 mg/dL, follow with a three-hour glucose tolerance test. Repeat hemoglobin/hematocrit.
28 weeks	**RhoGAM** injection for Rh-⊖ patients. Start fetal kick counting (the patient should count 10 fetal movements in less than one hour.).
35–37 weeks	Screen for **group B streptococcus** (GBS) with a rectovaginal swab. Repeat hemoglobin/hematocrit. Cervical gonorrhea and chlamydia cultures, RPR, and HIV (in at-risk patients). Assess fetal position with Leopold maneuvers and ultrasound.

Triple-Marker Screen/Quadruple Test Quad Screen

- Measured between 15 and 20 weeks' gestation.
- Any maternal serum α-fetoprotein (MSAFP) result > 2.5 multiples of the mean (MoM) can signify an open neural tube defect, an abdominal wall defect, multiple gestation, incorrect dating, fetal death, or placental abnormalities.
- The sensitivity for detecting chromosomal abnormalities (trisomies 18 and 21) is ↑ through the addition of estriol and β-hCG (**triple-marker screen**) to MSAFP. See Table 2.13-2 for trends in the detection of genetic abnormalities.
- The addition of **inhibin-A** to the three markers above (**quadruple test**) will ↑ the sensitivity and ↓ the false-⊕ rate for Down syndrome.

Amniocentesis

- Performed primarily between 15 and 20 weeks to detect possible genetic diseases or congenital malformations.
- Risks include fetal-maternal hemorrhage (1–2%) and fetal loss (0.5%).
- Amniocentesis is used:
    - In conjunction with an **abnormal triple-marker screen/quadruple test.**
    - In **women > 35 years of age** at the time of delivery.
    - In **Rh-sensitized pregnancy** to ascertain fetal blood type or to detect fetal hemolysis.
    - For the evaluation of **fetal lung maturity** in the third trimester.

Chorionic Villus Sampling (CVS)

- Performed to evaluate possible genetic diseases at an earlier time than amniocentesis with comparable diagnostic accuracy.
- Done at **10–12 weeks' gestation via transabdominal or transvaginal** aspiration of chorionic villus tissue (a precursor of the placenta). Risks include fetal loss (1–5%) and an association with distal limb defects.

Nonstress Test (NST)

- Fetal heart rate is monitored externally by Doppler.
- A **normal response** is an acceleration of ≥ 15 bpm above baseline lasting > 15 seconds.

TABLE 2.13-2. Detection of Genetic Abnormalities with the Triple-Marker Test

	NEURAL TUBE DEFECT	TRISOMY 18	TRISOMY 21
MSAFP	↑	↓	↓
Estriol	Not used	↓	↓
β-hCG	Not used	↓	↑

- A normal or "reactive" test includes two such accelerations in a **20-minute** period.
- An abnormal or "nonreactive" NST warrants a biophysical profile or a contraction stress test (see below).
- A nonreactive NST can be due to fetal sleep cycle, GA < 30 weeks, a fetal CNS anomaly, or maternal sedative or narcotic use.

Contraction Stress Test (CST)

> *When performing a BPP, remember to—* **Test the Baby, MAN!**
>
> Fetal **T**one
> Fetal **B**reathing
> Fetal **M**ovements
> **A**mniotic fluid volume
> **N**onstress test

- Used to assess uteroplacental dysfunction.
- Fetal heart rate is monitored during spontaneous or induced (nipple stimulation or pitocin) contractions.
- A normal or "negative" CST has no late decelerations and is highly predictive of fetal well-being.
- An abnormal or "positive" CST is defined by late decelerations in conjunction with at least 50% of contractions. A minimum of three contractions within a 10-minute period must be present for an adequate CST.

Biophysical Profile (BPP)

An HbA$_{1c}$ > 6.5 prior to conception or during the first trimester will → a higher rate of fetal malformations.

- Ultrasound is used to assess five parameters (see the mnemonic **Test the Baby, MAN**).
- A score of 2 (normal) or 0 (abnormal) is given to each of the parameters.
- A normal or "negative" test (a score of 8–10) is reassuring for fetal well-being.
- An abnormal or "positive" test (a score < 6) is worrisome for fetal compromise.

Fetal Heart Rate Patterns

Table 2.13-3 outlines different types of heart rate patterns seen in near-term and term fetuses.

TABLE 2.13-3. Fetal Heart Rate Patterns

TYPE OF DECELERATION	DESCRIPTION	COMMON CAUSE
Early	Deceleration begins and ends at approximately the same time as maternal contractions.	Fetal head compression **(no fetal distress).**
Variable	Variable onset of abrupt (< 30-sec) slowing of fetal heart rate in association with contractions. The return is similarly abrupt in most situations.	Umbilical cord compression.
Late	Decelerations begin after onset of maternal contractions and persist until after the contractions are finished. The time from peak to nadir is > 30 sec.	Late decelerations indicate fetal hypoxia **(fetal distress).** If late decelerations are repetitive and severe, immediate delivery is necessary.

Diabetes Mellitus (DM)

The **most common** medical complication of pregnancy. See Table 2.13-4 for a comparison of pregestational and gestational DM.

Preeclampsia/Eclampsia

Preeclampsia is characterized by hypertension and proteinuria and is thought to be due to ↓ organ perfusion 2° to vasospasm and endothelial activation. Risk factors include nulliparity, African-American ethnicity, extremes of age, multiple gestations (i.e., twins), renal disease, and chronic hypertension. **Eclampsia** is defined as seizures in a patient with preeclampsia. Preeclampsia is further distinguished as follows:

- **Mild preeclampsia:** SBP > 140, DBP > 90, and 1+ on dipstick or > 300 mg on 24-hour urine.

TABLE 2.13-4. Pregestational vs. Gestational DM

	PREGESTATIONAL	GESTATIONAL
Definition	Diagnosed **prior to pregnancy.**	Diagnosed **during pregnancy.**
Risk factors	Family history; autoimmune disorders (type 1), obesity (type 2).	Obesity, family history (in a first-degree relative), prior history of DM in pregnancy.
Diagnosis	See above.	Diagnosed if the one-hour glucose test is ≥ 140 mg/dL **and** the follow-up three-hour glucose test has at least two ↑ levels.

Treatment	Strict control of blood glucose levels with diet, exercise, and **insulin:**
	    ■ **Fasting morning:** < 90 mg/dL.
	    ■ **Two-hour postprandial:** < 120 mg/dL.
		ADA diet and regular exercise. If blood sugars are ↑ after one week, initiate **insulin** therapy. Can consider glyburide.

Labor	Fingersticks every 1–2 hours while in active labor with dextrose infusion +/– insulin drip to maintain tight glycemic control.	Diet controlled (A1): Fingersticks on admission and every four hours in labor. A2: Same as pregestational.
Postpartum	Continue glucose monitoring; body's insulin requirements quickly ↓.	Resume normal diet; no insulin is required.

Complications
  Fetus
 	
  Mother
	Congenital malformations, stillbirth, macrosomia, IUGR, hypoglycemia, birth trauma.
	Hypoglycemia, DKA, spontaneous abortion, polyhydramnios, preterm labor, worsening end-organ dysfunction, ↑ risk of preeclampsia.
		Hypoglycemia from hyperinsulinemia; macrosomia; birth trauma.
		Perineal trauma from macrosomic infant; ↑ lifetime risk of developing DM.

- **Severe preeclampsia:** SBP > 160, DBP > 110, and 3+ on dipstick or > 5 g on 24-hour urine.

SYMPTOMS/EXAM

Table 2.13-5 outlines key differences in the presentation of mild preeclampsia, severe preeclampsia, and eclampsia.

DIAGNOSIS

- Check UA, 24-hour urine for protein and creatinine clearance, CBC, BUN, creatinine, uric acid, LFTs, PT/PTT, fibrinogen, and a toxicology screen.
- Determine the precise GA; consider amniocentesis to assess fetal lung maturity for mild preeclampsia.
- Diagnosis is based on **clinical findings** as described in Table 2.13-5.

TREATMENT

Definitive treatment is **delivery.** See Table 2.13-5 for management.

Maternal Hyperthyroidism

- Although the most common etiology is Graves' disease, maternal hyperthyroidism may also be caused by subacute thyroiditis, toxic nodular goiter, and toxic adenoma.

TABLE 2.13-5. Mild and Severe Preeclampsia vs. Eclampsia

	MILD PREECLAMPSIA	SEVERE PREECLAMPSIA	ECLAMPSIA
Symptoms/exam	**SBP > 140** or **DBP > 90** on ≥ 2 occasions. **Proteinuria** (> 300 mg/24 hrs or 1+ on urine dipstick).	**SBP > 160** or **DBP > 110** on ≥ 2 occasions. **Proteinuria** (> 5 g/24 hrs or > 3+ on urine dipstick). HELLP syndrome (see mnemonic). Oliguria (< 500 mL/24 hrs). Pulmonary edema.	**Seizures with the diagnosis of preeclampsia.**
Treatment	Deliver if near term, fetal lungs are mature, or preeclampsia worsens. If far from term, treat with bed rest and conservative management. Use of magnesium sulfate for seizure prophylaxis is controversial.	Magnesium sulfate for seizure prophylaxis. Hydralazine +/− labetalol for BP control. When stable, deliver. Postpartum: Continue magnesium sulfate for atleast 12–24 hours after delivery. Watch for Mg^+ toxicity; treat life-threatening toxicity with IV calcium gluconate.	**Magnesium sulfate to control seizures.** Monitor ABCs closely. When stable, deliver. Seizures may occur before delivery, during delivery, and up to six weeks postpartum.
Complications	Fetal distress, stillbirth, placental abruption, DIC, seizures, fetal/maternal death, cerebral hemorrhage.	Same as with mild preeclampsia.	Fetal/maternal death.

- **Sx/Exam:** Symptoms include restlessness, heat intolerance, weight loss, frequent stools, and chest palpitations. Look for tachycardia, resting tremor, and the presence of goiter.
- **Dx: TFTs** show ↓ TSH and ↑ free T_4.
- **Tx:**
  - Start **propylthiouracil** (PTU) until the patient becomes euthyroid; then ↓ the dose. Check TFTs every 4–6 weeks.
  - **Subtotal thyroidectomy** is appropriate for refractory or noncompliant patients.
- **Complications: Thyrotoxicosis or thyroid storm** can be precipitated by delivery, acute illness, infection, trauma, or surgery. Early recognition is key; treat with supportive care and give a large loading dose of PTU, potassium iodide, propranolol, and IV fluids.

Hyperemesis Gravidarum

- Defined as refractory vomiting → **weight loss,** poor weight gain, dehydration, ketosis from starvation, and metabolic alkalosis. Typically persists beyond 14–16 weeks' gestation.
- Risk factors include nulliparity, multiple pregnancies, and trophoblastic disease.
- **DDx:** Rule out molar pregnancy, hepatitis, gallbladder disease, reflux, and gastroenteritis.
- **Dx:** Labs will show **hyponatremia** and a hypokalemic/hypochloremic **metabolic acidosis.** Ketonuria on UA suggests starvation ketosis.
- **Tx:** If there is evidence of weight loss, dehydration or altered electrolytes, **hospitalize** and give antiemetics, IV hydration, and vitamin and electrolyte replacement. Advance the diet slowly and avoid fatty foods.

PUERPERIUM

Postpartum Hemorrhage (PPH)

- Defined as blood loss of > 500 mL during a vaginal delivery or > 1000 mL during a cesarean section occurring before, during, or after delivery of the placenta. Table 2.13-6 summarizes common causes.
- Complications include **Sheehan's syndrome.**

Intrapartum and Postpartum Fevers

- Most commonly due to **infections** (see Table 2.13-7).
- Other causes include hematoma, atelectasis, breast engorgement, pelvic abscess, and septic pelvic thrombophlebitis.
- See the mnemonic **the 7 W's** for the causes of postpartum fever.

Mastitis

- Cellulitis of the periglandular tissue in breast-feeding mothers, typically due to *S. aureus*, occurring at about 2–4 weeks postpartum.
- **Sx/Exam:** Symptoms include breast pain and redness along with **high fever,** chills, and flulike symptoms. Look for **focal** breast erythema, swelling, and tenderness. **Fluctuance** indicates a breast abscess.

For all uterine causes of postpartum hemorrhage, when bleeding persists after conventional therapy, uterine/internal iliac artery ligation or hysterectomy can be lifesaving.

The 7 W's of postpartum fever:

Womb—endomyometritis
Wind—atelectasis, pneumonia
Water—UTI
Walk—DVT, pulmonary embolism
Wound—incision, lacerations
Weaning—breast engorgement, mastitis, breast abscess
Wonder drugs—drug fever

TABLE 2.13-6. Common Causes of Postpartum Hemorrhage

	UTERINE ATONY	GENITAL TRACT TRAUMA	RETAINED PLACENTAL TISSUE
Risk factors	Uterine overdistention, exhausted myometrium, uterine infection, grand multiparity.	Precipitous delivery, operative vaginal delivery, large infant, laceration.	Placenta accreta/increta/percreta, placenta previa, prior C-section, curettage, accessory placental lobe, retained membranes.
Diagnosis	Palpation of a soft, enlarged, "boggy" uterus.	Inspection of the cervix, vagina, and vulva for lacerations or hematoma.	Inspection of the placenta and uterine cavity. Ultrasound to look for retained placenta.
Treatment	Vigorous bimanual massage. Oxytocin infusion. Methylergonovine if not hypertensive; PGF_{2a} if not asthmatic; misoprostol.	Surgical repair of the defect.	Removal of remaining placental tissue.

TABLE 2.13-7. Common Infections During Labor and After Delivery

	CHORIOAMNIONITIS	ENDOMETRITIS
Definition	Infection of the **chorion, amnion,** and **amniotic fluid,** diagnosed **during labor.**	Infection of the **uterus,** diagnosed **after delivery.**
Symptoms/exam	Fever with no other obvious source **and** one of the following: ■ Fetal **or** maternal tachycardia ■ Abdominal tenderness ■ Foul-smelling amniotic fluid ■ Leukocytosis	**Two fevers within 24 hours postpartum** or any fever $\geq 38.6°C$ (101.5°F) without an obvious source.
Risk factors	**Prolonged rupture of membranes (ROM);** multiple vaginal exams while being ruptured in labor.	**C-section,** prolonged ROM, multiple vaginal exams while being ruptured in labor.
Diagnosis	Clinical; CBC with differential.	Pelvic exam to rule out hematoma or retained membranes. CBC with differential, UA, urine culture, and blood cultures as indicated.
Treatment	■ Delivery of the fetus (chorioamnionitis is **not** an indication for cesarean delivery). ■ Antibiotics until the patient is afebrile for 24 hours after delivery. Some stop antibiotics after delivery.	Antibiotics until the patient is afebrile 24 hours (vaginal) or 48 hours (cesarean) after delivery.

- **DDx:** Distinguish from simple breast engorgement, which can present as a swollen, firm, tender breast with low-grade fever.
- **Dx:** Diagnosis includes breast milk cultures and CBC.
- **Tx:** Treat with **dicloxacillin** or **erythromycin.** Continue nursing or manually expressing milk to prevent milk stasis. Incision and drainage of abscess if present.

Sheehan's Syndrome (Postpartum Hypopituitarism)

- The most common cause of anterior pituitary insufficiency in adult females. It occurs 2° to **pituitary ischemia,** usually as a result of postpartum blood loss and hypotension.
- **Sx/Exam:**
    - The most common presenting symptom is **failure to lactate** as a result of ↓ prolactin levels.
    - Other symptoms include lethargy, anorexia, weight loss, amenorrhea, and loss of sexual hair, but may not be recognized for many years.

Breast-feeding contraindications include HIV infection, active hepatitis, and certain drugs (e.g., tetracycline, chloramphenicol, warfarin).

TERATOGENS IN PREGNANCY

- **Radiation:** Diagnostic and nuclear medicine studies pose no risk of fetal teratogenicity if overall exposure during pregnancy is < 5000 mrads (e.g., 0.05 Gy). Table 2.13-8 outlines radiation exposure levels associated with such procedures.
- **Medications:** See Table 2.13-9 for medications that are safe during pregnancy.

Treatment of mastitis includes antibiotics and continued breast-feeding.

OBSTETRIC COMPLICATIONS OF PREGNANCY

Intrauterine Growth Restriction (IUGR)

- Defined as an estimated fetal weight at or below the 10th percentile for GA. See Table 2.13-10 for common causes of IUGR.
- **Sx/Exam:** Suspect IUGR clinically if the difference between fundal height and GA is > 2 cm.
- **Tx:** Focus on **prevention**—e.g., smoking cessation, BP control, and dietary changes. Order an ultrasound every 3–4 weeks to assess interval growth. Deliver once pregnancy reaches term.

TABLE 2.13-8. Radiation Exposure Resulting from Common Radiologic Procedures

RADIOLOGICAL FILM	EXPOSURE (MRAD)
Abdominal x-ray (1 view)	100
Chest x-ray (2 views)	0.02–0.07
CT head/chest	< 1000
CT abdomen/lumbar spine	3500
MRI	0

TABLE 2.13-9.   Safe vs. Teratogenic/Unsafe Medications During Pregnancy

INDICATION	SAFE TO USE	CONTRAINDICATED
Acne	Benzoyl peroxide.	Vitamin A and derivatives (e.g., isotretinoin, etretinate) → heart and great vessel defects, craniofacial dysmorphism, and deafness.
Antibiotics	Penicillins, cephalosporin, macrolides.	Tetracycline → discoloration of deciduous teeth. Quinolone → cartilage damage. Sulfonamide late in pregnancy → kernicterus. Streptomycin → CN VIII damage/ototoxicity.
Cancer	Alkylating agents can be used in the second and third trimesters.	Folic acid antagonists → abnormalities of the cranium.
Nausea/vomiting	Pyroxidine (B_6), doxylamine, prochlorperazine, metoclopramide, ondansetron, granisetron, promethazine.	Thalidomide → limb reduction and malformation of the ear, kidney, and heart.
Bipolar disorder	Need to assess risks vs. benefits of medications.	Lithium → congenital heart disease and Ebstein's anomaly (also avoid if the mother is breast-feeding).
Depression	Risks vs. benefits; TCAs, SSRIs.	SSRIs may cause persistent pulmonary hypertension of the newborn, poor feeding, and/or jitteriness.
Contrast studies	Indigo carmine.	Methylene blue → jejunal and ileal atresia.
GERD	OTC antacids (calcium carbonate, milk of magnesia), ranitidine, cimetidine, omeprazole.	Alka-Seltzer (has aspirin).
Headache/migraine	Acetaminophen, codeine, caffeine.	Avoid aspirin in late pregnancy because of risk of bleeding to mother and fetus at birth. Ergotamines have abortifacient potential and a theoretical risk of fetal vasoconstriction.
Hypertension	Labetalol, hydralazine, nifedipine, methyldopa, clonidine.	ACEIs and angiotensin receptor blockers → fetal renal damage and oligohydramnios.
Hyperthyroidism	PTU.	Methimazole → aplasia cutis.
Hypothyroidism	Levothyroxine.	
Pain	Acetaminophen, menthol, topical patches, morphine, hydrocodone, propoxyphene, meperidine; these medications should not be used continuously.	Avoid NSAIDs in late pregnancy for > 48 hours. When used over a long period, will → premature closure of the ductus arteriosus.

INDICATION	SAFE TO USE	CONTRAINDICATED
Seizure	Use an anticonvulsant that works best to control maternal seizures. Monotherapy at the lowest dose is preferred. Folate supplementation should be started three months prior to conception.	Phenytoin → dysmorphic facies, microcephaly, mental retardation, hypoplasia of the nails and distal phalanges, and neural tube defects (NTDs). Valproic acid → craniofacial defects and NTDs. Carbamazepine → craniofacial defects, mental retardation, and NTDs. Phenobarbital → **cleft palate, cardiac defects.** Trimethadione and paramethadione have strong teratogenic potential and → mental retardation, speech difficulty, and abnormal facies.
Thromboembolic disease	Heparin, low-molecular-weight heparin. Must use warfarin in cases of highly thrombogenic artificial heart valves.	Warfarin → fetal nasal hypoplasia and bony defects (chondrodysplasia).
URI	Pseudoephedrine (Sudafed), guaifenesin (Robitussin), acetaminophen, diphenhydramine, loratadine (Claritin).	

Oligohydramnios and Polyhydramnios

Table 2.13-11 contrasts oligohydramnios with polyhydramnios.

Rhesus (Rh) Isoimmunization

When fetal Rh-⊕ RBCs leak into Rh-⊖ maternal circulation, **maternal anti-Rh IgG antibodies** can form. These antibodies can cross the placenta and react with fetal Rh-⊕ RBCs → fetal hemolysis (erythroblastosis fetalis).

SYMPTOMS/EXAM

Inquire about prior events that may have exposed the mother to Rh-⊕ blood (ectopic pregnancy, abortion, blood transfusion, prior delivery of an

Oligohydramnios almost always indicates the presence of a fetal abnormality.

TABLE 2.13-10. **Causes of IUGR**

FETAL CAUSES	MATERNAL CAUSES
Chromosomal abnormalities: Trisomy 21 is most common, followed by trisomies 18 and 13.	**Hypertension.**
Infection: CMV is most common; then toxoplasmosis.	**Drugs: Cigarette** smoking is most common; also alcohol, heroin, methamphetamines and cocaine.
Placental abnormalities, uterine abnormalities, multiple gestations.	**SLE.**
	Maternal thrombophilia.
	Malnutrition, malabsorption (i.e., cystic fibrosis).
	Ethnic/genetic variation.

TABLE 2.13-11. Oligohydramnios vs. Polyhydramnios

	OLIGOHYDRAMNIOS	**POLYHYDRAMNIOS**
Definition	Amniotic fluid index (AFI) ≤ 5 cm on ultrasound.	AFI ≥ 25 cm on ultrasound.
Causes	**Fetal urinary tract abnormalities** (renal agenesis, polycystic kidneys, GU obstruction). Chronic uteroplacental insufficiency. ROM.	Normal pregnancy. Uncontrolled maternal DM. Multiple gestations. Pulmonary abnormalities. Fetal anomalies (duodenal atresia, tracheoesophageal fistula).
Diagnosis	Ultrasound for anomalies. Rule out ROM with ferning test, nitrazine paper.	Ultrasound for fetal anomalies. Glucose testing for DM.
Treatment	Possible amnioinfusion during labor to prevent cord compression.	Depends on the cause; therapeutic amniocentesis.
Complications	**Cord compression** → fetal hypoxia. Musculoskeletal abnormalities (facial distortion, clubfoot). Pulmonary hypoplasia, IUGR.	Preterm labor, placental abruption, fetal malpresentation, cord prolapse.

Rh-⊕ child, amniocentesis, traumatic procedures during pregnancy, recent RhoGAM).

TREATMENT

- **Give RhoGAM to Rh-⊖ women:**
  - If the father is Rh ⊕, Rh status is unknown, or paternity is uncertain.
  - If the baby is Rh ⊕ at delivery.
  - If the woman has had an abortion (therapeutic or spontaneous), an ectopic pregnancy, amniocentesis, vaginal bleeding, external cephalic version, or placental abruption.
- Sensitized Rh-⊖ women with titers > 1:16 should be closely monitored for evidence of fetal hemolysis with serial ultrasound and amniocentesis or middle cerebral artery Doppler velocimetry.
- In severe cases, intrauterine blood transfusion via the umbilical vein or preterm delivery is indicated.

Third-Trimester Bleeding

- Describes any bleeding after 20 weeks' gestation.
- The most common causes are placental abruption and placenta previa (see Table 2.13-12).
- Other causes of bleeding include bloody show, preterm/early labor, vasa previa, genital tract lesions, and trauma (e.g., intercourse).

Gestational Trophoblastic Disease (GTD)

Can range from benign (e.g., hydatidiform mole) to malignant (e.g., choriocarcinoma). Hydatidiform mole accounts for approximately 80% of cases of GTD.

TABLE 2.13-12.   Common Causes of Third-Trimester Bleeding

	PLACENTAL ABRUPTION	PLACENTA PREVIA	UTERINE RUPTURE
Pathophysiology	**Placental separation** from the site of uterine implantation before delivery of the fetus.	**Abnormal placental implantation** near or covering the os.	**A complete rupture disrupts the entire thickness of the uterine wall.**
Risk factors	**Hypertension,** abdominal/pelvic trauma, tobacco or **cocaine use,** uterine distention.	**Prior C-section,** grand multiparas, multiple gestations, prior placenta previa.	**Prior uterine scar,** trauma (e.g., motor vehicle accident), uterine anomalies, grand multiparity.
Symptoms	Abdominal pain; vaginal bleeding that does not spontaneously cease. Prolonged tightening of the abdomen coupled with prolonged contraction. **Fetal distress.**	Painless vaginal bleeding that ceases spontaneously with or without uterine contractions. The first bleeding episode usually occurs in the second or third trimester. **Usually no fetal distress.**	Severe abdominal pain, usually during labor, typically at the scar site. Change in the shape of the abdomen. **Fetal distress.** Loss of fetal station.
Diagnosis	**Primarily clinical.** Ultrasound to look for retroplacental hemorrhage (low sensitivity).	**Ultrasound** for placental position.	**Primarily clinical; based on symptoms and fetal distress.**
Treatment	**Mild abruption or premature infant:** Hospitalization, fetal monitoring, type and cross, bed rest. **Moderate to severe abruption:** ABCs, type and cross, immediate delivery.	**No cervical exams!** Stabilize patients with premature fetus. Serial ultrasound to assess fetal growth and resolution of previa. C-section for total or partial previa or if the patient/infant is in distress.	**Immediate C-section** with delivery of the infant and repair of the rupture.
Complications	Hemorrhagic shock; DIC; fetal death with severe abruption.	↑ risk of placenta accreta. Persistent hemorrhage requiring hysterectomy.	Fetal and maternal death.

SYMPTOMS/EXAM

- Suspect in patients with **first-trimester uterine bleeding** and excessive nausea and vomiting.
- Look for patients with **preeclampsia or eclampsia at < 24 weeks.**
- Other findings include uterine size greater than dates and hyperthyroidism.
- **No fetal heartbeat** is detected.
- Pelvic exam may show enlarged ovaries and possible expulsion of **grape-like molar clusters** into the vagina or blood in the cervical os.

HIGH-YIELD FACTS

OBSTETRICS

DIAGNOSIS

- β-hCG levels are markedly ↑ (usually > 100,000 mIU/dL).
- Pelvic ultrasound shows a **"snowstorm" appearance** with no gestational sac and no fetus or heart tones present.
- CXR to look for metastases.

TREATMENT

- D&C.
- Carefully monitor β-hCG levels after D&C for possible progression to malignant disease.
- Pregnancy prevention (contraception) is needed for one year to ensure accurate monitoring of β-hCG levels.
- Treat malignant disease with chemotherapy and residual uterine disease with hysterectomy.

ABNORMAL LABOR AND DELIVERY

Preterm Premature Rupture of Membranes (PPROM)

Defined as spontaneous ROM at < 37 **weeks,** prior to the onset of labor. Distinguished from premature rupture of membranes (PROM), which refers to loss of fluid at term prior to onset of contractions. Risk factors include low socioeconomic status, young maternal age, smoking, and STDs.

SYMPTOMS/EXAM

- Sterile speculum exam shows pooling of amniotic fluid in the posterior vaginal vault.
- Look for cervical dilation.

DIAGNOSIS

- **Nitrazine paper test:** Paper turns blue in alkaline amniotic fluid.
- **Fern test:** A ferning pattern is seen under the microscope after amniotic fluid dries on glass slide.
- Determine AFI by ultrasound to assess amniotic fluid volume.

TREATMENT

- Obtain cultures and/or wet mounts to look for infectious causes. If signs of infection are present, assume **amnionitis** (maternal fever, fetal tachycardia, foul-smelling amniotic fluid). Give antibiotics (ampicillin +/− gentamicin) and **induce labor** regardless of GA.
- If no signs of infection are present and GA is **24–32 weeks,** treat with **antibiotics (ampicillin and erythromycin)** to prolong pregnancy and **steroids** for fetal lung maturation +/− **tocolytics.**
- If no signs of infection are present and GA is ≥ **33 weeks,** hospitalize and treat expectantly until labor begins, signs of infection are seen, or 34 weeks' gestation is achieved.

Preterm Labor

Labor from 20 weeks up to 36 **completed** weeks' gestation.

- Patients may complain of menstrual-like cramps, uterine contractions, low back pain, pelvic pressure, new vaginal discharge, or bleeding.
- Rule out cervical insufficiency (treated with cerclage if early enough) and **preterm contractions** (no cervical dilation).
- Can → fetal respiratory distress syndrome, intraventricular hemorrhage, retinopathy of prematurity, necrotizing enterocolitis, or fetal death.

DIAGNOSIS

- Obtain an **ultrasound** to verify GA, fetal presentation, and AFI.
- Look for **regular** uterine contractions (≥ 3 contractions lasting 30 seconds each over a 30-minute period) coupled with a concurrent cervical change at < 37 weeks' gestation.

TREATMENT

- Begin with **hydration** and **bed rest.**
- Unless contraindicated, **administer steroids (to accelerate fetal lung maturity)** +/– tocolytics.
- Give **penicillin or ampicillin** for group B streptococcus prophylaxis if preterm delivery is likely.

Fetal Malpresentation

Defined as any presentation other than cephalic (head down). Breech presentation is the most common fetal malpresentation (affects 3% of all pregnancies).

DIAGNOSIS

- Perform Leopold maneuvers to identify fetal lie.
- Check by ultrasound if there is **any** doubt.

TREATMENT

- **Follow:** Up to 75% spontaneously change to cephalic presentation by 38 weeks.
- **External cephalic version** can be attempted at 36–37 weeks' gestation in the setting of persistent malpresentation.
  - Involves pressure applied to the maternal abdomen to turn the infant.
  - Risks of the procedure are placental abruption and cord compression; the infant **must** be monitored after the procedure, and consent must be obtained for emergent C-section.

Shoulder Dystocia

Defined as difficult delivery due to entrapment of the fetal shoulder at the level of the pubic bone. Risk factors include the following:

- Prior history of a shoulder dystocia.
- Fetal macrosomia or inadequate pelvis.

HIGH-YIELD FACTS

OBSTETRICS

TABLE 2.13-13. Indications for Cesarean Section

MATERNAL FACTORS	FETAL AND MATERNAL FACTORS	FETAL FACTORS
Any prior C-section regardless of uterine scar	**Cephalopelvic disproportion** (the most common cause of 1° C-section)	Fetal malposition
Active genital herpes infection	Placenta previa/placental abruption	Fetal distress
Cervical carcinoma	Failed operative vaginal delivery	Cord prolapse
Maternal trauma/demise		Erythroblastosis fetalis (Rh incompatibility)

DIAGNOSIS

- Prolonged second stage of labor with retraction of the head (turtle sign) back into the vaginal canal after pushing.
- After delivery of the head, difficulty delivering the anterior shoulder without performing additional maneuvers.

TREATMENT

- Flex and open the maternal hips (McRoberts amneuver), followed by suprapubic pressure. Most dystocias will be relieved with these two maneuvers:
  - Delivery of the posterior fetal arm or internal rotation of the fetal shoulders to lessen the shoulder diameter.
  - Replacement of the fetal head into the vaginal canal, followed by cesarean section (Zavanelli maneuver).

Indications for Cesarean Section

Table 2.13-13 outlines indications for C-section.

SPONTANEOUS AND RECURRENT ABORTION

Spontaneous Abortion (SAB)

Defined as **nonelective** termination of pregnancy at < 20 weeks' gestation. Also known as "miscarriage." Occurs in 10–15% of clinically recognizable pregnancies.

SYMPTOMS/EXAM

Differentiate types of SABs with symptoms, cervical exam, and ultrasound (see Table 2.13-14).

DIFFERENTIAL

Common causes of first-trimester bleeding include normal pregnancy (implantation bleeding), postcoital bleeding, ectopic pregnancy, vaginal or cervical lesions, pedunculated myomas or polyps, and extrusion of molar pregnancy.

TREATMENT

- Hemodynamic monitoring for significant bleeding.
- Check β-hCG to confirm pregnancy and transvaginal ultrasound to estab-

TABLE 2.13-14.   Types of Spontaneous Abortions

TYPE	SYMPTOMS	CERVIX/ULTRASOUND	TREATMENT
Threatened abortion	Minimal bleeding +/– cramping. Most cases are thought to be due to implantation bleed. **No products of conception (POC) are expelled.**	Closed os; ⊕ gestational sac.	Expectant management; consider pelvic rest for several weeks.
Inevitable abortion	Cramping with bleeding. **No POC are expelled.**	Open os; normal ultrasound.	D&C.
Incomplete abortion	Cramping with bleeding. **Some POC are expelled.**	Open os; normal ultrasound.	D&C.
Complete abortion	Slight bleeding; pain has usually ceased. **All POC are expelled.**	Closed os; empty uterus on ultrasound.	None.
Missed abortion	Often no symptoms. **No POC expelled.**	Closed os; no fetal cardiac activity; retained fetal tissue on ultrasound.	Allow up to four weeks for POC to pass; offer medical management with misoprostol or D&C.
Septic abortion	Constitutional symptoms; malodorous discharge. Often a recent history of therapeutic abortion; maternal mortality 10–50%.	Cervical motion tenderness.	Monitor ABCs; D&C, IV antibiotics, supportive care.

lish GA and rule out ectopic pregnancies; assess fetal viability or check for remaining tissue if completed abortion.
- Check blood type and antibody screen; give RhoGAM if appropriate.

Recurrent Abortion

- Defined as three or more consecutive pregnancy losses before 20 weeks' gestation.
- Usually due to **chromosomal** or **uterine abnormalities,** but can also result from hormonal abnormalities, infection, or systemic disease.
- **Dx:** Based on clinical and lab findings:
  - Perform pelvic exam (to look for anatomic abnormalities).
  - Check cervical cultures for chlamydia and gonorrhea.
  - Perform a maternal and paternal genetic analysis.
  - Obtain a sonohysterogram to look for uterine abnormalities.
  - Obtain TFTs, progesterone, lupus anticoagulant, and anticardiolipin antibody.
  - **Tx:** Treatment is based on the diagnosis.

All women with potential SABs should receive RhoGAM if appropriate.

HIGH-YIELD FACTS

OBSTETRICS

HIGH-YIELD FACTS

OBSTETRICS

SECTION II

Gynecology

Characterized by abnormalities in the frequency, duration, volume, and/or timing of menstrual bleeding. Defined as follows:

- **Menorrhagia:** Heavy or prolonged menstrual flow.
- **Metrorrhagia:** Bleeding between menses.
- **Metromenorrhagia:** Heavy bleeding at irregular intervals.

There are multiple causes of abnormal bleeding (see Table 2.14-1).

EXAM/DIAGNOSIS

- Determine if the bleeding is **ovulatory** or **anovulatory**.
  - **Ovulatory:**
    - Characterized by midcycle bleeding or changes in menstrual flow.
    - Can present with premenstrual syndrome symptoms (weight gain, breast tenderness, dysmenorrhea).
  - **Anovulatory:**
    - Characteristically acyclic with an unpredictable bleeding patterns.
    - Marked by excessive and prolonged bleeding due to unopposed estrogen on the endometrium.
    - Most often seen in adolescent and perimenopausal women.
    - Associated with an ↑ risk of endometrial hyperplasia and cancer.
- Look for a cervical lesion on speculum exam or an enlarged uterus on bimanual exam.
- Check a β-hCG and a CBC on each patient.

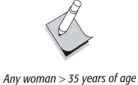

Any woman > 35 years of age with unexplained bleeding needs an endometrial biopsy to rule out malignancy.

HIGH-YIELD FACTS

GYNECOLOGY

TABLE 2.14-1. Types of Abnormal Bleeding

CATEGORY	ETIOLOGY	DIAGNOSIS
Anatomical	Leiomyoma, endometrial hyperplasia or polyps.	Transvaginal ultrasound, sonohysterogram, hysteroscopy.
Malignancy	Endometrial and cervical malignancies are most common, but may occur anywhere along the genital tract (rarely the vagina or due to an estrogen-producing ovarian tumor).	Endometrial biopsy, Pap smear/cervical biopsy, D&C (gold standard).
Systemic	1° bleeding disorders (e.g., von Willebrand's disease), endocrine abnormalities.	Coagulation profile, bleeding time, endocrine tests (FSH, LH, TSH, and prolactin).
Dysfunctional uterine bleeding (DUB)	A **diagnosis of exclusion.** Ninety percent of cases are due to unopposed estrogen in anovulation → proliferative endometrium; 10% of cases are ovulatory.	Other causes must be ruled out.
Postmenopausal bleeding	Endometrial cancer, vaginal atrophy, exogenous hormones.	By definition, occurs one or more years after menopause. Must rule out malignancy!

TREATMENT

- Treat the underlying cause.
- Acute, profuse bleeding can be treated with high-dose IV estrogen, D&C, uterine artery embolization, or hysterectomy.
- Surgical options include endometrial ablation and hysterectomy.
- DUB and anovulatory bleeding are treated with OCPs or NSAIDs.

AMENORRHEA

Defined as either 1° or 2° amenorrhea.

- **1° amenorrhea:** Absence of menses and lack of 2° sexual characteristics by age 14 **or** absence of menses by age 16 with or without 2° sexual characteristics. Associated with gonadal failure, congenital absence of the vagina, and constitutional symptoms.
- **2° amenorrhea:** Absence of menses for three cycles or for six months with prior normal menses. Etiologies include pregnancy, anorexia nervosa, stress, strenuous exercise, intrauterine adhesions, chronic anovulation, hypothyroidism, and hyperprolactinemia.

DIAGNOSIS

- **Check β-hCG** to make sure that the patient is not pregnant.
- **1° amenorrhea:** See Figure 2.14-1.
- **2° amenorrhea:** See Figure 2.14-2.

Always rule out pregnancy in a patient with amenorrhea.

Amenorrhea is a symptom, not a diagnosis. An etiology must be established to effectively treat amenorrhea.

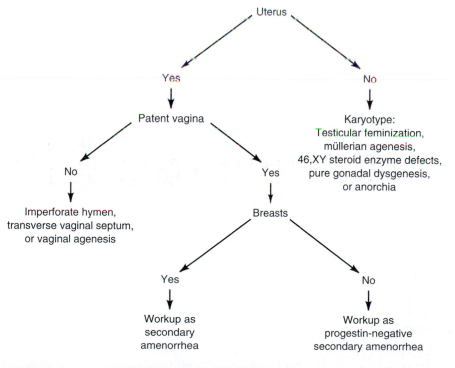

FIGURE 2.14-1.   Workup for patients with 1° amenorrhea.

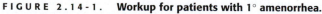

(Reproduced, with permission, from DeCherney AH, Nathan L. *Current Obstetric & Gynecologic Diagnosis & Treatment*, 9th ed. New York: McGraw-Hill, 2003: 995.)

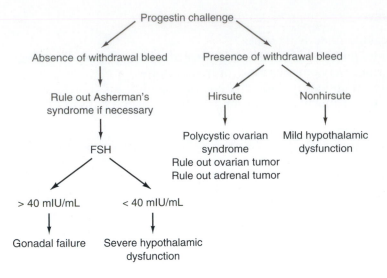

FIGURE 2.14-2. **Workup for patients with 2° amenorrhea.**

(Adapted, with permission, from DeCherney AH, Nathan L. *Current Obstetric & Gynecologic Diagnosis & Treatment*, 9th ed. New York: McGraw-Hill, 2003: 996.)

TREATMENT

Depends on the etiology; may include surgery or hormone therapy +/– drug therapy.

Always rule out a breast malignancy with a biopsy in anyone who is high risk.

BENIGN BREAST DISORDERS

Include **fibrocystic change** (the most common), fibroadenoma, intraductal papilloma (a common cause of bloody nipple discharge), duct ectasia, fat necrosis, mastitis, and breast abscess. See Table 2.14-2 for a list of common examples.

ENDOMETRIOSIS

Abnormal growth of tissue histologically resembling the endometrium in locations other than the uterine lining, usually in the ovaries (called endometriomas or "chocolate cysts"), cul-de-sac, and broad ligament. Associated with premenstrual pelvic pain due to stimulation from estrogen and progesterone during the menstrual cycle.

SYMPTOMS/EXAM

- Presents with pelvic pain, dysmenorrhea, dyspareunia, and infertility.
- On pelvic exam, patients may have tender nodularity along the uterosacral ligament +/– a fixed, retroflexed uterus or enlarged ovaries.

DIAGNOSIS

Diagnosis can be made by the history and physical, but the gold standard is direct visualization during laparoscopy with biopsy showing endometrial glands.

TABLE 2.14-2.   Benign Breast Disease

Disease Type	Symptoms/Exam	Treatment	Associated with Carcinoma
Fibrocystic changes	Mild to moderate pain in the breasts +/– lumps premenstrually; multifocal, bilateral nodularity. Most common in women 20–50 years of age.	OCPs.	Patients are at ↑ risk of breast cancer only in the presence of cellular atypia. Cancer must be excluded in high-risk groups.
Fibroadenoma	**The most common tumor in menstruating women** < 25 years of age. Presents as a small, firm, unilateral, nontender mass that is freely movable and slow growing. Ultrasound can be used to differentiate from a cyst.	Thirty percent will spontaneously disappear. Removal is not necessary, but surgical excision is both diagnostic and curative. Biopsy if the patient is in a high-risk group. Recurrence is common.	Risk is twice as high as that of control patients.
Intraductal papilloma	Clear, bloody, or discolored fluid from a single duct opening. Milking of the breast shows drainage from one duct opening.	Drainage and surgical exploration of the duct. **A malignant process must always be excluded.**	Risk is twice as high as that of control patients.
Mastitis	Seen in breast-feeding women; presents as a hard, red, tender, swollen area of breast accompanied by fever, myalgias, and general malaise.	Continued breast-feeding; NSAIDs, and antibiotics to cover common etiologies (staph, strep, *E. coli*).	None.
Abscess	Can develop if mastitis is inadequately treated. Examination reveals a fluctuant mass accompanied by systemic symptoms similar to those seen in mastitis.	Needle aspiration or surgical drainage in addition to antibiotics.	None.
Fat necrosis	Firm, tender, and ill-defined with surrounding erythema; related to trauma/ischemia.	Analgesia. An excisional biopsy may be done to rule out malignancy.	None.

HIGH-YIELD FACTS

GYNECOLOGY

TREATMENT

Treatment depends on the patient's symptoms, age, desire for future fertility, and disease stage.

- If the patient's main complaint is **infertility, operative laparoscopy** should be performed to excise the endometriosis and restore the pelvic anatomy. The patient can then undergo assisted reproductive procedures or wait to see if spontaneous pregnancy occurs.
- If the patient's main complaint is **pain,** the goal is to induce a state of anovulation.
  - For mild pain, first-line treatment is NSAIDs and/or continuous OCPs.

- For moderate to severe pain, options include medical treatment to induce anovulation (GnRH agonists) or **operative laparoscopy.**
- Hysterectomy with bilateral oophorectomy is curative.

Defined as pain with menstrual periods that requires medication and prevents normal activity. It is divided into 1° and 2° dysmenorrhea.

- **1° dysmenorrhea:** No clinically detectable pelvic pathology. Most likely due to ↑ uterine prostaglandin production.
- **2° dysmenorrhea:** Menstrual pain due to pelvic pathology, most commonly endometriosis, adenomyosis (endometrial glands and stroma within the myometrium), myomas, or PID.

Oral Contraceptives (OCPs)

The long-term consequences of OCP use include a ↓ in ovarian and endometrial cancers, a ↓ incidence of breast disease (but not breast cancer), ↓ menstrual flow, and dysmenorrhea. Contraindications to OCP use include the following:

- Pregnancy.
- Previous or active thromboembolic disease.
- Undiagnosed genital bleeding.
- Age > 35 years in patients who smoke.
- Estrogen-dependent neoplasms.
- Hepatocellular carcinoma.

Medroxyprogesterone Acetate (Depo-Provera)

Administered intramuscularly every three months.

- **Advantages:** Highly effective, and there is no need to remember a pill every day. Can be used in women who have a history of thromboembolic disease.
- **Disadvantages:** Associated with weight gain and menstrual effects (irregular menses and spotting initially with amenorrhea in 50% of women at 1 year); prolonged use can → ↓ bone mineralization.

Emergency Contraception

- Can be offered up to five days after unprotected intercourse; ↓ the risk of pregnancy to 1%.
- The **progestin-only regimen** is a newer method consisting of levonorgestrel 0.75 μg (the trade name is **Plan B**). It is given PO within 72 hours of unprotected intercourse and repeated 12 hours later.

Intrauterine Devices (IUDs)

Two types of IUDs are approved for use in the United States. Both are highly effective, with > 99% efficacy during the first year of use.

- **Copper IUD** (trade name ParaGard):
  - Lasts 10 years.
  - Nonhormonal; a good choice for women who cannot use hormonal contraceptive methods.
  - The main side effects are dysmenorrhea and ↑ menstrual bleeding.
- **Levonorgestrel IUD** (trade name Mirena):
  - Lasts 5 years.
  - ↓ amount of menstrual bleeding and dysmenorrhea—good choice to treat menorrhagia.
  - The main side effect is irregular menstrual bleeding or amenorrhea.

VULVOVAGINITIS

The most common outpatient gynecologic problem. Vulvovaginitis can be bacterial (bacterial vaginosis [BV]), fungal (*Candida*), or protozoal (*Trichomonas vaginalis*). Figure 2.14-3 shows the histologic appearance of two common causes of vulvovaginitis.

Sexual abuse must be considered in any child with vulvovaginitis.

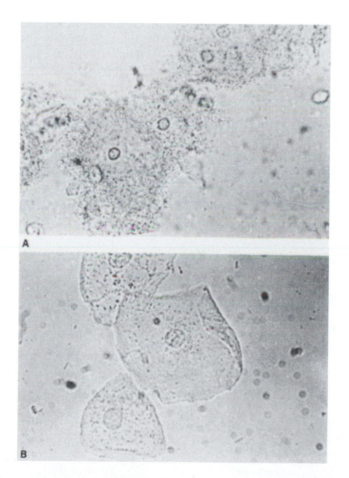

FIGURE 2.14-3. **Causes of vaginitis.**

(A) Candidal vaginitis. Branches to budding *Candida albicans* are evident on KOH preparation of vaginal discharge. (B). Saline wet mount of vaginal fluid reveals granulations on vaginal epithelial cells ("clue cells") due to adherence of BV-causing organisms to the cell surface. The presence of clue cells is just one of the diagnostic criteria for BV. (Reproduced, with permission, from Kasper DL et al. *Harrison's Principles of Internal Medicine*, 16th ed. New York: McGraw-Hill, 2005: 767.)

SYMPTOMS/EXAM

- Presents with ↑ vaginal discharge or a change in vaginal discharge.
- Patients may also complain of vulvovaginal pruritus with or without burning and/or odor.
- Perform a complete examination of the vulva, vagina, and cervix. Look for vulvar edema, erythema, and discharge.

DIAGNOSIS/TREATMENT

Obtain swabs from the vagina to perform a wet mount and cultures for gonorrhea, chlamydia, and HSV, depending on the exam (see Table 2.14-3).

POLYCYSTIC OVARIAN SYNDROME (PCOS)

The most common cause of female hirsutism (male-pattern hair growth). Typically affects women in the teenage years who are obese and hirsute. The cause is unknown; hyperinsulinemia with insulin resistance is usually seen.

SYMPTOMS

Look for an obese woman with hirsutism, oligo- or amenorrhea, infertility, acne, and diabetes or insulin resistance.

EXAM

- Exam may reveal evidence of hirsutism without evidence of cortisol or adrenal androgen excess.
- Pelvic exam may reveal palpably enlarged ovaries.

TABLE 2. 1 4 - 3.   **Common Causes of Vulvovaginitis**

	BACTERIAL VAGINOSIS	YEAST (USUALLY CANDIDA)	TRICHOMONAS VAGINALIS
Exam	Can be unremarkable except for discharge.	Erythema and irritating, curdlike discharge.	Malodorous discharge; the vagina and cervix can be swollen and red.
Discharge	Grayish or white, having a **fishy odor;** pronounced after intercourse.	White, curdlike discharge.	Yellow-green discharge.
Saline smear	> 20% of epithelial cells with indistinct cell margins (clue cells; see Figure 2.14-3).	Nothing.	Motile, flagellated protozoans.
KOH prep	⊕ **"whiff test"** when KOH is placed on slide → a fishy odor.	Pseudohyphae and spores (see Figure 2.14-3).	**Nothing.**
pH	Elevated (i.e., > 7)	Normal or < 7	Elevated or > 7
Treatment			
Nonpregnant	Metronidazole.	Topical antifungal for 3–7 days or fluconazole × 1 dose.	Metronidazole.
Pregnant	Metronidazole.	Use only topical antifungals for seven days.	Metronidazole.

DIAGNOSIS

- Two out of three of the following clinical signs must be present to diagnose PCOS:
  - Oligo- or anovulation.
  - Hyperandrogenism (acne, hirsutism, or elevated testosterone).
  - Polycystic ovaries (ultrasound may show ovaries with multiple small follicles).
- An ↑ LH/FSH ratio (> 2) may be present.
- Perform a glucose tolerance test to evaluate for diabetes.

TREATMENT

- Treat the specific symptoms.
  - **Infertility:** Induce ovulation with clomiphene and/or metformin.
  - **Hirsutism:** Start combination OCPs to suppress ovarian steroidogenesis.
- Weight loss will help with insulin resistance; treat diabetes with metformin, which may improve response to ovulation induction.

MENOPAUSE

Cessation of menstruation for > 12 months; average age is 51. Surgical menopause occurs after removal or irradiation of the ovaries. Postmenopausal women are at ↑ risk for developing **osteoporosis** and **heart disease.**

SYMPTOMS/EXAM

- Patients may complain of menstrual irregularities, hot flashes, sweating, sleep disturbances, mood changes, ↓ libido, and vaginal dryness.
- Exam can reveal vaginal dryness, ↓ breast size, and genital tract atrophy.

DIAGNOSIS

- Requires **one year** without menses without other known cause.
- ↑↑ **serum FSH** (**> 30 IU/L**) is suggestive.

TREATMENT

- The use of hormone therapy with estrogen (in woman without a uterus) or combined estrogen and progesterone (in woman with an intact uterus) can be used for short-term symptomatic relief.
- Absolute contraindications to hormone therapy include undiagnosed vaginal bleeding, active liver disease, recent MI, recent or active vascular thrombosis, and a history of endometrial or breast cancer.
- Alternatives to hormone therapy include the following:
  - Venlafaxine and some SSRIs for vasomotor instability.
  - Vaginal lubricants or topical estrogens for vaginal atrophy.
  - Calcium, vitamin D, calcitonin, bisphosphonates (alendronate), and selective estrogen receptor modulators (raloxifene) for osteoporosis.
- Unopposed estrogen (without progesterone therapy) can → endometrial hyperplasia and/or carcinoma.

URINARY INCONTINENCE

Involuntary loss of urine that is a social or hygienic problem. See Table 2.14-4 for an outline of stress, urge, and mixed incontinence.

Premature menopause occurs before age 40 and is often due to idiopathic premature ovarian failure.

Use the lowest possible dose of hormone therapy for the shortest duration to treat symptoms.

TABLE 2.14-4. Types of Urinary Incontinence

	STRESS INCONTINENCE	URGE INCONTINENCE (DETRUSOR INSTABILITY)	MIXED INCONTINENCE
History	Loss of urine with exertion (running) or straining (coughing, laughing).	Loss of urine with strong desire to void. Often associated with urinary frequency and urgency.	Stress and urge incontinence present simultaneously.
Mechanism	Poor support or poor function of the urethral sphincter.	Involuntary detrusor muscle contractions.	A combination of both mechanisms.
Etiology	Urethral hypermobility, weakened urethral closing mechanisms.	Idiopathic. Neurologic (Alzheimer's, diabetes, MS).	As for both conditions.
Diagnosis	Patient history. Demonstrable leakage with stress (cough).	Patient history. Cystometry reveals involuntary detrusor muscle contraction associated with urinary leakage.	As for both conditions.
Treatment	Pelvic floor strengthening exercises (Kegel) with or without biofeedback, pessaries, weight loss, surgery to restore bladder neck support.	Behavior modification (e.g., avoiding caffeinated or alcoholic beverages). Bladder retaining (contracting pelvic floor instead of running to bathroom). Medical therapy (anticholinergic).	Based on the patient's worst symptom; some treatments overlap (e.g., Kegels).

UTI must be ruled out in all women complaining of urinary incontinence.

EXAM/DIAGNOSIS

- Voiding diaries help quantify the frequency and volume of urine lost, circumstances of leakage (to diagnose stress or urge types of incontinence), voiding patterns, and the amount and type of fluid taken in.
- Patients with incontinence should have a screening neurologic exam to rule out neurologic causes.
- A standing cough stress test can be used to diagnose stress incontinence; cystometry can be used to diagnose urge incontinence.
- Urinary retention with overflow can be a cause of urinary incontinence and can be diagnosed with an elevated postvoid residual.

TREATMENT

Table 2.14-4 outlines treatment measures for urinary incontinence.

ECTOPIC PREGNANCY

Any pregnancy implanted outside the uterine cavity. The most common location is the fallopian tube (95%). Risk factors include a history of PID, prior ectopic pregnancy, tubal/pelvic surgery, DES exposure in utero → abnormal tubal development, and IUD use.

SYMPTOMS/EXAM

- Patients may complain of lower abdominal or pelvic pain as well as abnormal vaginal spotting or bleeding and amenorrhea.
- The abdomen may be tender to palpation with or without cervical motion tenderness and an adnexal mass on bimanual exam.
- A ruptured ectopic may present with unstable vital signs, generalized abdominal pain, rebound tenderness, shoulder pain, and shock.

DIFFERENTIAL

Spontaneous abortion, molar pregnancy, ruptured corpus luteum cyst, PID, ovarian torsion, appendicitis, pyelonephritis, diverticulitis, regional ileitis, ulcerative colitis.

DIAGNOSIS

- An ↑ β-hCG in the absence of an intrauterine pregnancy on ultrasound is highly suspicious for an ectopic pregnancy.
    - An ↑ serum β-hCG will not determine the location of the pregnancy.
    - An ectopic pregnancy usually has lower levels and abnormal rising patterns of β-hCG than expected for estimated gestational age (GA) (β-hCG levels should double every two days in a normal pregnancy).
- Do an **ultrasound** to look for **intrauterine** pregnancy.
    - The gestational sac may be visualized on:
        - Transvaginal ultrasound when β-hCG is approximately 1000–2000 mIU/mL, or at about 4–5 weeks' GA.
        - **Transabdominal** ultrasound when β-hCG is > 1800–3600 mIU/mL.
    - Fetal heart motion of the embryo can be seen after 5–6 weeks' GA.
- Definitive diagnosis is made by laparoscopy, laparotomy, or ultrasound visualization of a pregnancy outside the uterus.

TREATMENT

- For **hemodynamically unstable** patients, immediate surgery is required.
- Treatment measures for **hemodynamically stable** patients include the following:
    - Follow serial β-hCG levels closely with or without ultrasound studies.
    - **Methotrexate** is used for small (< 3.5-cm), unruptured ectopic pregnancies in asymptomatic women until levels are undetectable.
    - **Laparoscopy or laparotomy for removal of ectopic pregnancy.**
    - Expectant management is appropriate for asymptomatic, compliant patients with decreasing β-hCG levels or β-hCG < 200 mIU/mL, and if the risk of rupture is low.
- All women should be typed and screened and given **RhoGAM if Rh is ⊖**.
- Prevention of ectopic pregnancies includes thorough **treatment of STDs**.

INFERTILITY

Defined as the inability of a couple to conceive after one year of unprotected intercourse. It affects 10–15% of couples. Causes include the following:

Any woman with abdominal pain needs a urine pregnancy test.

↑ β-hCG in the absence of an intrauterine pregnancy on ultrasound is suspicious for an ectopic pregnancy.

Endometriosis is the leading cause of female infertility, followed by PID.

- **Male dysfunction (35%):** Defects in spermatogenesis (male factor); varicoceles.
- **Female dysfunction (50%):**
  - **Uterine/tubal factors: Endometriosis,** infection or myomas that distort the endometrium or fallopian tubes, PID, congenital genital tract abnormalities.
  - **Ovulatory dysfunction:** Ovarian failure, prolactinoma.
  - **Endocrine dysfunction:** Thyroid/adrenal disease, PCOS.
- **Unexplained infertility and rare problems (15%).**

DIAGNOSIS

- Semen analysis to rule out male factors.
- Serum FSH/LH/TSH/prolactin to rule out endocrine dysfunction.
- Hysterosalpingography to rule out tubal and uterine cavity abnormalities.
- Basal body temperatures or ovulation kits to rule out ovulatory dysfunction.

TREATMENT

- Treat the underlying cause.
- Fertility rates in endometriosis can be improved through laparoscopic removal of implants.
- Ovulation can be induced with **clomiphene,** but this can → ovarian hyperstimulation and multiple gestations.
- Assisted reproductive technologies such as in vitro fertilization can be used for refractory cases.

SECTION II

Pediatrics

Developmental Milestones

Table 2.15-1 highlights major developmental milestones. Red flags include the following:

- Persistent primitive reflexes by 6 months.
- Handedness before 1 year.
- No pointing by 18 months.

Immunizations

Table 2.15-2 summarizes the recommended timetable for childhood immunizations. Schedules may vary for children who are behind and require catch-up immunizations.

TABLE 2.15-1.   Developmental Milestones

AGE	GROSS MOTOR	FINE MOTOR	LANGUAGE	SOCIAL/COGNITIVE
2 months	Lifts head/chest when prone.	Tracks past midline.	Alerts to sound; coos.	Recognizes parent; **social smile.**
4–5 months	**Rolls** front to back and back to front (5 months).	Grasps rattle.	Orients to voice; "ah-goo"; razzes.	Enjoys looking around; laughs.
6 months	**Sits unassisted** (7 months).	**Transfers objects;** raking grasp.	Babbles.	**Stranger anxiety.**
9–10 months	Crawls; pulls to stand.	Uses three-finger pincer grasp.	**Says mama/dada** (nonspecific).	Waves bye-bye; plays pat-a-cake.
12 months	Cruises (11 months); **walks alone.**	Uses two-finger pincer grasp.	Says mama/dada (specific).	Imitates actions.
15 months	Walks backward.	Uses cup.	Uses 4–6 words.	Temper tantrums.
18 months	Runs; kicks a ball.	Builds tower of 2–4 cubes.	Names common objects.	Copies parent in tasks (e.g., sweeping).
2 years	Walks up/down steps with help; jumps.	Builds tower of six cubes.	Uses **two-word** phrases.	Follows **two-step** commands; removes clothes.
3 years	Rides **tricycle;** climbs stairs with alternating feet (3–4 years).	Copies a circle; uses utensils.	Uses **three-word** sentences.	Brushes teeth with help; washes/dries hands.
4 years	Hops.	Copies a cross.	Counts to 10.	Cooperative play.

Reproduced, with permission, from Le T et al. *First Aid for the USMLE Step 2 CK,* 6th ed. New York: McGraw-Hill, 2007: 360.

TABLE 2.15-2. Immunization Timetable

VACCINE	AGES ADMINISTERED	NOTES
Diphtheria, tetanus, acellular pertussis (DTaP)	2, 4, 6 months; 15–18 months; 4–6 years; tetanus booster at 11–12 years and then every 10 years thereafter.	Common adverse events include fever and local reactions at the injection site. Consider deferring in children with neurologic disorders.
Polio (IPV)	2, 4 months; 6–8 months; 4–6 years.	Generally well tolerated.
Hepatitis B	First given at birth **or** at 1–4 months; second given 4 weeks after first dose; third given 16 weeks after first dose.	In addition to receiving the vaccine, infants who may be exposed to hepatitis B perinatally may require IVIG.
H. influenzae type b (Hib)	2, 4, 6 months; 12–15 months.	Prior to the vaccine, Hib was the most common cause of bacterial meningitis in children.
Measles, mumps, rubella (MMR)	12–15 months; 4–6 years.	A **live vaccine**—avoid in immunocompromised patients.
Rotavirus	2, 4, 6 months.	The first dose must be given prior to 12 weeks of age, or the child cannot have any of the series.
Varicella	> 12 months.	A **live vaccine**—avoid in immunocompromised patients.
Pneumococcal conjugate vaccine	2, 4, 6 months; 12–15 months.	Children with fever, particularly those < 3 months of age, are much more likely to have a serious bacterial infection if they are unvaccinated against pneumococcus.
Influenza	> 6 months, yearly, October through April.	It is recommended that children getting the shot for the first time at 6 months to 9 years of age receive it in two installments.

Routine Health Screening

Routine screening should be conducted at the following intervals:

- **Metabolic/genetic diseases:** At one day of life, a state newborn screen is drawn. The exact tests vary by state, but all include testing for phenylketonuria and congenital hypothyroidism.
- **Growth parameters/development/behavior:** Screen at each visit every 2–6 months for the first three years; then screen annually.
- **Lead/anemia:** Screen at 9–15 months. Lead screening should be repeated at two years of age, especially in high-risk communities. Consider repeating anemia screening in menstruating adolescents.
- **BP:** Screen with every medical exam starting at three years of age.

- **Vision and hearing screening:** Conduct subjective testing at each visit; red reflex testing at all infant visits; and objective hearing and vision screening at birth and annually starting at three years of age.
- **TB:** Conduct a risk assessment at each well-child check. PPD placement is appropriate for high-risk children.
- **High-risk behaviors/STD screening:** Screen at each adolescent visit (at approximately 10–11 years of age).
- **Anticipatory guidance:** Provide nutrition and sleep counseling as well as injury/violence prevention counseling at each health maintenance visit.

COLIC

- Severe and paroxysmal crying, mainly in the late afternoon.
- **Sx/Exam:** Suspect in a well-fed infant who cries > 3 hours a day > 3 days a week for > 3 weeks. Occurs between three weeks and three months of age, with spontaneous resolution.
- **Tx:** Offer reassurance and parental education/soothing skills.

All infants go "back" to sleep to ↓ the risk of sudden infant death syndrome (SIDS).

GROWTH DEFICIENCY/FAILURE TO THRIVE (FTT)

Defined as follows:

- **Failure to grow:** Growth is significantly slower than that of children of the same age. Height and weight are both slow (e.g., growth hormone deficiency, genetic disease).
- **Failure to gain weight:** The child is or was previously able to maintain normal height velocity, but weight is disproportionately low or has "fallen off" the growth curve. Height velocity may subsequently slow if the child has been underweight for a prolonged period of time. Head circumference is the last to fall off the curve.

SYMPTOMS/EXAM

- Obtain a thorough feeding/nutrition history.
- Ask about malabsorption and/or systemic symptoms.
- Obtain a detailed social history (family stressors) and family history (CF, genetic diseases, HIV).
- Plot height, weight, and head circumference since birth.
- Conduct a complete physical exam.

DIFFERENTIAL

- **Inadequate intake:** The most common cause (i.e., overdiluting formula). Often 2° to psychosocial issues, with no underlying medical condition.
- **Increased output:** Malabsorption.
- **Increased metabolic demand:** Examples include inborn errors of metabolism, CF/lung disease, HIV/infection, endocrine disorders, and congenital heart disease.

DIAGNOSIS

- The H&P will dictate the extent of lab workup.
- First-line lab evaluation includes CBC, electrolytes, BUN/creatinine, and UA.

TREATMENT

- Treat the underlying cause.
- If the H&P does not suggest an organic cause, start a calorie count and consider nutritional supplementation.
- Hospitalization may be necessary in the setting of severe malnourishment or when there is concern for neglect.

SAFETY

Car Seats

- Seats should be placed in the rear of the car.
- Seats should be rear-facing until the child is 20 lbs **and** one year of age. A car seat should never be placed in a seat that is equipped with an active airbag.

Child Abuse

Includes physical, sexual, and emotional abuse/neglect. Diagnosis is based on a **history that is discordant with physical findings.**

SYMPTOMS/EXAM

Presentation may include the following:

Consider nonaccidental trauma when the history of an injury is discordant with physical findings.

- Multiple injuries in **various stages of healing.**
- Irritability/lethargy.
- Growth failure.
- **Oddly situated bruises** (not over bony prominences) or bruises on a child who is not yet mobile.
- **Pattern injuries** (cigarette/immersion burns).
- **Skeletal trauma** (spiral fracture of long bones, multiple/old/posterior rib fractures, corner fractures).
- **Retinal hemorrhage** in infants.
- **Intracranial hemorrhage.**
- Signs/symptoms of STDs or genital trauma.

DIAGNOSIS

Skeletal survey, head CT, ophthalmologic exam.

TREATMENT

- Physicians are mandated reporters of **any suspected abuse or nonaccidental trauma** and should immediately notify social services or Child Protective Services.
- Consider hospitalization to ensure the safety of the child.

NEONATOLOGY

Respiratory Distress

- Causes of neonatal respiratory distress include those listed in Table 2.15-3.
- Also consider congenital heart disease (if O_2 sats fail to improve with supplemental oxygen), anatomic airway anomalies (e.g., choanal atresia, in

which an NG tube cannot be passed at birth), pneumothorax (especially in an infant who suddenly decompensates), neurologic abnormalities, pneumonia, and **sepsis**.

- **Dx/Tx:** The diagnosis and treatment of common pediatric respiratory disorders are outlined in Table 2.15-3.

Neonatal Sepsis

Serious bacterial infections are relatively common in infants < 2 months of age. The most frequent infections are UTIs, followed by bacterial sepsis, meningitis, and pneumonia. Risk factors include maternal group B strep (GBS) positivity, rupture of membranes > 18 hours, maternal fever, chorioamnionitis, and premature labor. The most common pathogens are *E. coli*, GBS, and other gram-$\ominus$ rods. *Listeria monocytogenes* may also be implicated.

A fever in the first month of life is an indication for a full sepsis workup, admission, and IV antibiotics.

SYMPTOMS/EXAM

- **Never trust a neonate to look or act sick.**
- Temperature may be high or low, and the infant may or may not have additional vital sign instability.
- Infants often present with poor feeding and may also present with respiratory distress.

DIAGNOSIS

Evaluation should include a CBC, a blood culture, a UA/urine culture, and an LP for CSF culture. Consider a CXR.

TREATMENT

- **Initial treatment:** Begin IV **ampicillin** (to cover *Listeria*) plus **gentamicin** or ampicillin plus a third-generation cephalosporin.
- **Subsequent therapy:** If the cause of sepsis was a UTI, a renal ultrasound and VCUG must be obtained to evaluate the infant for hydronephrosis and vesicoureteral reflux (VUR).

PREVENTION

- Screen the mother for GBS at 36 weeks, and treat with prophylactic antibiotics during delivery.
- If VUR is present, the infant must be started on daily antibiotic prophylaxis.

TORCHeS Infections

Many congenital infections present with jaundice, hepatosplenomegaly, and thrombocytopenia. Table 2.15-4 outlines the diagnosis and treatment of each.

Congenital Anomalies

Table 2.15-5 outlines the clinical presentation and treatment of common congenital anomalies and malformations.

With Down syndrome, look for the "double bubble" sign of duodenal atresia.

TABLE 2.15-3. **Common Pediatric Respiratory Disorders**

DISORDER	DESCRIPTION	HISTORY	EXAM/CXR FINDINGS	TREATMENT	COMPLICATIONS
Respiratory distress syndrome/hyaline membrane disease	**Surfactant deficiency** → poor lung compliance and respiratory failure.	Usually occurs in **premature infants.**	↓ air movement; CXR shows ↓ lung volumes and ground-glass appearance.	Maternal antenatal steroids for prevention; surfactant administration at time of delivery; respiratory support.	Chronic lung disease.
Transient tachypnea of the newborn	**Retained fetal lung fluid** → brief, mild respiratory distress. Diagnosis of exclusion.	Term or near-term infants; nonasphyxiated; born following short labor or often via C-section without labor.	CXR shows perihilar streaking and fluid in interlobar fissures.	Usually only mild to moderate O_2 requirement for support.	None.
Meconium aspiration syndrome	Inhalation of meconium at or near time of birth → **aspiration pneumonitis.**	**Term infants;** meconium present at time of delivery.	**Barrel chest;** coarse breath sounds; CXR shows coarse irregular infiltrates, hyperexpansion, and lobar consolidation.	Nasopharyngeal suctioning at perineum; tracheal suctioning at birth; ventilatory support.	Pulmonary hypertension. Suspect CF.
Congenital diaphragmatic hernia	Defect in diaphragm → herniation of abdominal contents into the chest cavity; limitation of lung growth → **pulmonary hypoplasia.**	Severe respiratory distress at birth; may be diagnosed by prenatal ultrasound.	Scaphoid abdomen; CXR may show bowel loops in chest.	Immediate intubation, ventilatory support, and surgical correction after stabilization. Patients may require extracorporeal membrane oxygenation (ECMO).	Severe pulmonary hypertension. Mortality 25–40%.

Jaundice

PHYSIOLOGIC JAUNDICE

Indirect hyperbilirubinemia.

SYMPTOMS/EXAM

- A common neonatal problem that usually presents within the first 36–48 hours of life. It starts at the head (or eyes) and travels down the body.

250

TABLE 2.15-4. TORCHeS Infections

INFECTION	DESCRIPTION	TREATMENT	PREVENTION
Toxoplasmosis	Hydrocephalus, seizures, intracranial calcifications, and ring-enhancing lesions on head CT.	Pyrimethamine, sulfadiazine, spiramycin.	Avoid exposure to cats and cat feces during pregnancy; avoid raw/undercooked meat; treat women with 1° infection.
Other	Includes HIV, parvovirus, varicella, *Listeria*, TB, malaria, and fungi.	Disease specific.	For HIV-⊕ mothers, treatment of mother pre- and perinatally as well as prophylaxis of infant for six weeks after birth will ↓ transmission.
Rubella	"Blueberry muffin" rash, cataracts, hearing loss, PDA and other cardiac defects, encephalitis.	None.	Immunize mothers prior to pregnancy.
Cytomegalovirus (CMV)	Petechial rash, periventricular calcifications, microcephaly, chorioretinitis.	Ganciclovir.	Avoid exposure.
Herpes	Skin, eye, and mouth vesicles; can progress to severe CNS/systemic infection.	Acyclovir.	Perform a C-section if mother has active lesions at time of delivery. Highest risk is from mother with 1° infection.
Syphilis	Maculopapular skin rash, lymphadenopathy, "snuffles," osteitis.	Penicillin.	Treat seropositive mothers with penicillin.

- Indirect hyperbilirubinemia can cross the blood-brain barrier and deposit in the basal ganglia, causing **kernicterus,** an irreversible, potentially fatal encephalopathy.

DIFFERENTIAL

Jaundice is **not** physiologic if it is severe or prolonged, occurs within the first 24 hours of life, or is associated with a direct component.

TREATMENT

- UV **phototherapy.** Phototherapy is more likely to be necessary if the mother's blood type is O ⊖ or if the infant suffered birth trauma, is of Asian descent, was born preterm, or is infected.
- Exchange transfusion for severe jaundice.

Ceftriaxone displaces bilirubin and should not be used in neonates.

TABLE 2.15-5.   Common Congenital Anomalies and Malformations

LESION	DESCRIPTION	AGE OF PRESENTATION	SYMPTOMS	TREATMENT
Cleft lip/palate	Abnormal ridge/division.	Presents at birth.	Poor feeding; severe, recurrent otitis media. May be associated with other anomalies.	Surgical repair of the lip/palate.
Tracheoesophageal fistula	Blind esophageal pouch; fistula between the distal esophagus and trachea (most common).	Usually presents in the first few hours of life, but other types can present later in infancy.	Copious secretions, choking, cyanosis, respiratory distress.	Suctioning of the pouch with an NG tube, reflux precautions, supportive care, surgical repair.
Abdominal wall defects	Gastroschisis (the intestine extrudes through the defect); omphalocele (a membrane-covered herniation of abdominal contents).	Presents antenatally or at birth.	Visible defect. Associated anomalies are common in omphalocele but are rare in gastroschisis.	Coverage of abdominal contents with sterile dressing. NG decompressions, antibiotics, supportive care, and stabilization followed by 1° or staged closure.
Intestinal atresias	Intestinal obstruction.	Present antenatally or at birth.	Abdominal distention, bilious vomiting, obstipation/failure to pass meconium, polyhydramnios.	Surgical resection.
Hirschsprung's disease	Absence of ganglion cells in the colon → narrowing of the aganglionic segment with dilation of the proximal normal colon. Can be a short (75%) or long segment.	Presents at infancy or within the first two years of life.	Failure to pass meconium, vomiting, abdominal distention, chronic constipation.	Diagnose by rectal biopsy at the anal verge to look for ganglion cells. Staged procedure with initial diverting colostomy and later resection when the infant is > 6 months old.
Neural tube defects	Includes anencephaly (incompatible with life) and spina bifida (myelomeningocele, meningocele).	Presents at birth, but may be detected prenatally. Associated with ↑ maternal and amniotic fluid α-**fetoprotein.**	Depends on defect. Ranges from incompatible with life to hydrocephalus, paralysis, and neurogenic bowel and bladder. ↑ risk of latex allergy.	Risk ↓ with folate ingestion during the first trimester. Surgical repair.

Breast Milk Jaundice

- **Sx/Exam:** Occurs at 2–3 weeks of age.
- **Dx:** A diagnosis of exclusion.
- **Tx:** Rarely requires phototherapy.

Pathologic Jaundice

Direct hyperbilirubinemia. Causes can be hepatic or extrahepatic and include biliary atresia (most common), hypothyroidism, CF, inborn errors of metabolism, neonatal hepatitis, Crigler-Najjar syndrome, Gilbert's syndrome, α_1-antitrypsin deficiency, and TPN cholestasis (affects premature infants on TPN).

Symptoms/Exam

- Look for hepatomegaly.
- **Kernicterus** presents with jaundice, lethargy, poor feeding, a high-pitched cry, hypertonicity, and seizures.

Diagnosis

- Order a CBC (to follow for anemia) and a peripheral blood smear (to rule out hemolysis).
- A Coombs' test can distinguish antibody-mediated disease (e.g., ABO incompatibility) from non-immune-related disorders (e.g., G6PD deficiency, hereditary spherocytosis).

Treatment

Phototherapy/transfusion.

INFECTIOUS DISEASE

Fever of Unknown Origin (FUO)

- Evaluation is age dependent:
  - **0–28 days:** See the discussion of neonatal sepsis.
  - **1–2 months:** Obtain a CBC, a blood culture, and a UA and urine culture. Consider an LP if the infant is irritable or lethargic.
  - **3–36 months:** Obtain a CBC and a UA and urine culture. If the WBC count is < 5 or > 15, obtain a blood culture. If the infant has been vaccinated and appears well, the risk of bacteremia and/or meningitis is low.
- **UTI** is a common cause of FUO and affects females more than males. Evaluate the first UTI in any male or any female < 5 years of age with renal ultrasound and VCUG (to rule out obstructive disease).

IMMUNOLOGY

Immunodeficiency Syndromes

Present as recurrent or severe infections. In general, the frequency is roughly 1 in 10,000. Table 2.15-6 outlines the clinical presentation, diagnosis, and treatment of common pediatric immunodeficiency disorders.

TABLE 2.15-6. Pediatric Immunodeficiency Disorders

Disorder	Description	Symptoms	Diagnosis	Treatment
B-cell (most common)		Present with recurrent **URIs** and **bacteremia with encapsulated organisms** (pneumococcus, *Staphylococcus, H. influenzae*) after six months of age (when maternal antibodies taper).	**Quantitative Ig levels** (subclasses) and specific antibody responses.	Prophylactic antibiotics and IVIG.
X-linked (**B**ruton's agamma-globulinemia)	A profound **B**-cell deficiency found only in **B**oys.	May present before six months of age. Patients are at risk for pseudomonal infection.		
Common variable immuno-deficiency (CVID)	Ig levels drop in the second and third decades of life.	Associated with an ↑ risk of lymphoma and autoimmune disease.		
IgA deficiency (most common)	Low IgA.	Usually asymptomatic. Recurrent infection may be seen.		
T-cell		**Viral infection, fungal infection, intracellular bacteria** (broader range of infections). Present at 1–3 months of age.	**Absolute lymphocyte count,** mitogen stimulation response, and delayed hypersensitivity skin testing.	
Thymic aplasia (DiGeorge syndrome)	Patients are unable to generate T cells owing to lack of a thymus.	**Tetany** (due to hypocalcemia) in the first few days of life.		Consider thymus transplant instead of bone marrow transplant (BMT).
Ataxia-telangiectasia	A DNA repair defect.	Oculocutaneous telangiectasias and progressive cerebellar ataxia.		**BMT** for severe disease; **IVIG** for antibody deficiency.
Combined			Absolute lymphocyte count and quantitative Ig levels.	
Severe combined immunodeficiency (SCID)	Severe lack of B and T cells.	Frequent and severe bacterial infections, chronic candidiasis, and opportunistic infections.		**BMT** or **stem-cell transplant;** IVIG for antibody deficiency. **PCP prophylaxis.**
Wiskott-Aldrich syndrome	An X-linked disorder with less severe B- and T-cell dysfunction.	**Eczema,** ↑ IgE, ↑ IgA, ↓ IgM, and **thrombocytopenia.**		**Supportive treatment:** IVIG and aggressive antibiotics. Patients rarely survive to adulthood.

TABLE 2.15-6. Pediatric Immunodeficiency Disorders (continued)

DISORDER	DESCRIPTION	SYMPTOMS	DIAGNOSIS	TREATMENT
Phagocytic		Commonly caused by catalase-⊕ (S. aureus) and enteric gram-⊖ organisms.	Absolute neutrophil count; adhesion, chemotactic, phagocytic, and bactericidal assays.	
Chronic granulomatous disease (CGD)	An X-linked or autosomal-recessive disorder with deficient superoxide reduction by PMNs and macrophages.	Chronic GI and GU infections; osteomyelitis, hepatitis. Anemia, lymphadenopathy, and hypergamma-globulinemia.	A **nitroblue tetrazolium** test is **diagnostic.**	**Daily TMP-SMX,** judicious use of antibiotics, gamma-interferon.
Chédiak-Higashi syndrome	An autosomal-recessive defect in neutrophil chemotaxis.	**Recurrent pyogenic skin** and **respiratory infections.** Oculocutaneous albinism, neuropathy, neutropenia.	Blood smear shows PMNs with **giant cytoplasmic granules.**	Aggressive treatment of bacterial infections; corticosteroids, splenectomy.
Complement		Recurrent **sinopulmonary** infections, bacteremia, and/or **meningitis** due to **encapsulated organisms** (*S. pneumoniae*, *H. influenzae* **type b,** *Neisseria meningitidis*).		
C1 esterase deficiency (hereditary angioneurotic edema)	An autosomal-dominant disorder with recurrent angioedema lasting 21–72 hours.	Presents in late childhood or early **adolescence.** Provoked by stress, trauma, or puberty/menses. Can → **life-threatening airway edema.**	Measurement of complement components.	Daily prophylactic antifibrinolytic agents or **danazol.** Purified C1 esterase and FFP prior to surgery.
Terminal complement deficiency (C5–C9)	A deficiency of components of the membrane attack complex (C5–C9). Associated with meningococcal and gonococcal infection.	**Mild, recurrent** infection by *Neisseria* spp. (**meningococcal** or **gonococcal**). Rarely, SLE or glomerulonephritis.	**Total hemolytic complement (CH_{50});** assess the quantity and function of complement pathway components.	Meningococcal vaccine and appropriate antibiotics.

Adapted, with permission, from Le T et al. *First Aid for the USMLE Step 2 CK,* 6th ed. New York: McGraw-Hill, 2007: 368–370.

HIGH-YIELD FACTS

PEDIATRICS

Kawasaki Disease (Mucocutaneous Lymph Node Syndrome)

A common vasculitis of childhood that predisposes to coronary artery aneurysms and to the subsequent development of myocardial ischemia. More common in children < 5 years of age and among those of **Asian**, particularly Japanese, ethnicity.

SYMPTOMS/EXAM

Presents as an acute illness characterized by the following (also see the mnemonic **CRASH and BURN**):

- Prolonged fever
- Bilateral, nonpurulent conjunctivitis
- Swelling of the hands and feet
- Rash
- Cervical lymphadenopathy
- Oropharyngeal changes ("strawberry tongue")

DIAGNOSIS

- A clinical diagnosis.
- Patients must have **fever for > 5 days** and meet **4–5 of the other criteria.**
- Labs reveal ↑ **ESR/CRP** and **thrombocytosis.**

TREATMENT

- Give anti-inflammatory, **high-dose aspirin** during the acute phase to ↓ the incidence of coronary abnormalities.
- Administer **IVIG** to prevent aneurysms and to preserve myocardial contractility (give a single infusion within the first 7–10 days of illness).
- During the convalescent phase, switch to low-dose aspirin for its antiplatelet effect.
- Follow patients with echocardiography.

COMPLICATIONS

Myocarditis; pericarditis; **coronary artery aneurysm** predisposing to myocardial ischemia.

CARDIOLOGY

The incidence of congenital heart disease is approximately 1%. The most common congenital lesion is VSD, followed by ASD. The most common cyanotic lesion is transposition of the great arteries (TGA).

Ventricular Septal Defect (VSD)

A hole in the ventricular septum. Can be membranous (least likely to close spontaneously), perimembranous, or muscular (most likely to close spontaneously).

SYMPTOMS/EXAM

- May be asymptomatic at birth if the lesion is small.
- Cardiac exam may reveal a **pansystolic, vibratory** murmur at the **left lower sternal border without radiation** to the axillae.
- May become symptomatic between two and six months of age.

- If the lesion is large, it may present with symptoms of **CHF** (shortness of breath, pulmonary edema), **frequent respiratory infection, FTT,** and **exercise/feeding intolerance** (sweating with feeds).
- Look for cardiomegaly and crackles on exam.

Diagnosis

- **ECG** shows RVH and LVH.
- **Echocardiography** is definitive.

Treatment

- Treat CHF.
- Follow small muscular VSDs annually.
- Surgically repair large or membranous VSDs to prevent heart failure and pulmonary hypertension.

Complications

If left untreated, VSD may → irreversible **Eisenmenger's syndrome** (pulmonary hypertension, RVH, and reversal of right-to-left shunt).

Atrial Septal Defect (ASD)

A hole in the atrial septum.

Symptoms/Exam

- May be asymptomatic until late childhood or early adulthood.
- Cardiac exam may reveal a **systolic ejection murmur** at the **left upper sternal border.**
- **A wide and fixed split S2** and a **heaving cardiac impulse** at the left lower sternal border are characteristic signs.
- Progression to CHF and cyanosis depends on the size of the lesion.

Diagnosis

- **ECG** shows left-axis deviation.
- **CXR** shows cardiomegaly and ↑ pulmonary vascularity.
- **Echocardiography** is definitive.

Treatment

Treat CHF; follow small ASDs. Surgically repair large ASDs in patients with CHF.

Complications

Eisenmenger's syndrome.

Patent Ductus Arteriosus (PDA)

Failure of the ductus arteriosus (the connection between the pulmonary artery and aorta) to close in the first few days of life. Results in **left-to-right** shunt. Risk factors include **prematurity,** high altitude, and maternal first-trimester **rubella** infection.

SYMPTOMS/EXAM

- Presentation ranges from asymptomatic to CHF.
- Cardiac exam may reveal a **wide pulse pressure; a continuous "machinery" murmur** at the **left upper sternal border;** and **bounding peripheral pulses.**
- A loud S2 is characteristic.

DIAGNOSIS

Echocardiography is definitive, showing shunt flow as well as LA and LV enlargement.

TREATMENT

- **Indomethacin** to close the PDA within days of birth.
- Surgical repair is indicated if the infant is > 6–8 months of age or if indomethacin fails.

COMPLICATIONS

Remember that some cyanotic heart lesions (e.g., TGA) are dependent on a patent ductus, so do not close the PDA in such cases.

Tetralogy of Fallot

Consists of four lesions (see the mnemonic **PROVe**).

> **Anatomy of tetralogy of Fallot—**
>
> **PROVe**
>
> **P**ulmonary stenosis (RV outflow obstruction)
> **R**VH
> **O**verriding aorta
> **V**SD

SYMPTOMS/EXAM

- Presentation ranges from acyanotic ("pink tet") to profoundly cyanotic. Most patients have some cyanosis, depending on the severity of pulmonary stenosis.
- Look for cyanotic "tet spells" in a child who needs to stop running or playing in order to squat.
- Cardiac exam may reveal a **systolic ejection murmur** at the **left sternal border** along with **RV lift.**
- A **single S2** is characteristic.

DIAGNOSIS

- **Echocardiography** is definitive.
- CXR shows a **boot-shaped heart.**

TREATMENT

- If the infant is cyanotic, administer **prostaglandin E** to maintain the PDA.
- Surgical repair is necessary.
- Treat tet spells with **O$_2$, squatting position, fluids, morphine,** propranolol, and phenylephrine if severe.

Transposition of the Great Arteries

The aorta arises from the right ventricle and the pulmonary artery from the left ventricle.

- Extreme cyanosis.
- May have no murmur.
- A **single, loud S2** is characteristic.

DIAGNOSIS

- **Echocardiography** is definitive.
- CXR shows a **egg-on-a-string.**

TREATMENT

- Administer **prostaglandin E** to maintain the PDA.
- Surgical repair is necessary.

Coarctation of the Aorta

Narrowing of the lumen of the aorta → ↓ blood flow below the obstruction and ↑ flow above it. Risk factors include **Turner's syndrome** and male gender; also associated with **bicuspid aortic valve.**

SYMPTOMS/EXAM

- Presents with dyspnea on exertion, syncope, and systemic hypoperfusion/shock.
- Cardiac exam may reveal **hypertension in the upper extremities** and **lower BP in the lower extremities.**
- ↓ **femoral** and **distal lower extremity pulses** are characteristic.

DIAGNOSIS

- **Echocardiography** or **catheterization** is definitive.
- CXR shows **rib notching** due to collateral circulation through the intercostal arteries.

TREATMENT

- Surgical repair or balloon angioplasty.
- Patients require prophylactic antibiotics prior to dental work even after surgical repair.

COMPLICATIONS

Often recurs.

GASTROENTEROLOGY

Pyloric Stenosis

Hypertrophy of the pylorus → gastric outlet obstruction.

SYMPTOMS/EXAM

- Occurs at **3–4 weeks** of life (range: two weeks to four months) in term, **first-born male** infants.
- Presents with progressively **projectile, nonbilious emesis** that may → dehydration.

- Exam reveals an **olive-shaped mass** in the epigastrium along with visible peristaltic waves.

DIAGNOSIS

- Electrolytes show **hypochloremic, hypokalemic metabolic alkalosis** 2° to emesis.
- Ultrasound is the gold standard and shows a **hypertrophied pylorus**.
- Barium studies show a **"string sign"** (a narrow pylorus) or a pyloric beak.

TREATMENT

- **First correct dehydration and electrolyte abnormalities.**
- Surgical repair consists of pyloromyotomy and is usually well tolerated.

Intussusception

Telescoping of a bowel segment into itself (see Figure 2.15-1) may → edema, arterial occlusion, gut necrosis, and death. Intussusception is the **most common** cause of bowel obstruction in the first two years of life. It is usually idiopathic in children < 2 years of age and often has an identifiable "lead point" (e.g., a lymph node) in children > 5 years of age. Ileoileal intussusception is likely due to a pathologic cause.

SYMPTOMS/EXAM

- Presents as a triad of **paroxysmal abdominal pain, "currant jelly" stool, and vomiting.** The child is **completely comfortable between paroxysms.**
- May also present with altered mental status (lethargy or even obtundation); may be preceded by a viral illness.
- Abdominal exam may reveal a **palpable, sausage-shaped mass.**

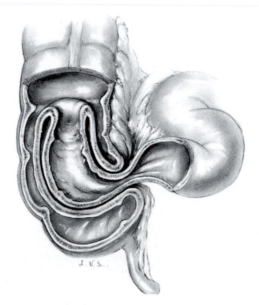

FIGURE 2.15-1.   Intussusception.

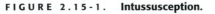

(Reproduced, with permission, from Way LW, Doherty GM. *Current Surgical Diagnosis & Treatment*, 11th ed. New York: McGraw-Hill, 2003: 1323.)

DIAGNOSIS

- Usually ileocecal.
- **Air-contrast enema** is both **diagnostic and therapeutic.**

TREATMENT

Following reduction, treat with supportive care.

COMPLICATIONS

Associated with **Henoch-Schönlein** purpura and **CF.**

Malrotation/Volvulus

Distinguished as follows:

- **Malrotation:** Failure of normal rotation as the gut returns to the abdominal cavity (during the tenth week of gestation).
- **Volvulus:** Incomplete fixation to the posterior abdominal wall, causing a malrotated gut to twist on itself.

SYMPTOMS/EXAM

- **First three weeks of life: Recurrent bilious emesis,** acute small bowel obstruction, or bowel necrosis.
- **Later in infancy/early childhood:** Intermittent intestinal obstruction, malabsorption, protein-losing enteropathy, diarrhea.

DIAGNOSIS

- An **upper GI series** shows the duodenojejunal junction on the **right side** of the spine.
- Contrast studies show a "bird's beak" where the gut is twisted.
- **Barium enema** shows a **mobile cecum** that is not in the RLQ.

TREATMENT

- **Volvulus is a surgical emergency** because gut may necrose as a result of SMA occlusion.
- Surgical repair is necessary in asymptomatic patients in view of the risk of volvulus.

COMPLICATIONS

- The 1° complication is "short bowel syndrome," which occurs when < 30 cm of short bowel is left.
- May also → malnutrition, TPN dependence, and liver failure.

Meckel's Diverticulum

A remnant of the omphalomesenteric duct that persists as an outpouching of the distal ileum. Can contain ectopic (usually gastric or pancreatic) mucosa.

SYMPTOMS/EXAM

- Often asymptomatic.
- Patients may present with **painless rectal bleeding** or **intussusception** (with Meckel's as the lead point).

DIAGNOSIS

- Perform a **technetium radionuclide** scan ("Meckel scan") to detect gastric mucosa.
- The gold standard is tissue obtained surgically.

TREATMENT

- Stabilize the patient with IV fluids; transfuse if needed.
- Surgical exploration is indicated if the patient is symptomatic.
- Bowel resection may be required with resection of diverticula depending on the location and complexity of the lesion.

Necrotizing Enterocolitis

Intestinal necrosis occurring primarily in watershed distributions. Constitutes the most common GI emergency in newborns. Risk factors include **prematurity** and **congenital heart disease.**

SYMPTOMS/EXAM

- **Nonspecific symptoms** include apnea, respiratory failure, lethargy, poor feeding, temperature instability, and hypotension/shock.
- Also presents with **abdominal distention,** gastric retention, tenderness, discoloration, and **bloody stools.**

DIAGNOSIS

AXR shows **pneumatosis intestinalis** and/or **hepatobiliary/portal air.**

TREATMENT

- Medical management with IV fluids (no enteral feeds) and antibiotics if the patient is hemodynamically stable and/or too small or sick to go to the OR.
- **Surgical** management (resection of necrotic bowel) is necessary in the setting of extensive disease and/or hemodynamic instability.

PULMONOLOGY

Croup (Laryngotracheobronchitis)

An acute viral inflammatory disease of the larynx/subglottic space (see Table 2.15-7). Most common in children three months to five years of age. Commonly caused by parainfluenza virus (PIV) type 1, but may also be caused by other PIVs as well as by RSV, influenza, rubeola, adenovirus, and *Mycoplasma pneumoniae.*

SYMPTOMS/EXAM

- Typically has a viral prodrome with URI symptoms.
- Also presents with low-grade fever, mild dyspnea, and inspiratory stridor that worsens with agitation and may improve with cool air or a warm shower.
- Listen for the characteristic **barky cough.**

TABLE 2.15-7.   **Characteristics of Croup, Epiglottitis, and Tracheitis**

	CROUP	EPIGLOTTITIS	TRACHEITIS
Age group	3 months to 3 years	3–7 years	3 months to 2 years
Incidence in children presenting with stridor	88%	8%	2%
Pathogen	PIV	*H. influenzae*	Often *S. aureus*
Onset	Prodrome (1–7 days)	Rapid (4–12 hours)	Prodrome (three days) → acute decompensation (10 hours)
Fever severity	Low grade	High grade	Intermediate grade
Associated symptoms	Barking cough, hoarseness	Muffled voice, drooling	Variable respiratory distress
Position preference	None	Seated, neck extended	None
Response to racemic epinephrine	Stridor improves	None	None
CXR findings	"Steeple sign" on AP films	"Thumbprint sign" on lateral film	Subglottic narrowing

Reproduced, with permission, from Le T et al. *First Aid for the USMLE Step 2 CK,* 6th ed. New York: McGraw-Hill, 2007: 374.

DIAGNOSIS

- Based on clinical findings.
- A **"steeple sign"** formed by subglottic narrowing may be seen on lateral neck x-ray (see Figure 2.15-2).

TREATMENT

- Mist therapy, O_2, aerosolized racemic epinephrine, dexamethasone.
- Following the administration of racemic epinephrine, observe for rebound symptoms.
- Hospitalize patients with stridor at rest.

Epiglottitis

A serious and rapidly progressive infection of the epiglottis and contiguous structures that can → **life-threatening airway obstruction.** It is increasingly rare owing to the Hib vaccine, as the disease is most commonly caused by *H. influenzae* type b. Other pathogenic organisms include *Streptococcus* spp. and nontypable *H. influenzae.*

In epiglottitis, throat examination may cause laryngospasm and airway obstruction.

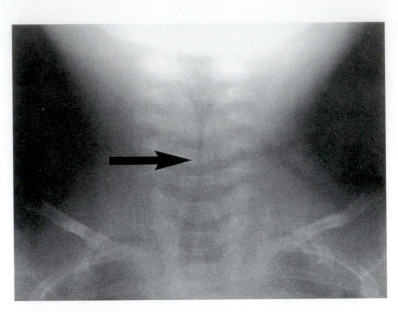

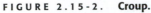

FIGURE 2.15-2. Croup.

The x-ray shows marked subglottic narrowing of the airway (arrow). (Reproduced, with permission, from Stone CK, Humphries RL. *Current Emergency Diagnosis & Treatment*, 5th ed. New York: McGraw-Hill, 2004: 648.)

SYMPTOMS/EXAM

- Maintain a high index of suspicion in children with sudden-onset high fever, dysphagia, drooling, a muffled voice, inspiratory retractions, cyanosis, and soft stridor.
- Patients may be in the "sniffing" position, with the neck hyperextended and the chin protruding.
- The disease can quickly progress to complete airway obstruction and respiratory arrest.

DIAGNOSIS

- Diagnosis is based on the clinical picture.
- Given the risk of laryngospasm and obstruction, **do not examine the throat until the patient is in the OR** with an anesthesiologist present.
- Lateral neck films show the characteristic **"thumbprint sign"** of a swollen epiglottis obliterating the valleculae (see Figure 2.15-3).

TREATMENT

- Keep the patient calm, call anesthesia immediately, and transfer to the OR.
- Treat with endotracheal intubation and IV antibiotics.

Pertussis

Commonly known as "whooping cough." The causative agent is *Bordetella pertussis* or *B. parapertussis*.

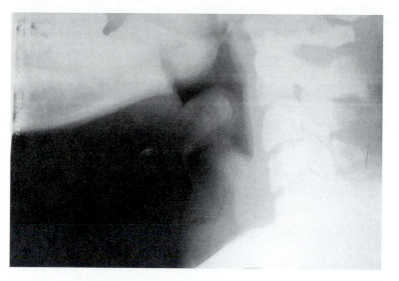

FIGURE 2.15-3. Epiglottitis.

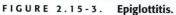

The classic swollen epiglottis ("thumbprint sign") and obstructed airway are seen on x-ray. (Reproduced, with permission, from Stone CK, Humphries RL. *Current Emergency Diagnosis & Treatment*, 5th ed. New York: McGraw-Hill, 2004: 1055.)

SYMPTOMS/EXAM

- The disease has three stages:
    - **Catarrhal:** Presents with nasal congestion, sneezing, and low-grade fever.
    - **Paroxysmal:** Presents with intense coughing paroxysms followed by a "whoop" in young children.
    - **Convalescent:** Characterized by a chronic cough that may last for weeks (also known as "hundred-day cough").
- Children may have posttussive emesis associated with coughing fits.

DIAGNOSIS

Diagnosed by a nasopharyngeal swab that is PCR ⊕ for *B. pertussis*.

TREATMENT

Treat with azithromycin before the convalescent phase, when the patient is no longer contagious.

Respiratory Syncytial Virus (RSV)

The leading cause of bronchiolitis/viral pneumonia in infants and young children. Peak incidence is 2–8 months. Symptoms are due to sloughing of epithelial cells → bronchiolar obstruction.

SYMPTOMS/EXAM

Presents with wheezing and a changing lung exam.

DIAGNOSIS

- Nasopharyngeal swab is PCR ⊕ for RSV.
- CXR shows a nonspecific bilateral, perihilar infiltrate.

TREATMENT

- Supportive care; O_2 as needed.
- Patients may or may not respond to albuterol.
- Endotracheal intubation in severe cases with respiratory failure.

NEUROLOGY

Febrile Seizures

Fever-associated seizures that occur in children six months to six years of age. A ⊕ family history is common. Seizures may present as two types:

- **Simple:** A generalized seizure characterized by a short duration (< 15 minutes), one seizure per 24-hour period, and a quick return to normal function with no residual focal neurologic deficit.
- **Complex:** A focal seizure that may or may not → a generalized seizure and is longer in duration (> 15 minutes). Patients may have > 1 seizure per 24-hour period and an incomplete or slow return to normal neurologic status.

DIAGNOSIS/TREATMENT

- **Simple:** No further evaluation is necessary beyond finding a source for the fever in infants and young children.
- **Complex:** Check electrolytes with glucose, blood cultures, UA, and CBC with differential.
- **Obtain an LP in all children < 1 year of age** as well as in children > 1 year of age in whom CNS infection is suspected.
- EEG and MRI for children with complex febrile seizures.
- Treat the underlying infection; acetaminophen for future illnesses.

Epilepsy Syndromes

Table 2.15-8 outlines the presentation and treatment of common epilepsy syndromes affecting the pediatric population.

ONCOLOGY

Wilms' Tumor

An embryonal tumor of renal origin. Wilms' tumor is the most common renal tumor in children and is usually seen in those 1–4 years of age. Risk factors include a ⊕ family history, neurofibromatosis, aniridia (WAGR syndrome), Beckwith-Wiedemann syndrome, and congenital GU anomalies (e.g., Denys-Drash syndrome).

SYMPTOMS/EXAM

- Patients may have abdominal pain or may present with a painless abdominal or flank mass.
- Hematuria and hypertension are commonly seen.
- Systemic symptoms include weight loss, nausea, emesis, bone pain, dysuria, and polyuria.

TABLE 2.15-8.   Common Pediatric Epilepsy Syndromes

SYNDROME	SYMPTOMS/EXAM	DIAGNOSIS	TREATMENT
Absence seizures	Multiple, brief staring episodes.	A generalized, **3-Hz, spike-and-wave** pattern on EEG.	Ethosuximide.
Infantile spasms (West syndrome)	Affects infants < 1 year of age, presenting with **"jackknife"** spasms and psychomotor arrest/**developmental regression.**	**Hypsarrhythmia** on EEG. Associated with tuberous sclerosis.	ACTH.
Lennox-Gastaut syndrome	The first seizure occurs between one and seven years of age. Presents with multiple, progressive, difficult-to-treat seizure types, including generalized tonic-clonic seizures (GTCS) and drop attacks.	An **atypical spike-and-wave** pattern, primarily in the frontal region, on EEG. Progressive mental retardation. Associated with refractory infantile spasms and tuberous sclerosis.	No effective treatment.
Juvenile myoclonic epilepsy	Affects healthy adolescents, presenting with myoclonic jerks or GTCS in the **early-morning hours/upon awakening.**	May have a genetic basis; patients often have ⊕ family history.	Easily treated with a variety of antiepileptic medications.
Benign partial epilepsy	Affects healthy children, presenting with partial seizures during wakefulness (oral, vocal, upper extremity symptoms). May spread to GTCS during sleep.	Classic **interictal** spikes from the centrotemporal (rolandic) region.	Seizures usually disappear by adolescence.
Landau-Kleffner syndrome	Those affected are developmentally normal children who **lose language ability** between three and six years of age. Often confused with autism.	A bilateral temporal spike and sharp waves on EEG.	Antiepileptic medications may improve the long-term prognosis but cannot reverse language loss.

Data from Hay WW et al. *Current Pediatric Diagnosis & Treatment,* 18th ed. New York: McGraw-Hill, 2007: 721–725.

DIAGNOSIS

- Initially, an abdominal CT or ultrasound should be obtained.
- CXR, chest CT, CBC, LFTs, and BUN/creatinine can be used to assess severity and spread.
- Excisional biopsy to confirm.

TREATMENT

- Transabdominal nephrectomy followed by postoperative chemotherapy (vincristine/dactinomycin).
- Flank irradiation is of benefit in some cases.
- The prognosis is usually good but depends on staging and tumor histology.

Neuroblastoma

A tumor of neural crest cell origin that most commonly affects children < 5 years of age; the most common tumor during infancy. Risk factors include neurofibromatosis, tuberous sclerosis, pheochromocytoma, and Hirschsprung's disease.

SYMPTOMS/EXAM

- Lesions can appear anywhere in the body (e.g., the skin or skull).
- Presentations include abdominal mass/distention/hepatomegaly, anorexia, weight loss, respiratory distress, fatigue, fever, diarrhea, irritability, or neuromuscular symptoms (if paraspinal).
- Other symptoms include leg edema, hypertension, and periorbital bruising ("raccoon eyes").

DIAGNOSIS

- Abdominal CT; 24-hour urinary catecholamines to look for ↑ VMA and HVA.
- Assess severity and spread with CXR, bone scan, CBC, LFTs, BUN/creatinine, and a coagulation screen.

TREATMENT

- Localized tumors are usually cured with excision.
- Chemotherapy includes cyclophosphamide and doxorubicin.
- Radiation can be used as an adjunct.
- The prognosis is improved if the diagnosis is made before one year of age. Staging is based on the Shimada classification.

GENETICS

Common Genetic Disorders

Table 2.15-9 outlines the presentation and diagnosis of genetic syndromes.

TABLE 2.15-9. **Common Genetic Syndromes**

SYNDROME	SYMPTOMS	EXAM	DIAGNOSIS	PROGNOSIS
Trisomy 21 (incidence 1:600)	Hypotonia, brachycephalic head, slanted palpebral fissures, dysplasia of the midphalanx of the fifth finger, single transverse palmar (simian) crease.	Mental retardation, cardiac defects, thyroid disease, GI atresias, atlantoaxial instability, leukemia.	Karyotype, baseline echocardiogram, TFTs, LFTs, CBC.	Fifty percent of those with congenital heart defects survive to 30 years; 80% of those without such defects survive to 30 years. Most who reach age 40 years develop Alzheimer's disease.
Trisomy 18 (incidence 1:4000; 3:1 female predominance)	Clenched hand/ overlapping fingers, intrauterine growth retardation, cardiac defects, rocker-bottom feet.	Profound mental retardation in survivors.	Karyotype with fluorescent in situ hybridization (FISH) analysis.	Fifty percent die by one week and 90% by one year.
Trisomy 13 (incidence 1:12,000)	CNS malformations, polydactyly, seizures, deafness, sloping forehead, aplasia cutis, cleft lip/cleft palate, microphthalmia/eye defects, cardiac defects.	Profound mental retardation in survivors.	Karyotype with FISH analysis.	Forty-four percent die within one month; > 70% die by one year.
22q11 syndrome (DiGeorge syndrome, velocardiofacial syndrome, Shprintzen syndrome, conotruncal anomaly face syndrome) (incidence 1:4000)	Congenital heart disease, palatal abnormalities, prominent/squared nose, thymic hypoplasia/ immune deficiency, absent parathyroid glands/ hypocalcemia.	Mild to moderate mental retardation. Most have speech and language delay, learning disabilities, and feeding difficulties. Psychosis.	FISH analysis for 22q11.2 deletion. Serum calcium, absolute lymphocyte count, renal ultrasound, baseline echocardiogram.	Parents should be tested for being carriers of the deletion.
Turner's syndrome (45,XO) (incidence 1:10,000)	Short female with shield chest, wide-spaced nipples, webbed neck, and congenital lymphedema.	Mental retardation, gonadal dysgenesis, renal anomalies, cardiac defects (coarctation of the aorta), hearing loss.	Karyotype for diagnosis. Baseline echocardiogram, renal ultrasound, BP, hearing screen.	Infertility; normal life span.

TABLE 2.15-9. **Common Genetic Syndromes** (continued)

SYNDROME	SYMPTOMS	EXAM	DIAGNOSIS	PROGNOSIS
Fragile X syndrome (incidence 1:1500 males)	Boys present with macrocephaly, large ears, macroorchidism, and tall stature. Girls may have only learning disabilities.	Mild to profound mental retardation, autism.	DNA analysis shows expansion of a CGG nucleotide repeat in the FMR1 gene. The size of the repeat correlates with disease severity.	Normal life span.
Marfan's syndrome (incidence 1:10,000)	Tall stature, low upper-to-lower-segment ratio, arachnodactyly, joint laxity, scoliosis, pectus excavatum or carinatum, lens dislocation, retinal detachment, dilation of aortic root, mitral valve prolapse, lumbosacral dural ectasia, high-arched palate.	Normal intelligence.	Slit-lamp examination, echocardiography, genetic evaluation. Diagnosis is made clinically.	With treatment/ corrective surgery of aortic root dilation, patients have a normal life span.

Data from Hay WW et al. *Current Pediatric Diagnosis & Treatment,* 18th ed. New York: McGraw-Hill, 2007: 721–725.

SECTION II

Psychiatry

Generalized Anxiety Disorder (GAD)

Lifetime prevalence is 5%; the male-to-female ratio is 1:2. Clinical diagnosis is usually made in the early 20s.

SYMPTOMS/EXAM

- Characterized by **excessive and pervasive worry** about a number of activities or events that → significant impairment or distress.
- Patients may seek medical care for somatic complaints.

DIFFERENTIAL

Substance-induced anxiety disorder, anxiety disorder due to a general medical condition (e.g., hyperthyroidism), panic disorder, OCD, depression, social phobia, hypochondriasis, somatization disorder.

DIAGNOSIS

Diagnostic criteria are as follows:

- Anxiety/worry on most days for at least six months.
- **Three or more somatic symptoms,** including restlessness, fatigue, difficulty concentrating, irritability, muscle tension, and sleep disturbance.

TREATMENT

- Pharmacologic therapy includes venlafaxine, SSRIs, benzodiazepines, and buspirone; second-line treatment with TCAs is appropriate if other antidepressants are ineffective or not tolerated.
- Benzodiazepines offers acute relief, but tolerance and dependence may result from their use.
- Psychotherapy and relaxation training are important adjuncts.

Obsessive-Compulsive Disorder (OCD)

Lifetime prevalence is 2–3%. Typically presents in late adolescence or early adulthood.

SYMPTOMS/EXAM

- Obsessions are **persistent, intrusive thoughts, impulses, or images.** Common themes are contamination and fear of harm to oneself or to others.
- Compulsions are **conscious, repetitive behaviors** (e.g., hand washing) or mental acts (e.g., counting) that patients feel driven to perform.

DIFFERENTIAL

Other anxiety disorders, Tourette's syndrome (multiple motor and vocal tics), depression, schizophrenia, obsessive-compulsive personality disorder (lacks severe functional impairment), medical conditions (e.g., brain tumor, temporal lobe epilepsy, group A β-hemolytic streptococcal infection).

DIAGNOSIS

Obsessions and/or compulsions are recognized at some point as **excessive or unreasonable,** cause marked distress, and are time-consuming (take > 1 hour/day).

TREATMENT

Pharmacotherapy (e.g., SSRIs or clomipramine) and **behavioral therapy** (e.g., exposure and response prevention).

Panic Disorder

More common in women, with a mean age of onset of 25. Lifetime prevalence is 1.5–3.5%. Often accompanied by **agoraphobia,** which is a fear of being in places or situations from which escape is difficult; of being outside the home alone; or of being in public places.

SYMPTOMS/EXAM

Presents as **panic attacks**—discrete periods of intense fear or discomfort in which at least four of the following symptoms develop abruptly and peak within 10 minutes:

- Palpitations
- Sweating
- Trembling
- Shortness of breath
- Chest pain
- Nausea
- Dizziness
- Numbness
- Depersonalization
- Fear of losing control

DIFFERENTIAL

Medical conditions (e.g., angina, hyperthyroidism, hypoglycemia), substance-induced anxiety disorder, other anxiety disorders.

DIAGNOSIS

Recurrent, unexpected panic attacks followed by at least **one month** of worry about attacks.

TREATMENT

- Cognitive-behavioral therapy (CBT).
- Pharmacotherapy includes SSRIs, alone or in combination with benzodiazepines. TCAs or MAOIs should be used only if SSRIs are not tolerated or are ineffective.
- Benzodiazepines (e.g., alprazolam, clonazepam) are effective for immediate relief but have abuse potential.

Phobias

The three categories of phobia are agoraphobia, social phobia, and specific phobia. Lifetime prevalence is 10%.

SYMPTOMS/EXAM

- Phobias are persistent, excessive, or unreasonable fear and/or avoidance of an object or situation that → significant distress or impairment.
- Exposure to the object or stimulus may precipitate **panic attacks.**

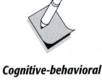

Cognitive-behavioral therapy is a type of therapy that helps patients learn new ways to cope by:
- *Identifying automatic thoughts, or "cognitive distortions."*
- *Testing the automatic thoughts.*
- *Identifying and testing the validity of maladaptive assumptions.*
- *Strategizing on alternative ways to deal with problems.*

DIFFERENTIAL

Other anxiety disorders, depression, avoidant and schizoid personality disorders, schizophrenia, appropriate fear, normal shyness.

DIAGNOSIS

- **Social phobia** is characterized by unreasonable, marked, and persistent **fear of scrutiny and embarrassment in social or performance situations** (also referred to as social anxiety disorder.).
- **Specific phobia** is immediately **cued by an object or a situation** (e.g., spiders, animals, heights).
- In adults, the **duration is six or more months.**

TREATMENT

- CBT and pharmacotherapy (e.g., SSRIs, benzodiazepines, β-blockers) are effective for social phobias.
- **Behavioral therapy** that uses exposure and desensitization is best for specific phobia.

Post-traumatic Stress Disorder (PTSD)

Results from exposure to a traumatic event that involved **actual or threatened death or serious injury** and evoked **intense fear, helplessness, or horror.** The lifetime prevalence is 8%.

SYMPTOMS/EXAM

- Examples of traumatic events include war, torture, natural disasters, assault, rape, and serious accidents.
- Patients with PTSD may have experienced the trauma personally, or they may have witnessed the event in a way that leads them to feel personally threatened, helpless, and horrified (e.g., a child witnessing a parent being assaulted).
- Watch for survival guilt, personality change, substance abuse, depression, and suicide.

DIFFERENTIAL

- **Acute stress disorder:** Symptoms are the same as similar to those of PTSD but last < 1 month and occur within one month of a trauma, and empahsizes dissociative symptoms.
- **Adjustment disorder with anxiety:** Emotional or behavioral symptoms within three months of a stressor; lasts < 6 months.
- **Other:** Depression, OCD, acute intoxication or withdrawal, factitious disorders, malingering, borderline personality disorder.

DIAGNOSIS

Symptoms persist for **> 1 month** and include the following:

- Reexperiencing of the event (e.g., nightmares, flashbacks).
- Avoidance of trauma-related stimuli or numbing of general responsiveness.
- Hyperarousal (e.g., hypervigilance, exaggerated startle, irritability, difficulty falling or staying asleep).

HIGH-YIELD FACTS

PSYCHIATRY

275

TREATMENT

- Pharmacotherapy includes first-line treatment with SSRIs; if SSRIs are not tolerated or are ineffective, use TCAs or MAOIs. Second-generation antipsychotics (e.g., risperidone, olanzapine, quetiapine), anticonvulsants (e.g., divalproex, topiramate), α_2-adrenergic agonists (clonidine), or β-blockers (propranolol) may be helpful for some patients.
- CBT and group therapy are also effective.

MOOD DISORDERS

Major Depressive Disorder (MDD)

Untreated episodes of MDD can last for four or more months, and the risk of recurrence is 50% after only one episode. The average age of onset is in the mid-20s; lifetime prevalence is 10–25% for females (the highest risk is in the childbearing years) and 5–12% for males. The **male-to-female ratio is 1:2.** MDD is often associated with a life stressor, and up to 15% of those affected die by suicide.

SYMPTOMS/EXAM

Diagnosis requires depressed mood OR loss of interest or pleasure. Patients have at least five of the following symptoms during a two-week period:

- Significant weight loss or weight gain, or change in appetite.
- Insomnia or hypersomnia.
- Psychomotor agitation or retardation.
- Fatigue or loss of energy.
- Feelings of worthlessness or excessive guilt.
- ↓ ability to concentrate, or indecisiveness.
- Recurrent thoughts of death or suicide.

DIFFERENTIAL

- **Dysthymia:** A milder, chronic depressed state of two or more years' duration.
- **Bereavement:** Does not involve severe impairment or suicidality; usually improves within two months.
- **Adjustment disorder with depressed mood:** Has fewer symptoms; occurs within three months of a stressor; lasts < 6 months.
- **Other:** Substance-induced mood disorder (e.g., illicit drugs, β-blockers); mood disorder due to a medical condition (e.g., hypothyroidism); dementia.

DIAGNOSIS

- Requires at least **five signs/symptoms,** one of which must be **depressed mood or anhedonia** (loss of interest or pleasure).
- Symptoms last ≥ 2 weeks and must → **significant dysfunction or impairment.**

TREATMENT

- **Pharmacotherapy:** The effectiveness of antidepressants is similar between and within classes (50–70% of patients), and these drugs take at least 3–4 weeks to have an effect. Thus, the selection of an antidepressant is based on side effect profiles, safety and tolerability of side effects, patient prefer-

---

Symptoms of depression—SIG E CAPS

Sleep (↓/↑)
Interest (↓)
Guilt
Energy (↓)
Concentration
Appetite (↓/↑)
Psychomotor agitation or retardation
Suicidal ideation

Cognitive decline is a common sign of major depressive disorder in the elderly ("pseudodementia").

Seasonal affective disorder (SAD), typified by fall/winter depression, is treated with bright-light therapy.

ence, cost, and the patient's previous response to specific antidepressants. Continue treatment for six or more months.

- **Electroconvulsive therapy (ECT):**
  - Safe and effective.
  - Best for refractory or catatonic depression, but may also be used for acute mania or acute psychosis and when the patient refuses to eat or drink (e.g., severely depressed elderly) or is suicidally depressed.
  - Adverse effects include postictal confusion, arrhythmias, headache, and **retrograde amnesia.**
  - Relative contraindications include intracranial mass, aneurysm, and recent MI/stroke. **Pregnancy is not a contraindication.**
- **Psychotherapy:** Psychotherapy combined with antidepressants is more effective than either modality alone.

Bipolar Disorder

A family history of bipolar illness significantly ↑ risk. Prevalence is 1%; the **male-to-female ratio is 1:1.** About 10–15% of those affected die by suicide.

SYMPTOMS/EXAM

- **A manic episode** is defined as follows:
  - **One week** of an abnormally and persistently **elevated ("euphoria"), expansive, or irritable mood.**
  - At least three of the following (**four if the mood is irritable**):
    - Inflated self-esteem or grandiosity
    - ↓ need for sleep
    - Pressured speech
    - Flight of ideas/racing thoughts
    - Distractibility
    - ↑ goal-directed activity/psychomotor agitation
- **A mixed episode** must meet the criteria for **both** manic and depressive episodes for one week or more.

DIFFERENTIAL

- **Cyclothymic disorder:** Chronic cycles of mild depression and mania for two or more years.
- **Other:** Substance-induced mood disorder, schizophrenia, schizoaffective disorder, personality disorders, medical conditions (e.g., temporal lobe epilepsy, hyperthyroidism), ADHD.

DIAGNOSIS

- **Bipolar I disorder:** One or more mixed or manic episodes. Depressive episodes are common **but are not required for diagnosis.**
- **Bipolar II disorder:** Characterized by **hypomanic** rather than manic episodes, where *hypomania* is defined as < 4 days of manic symptoms that **do not cause marked functional impairment, do not require hospitalization, and do not present with psychotic features.**

TREATMENT

- **Acute mania:** Lithium, anticonvulsants, antipsychotics, benzodiazepines, ECT.
- **Bipolar depression:** First-line treatment is lithium or lamotrigine. **Monotherapy with an antidepressant is not recommended.** If the patient does

Screen for bipolar disorder before starting antidepressants, which can induce acute mania or psychosis in bipolar patients.

Severe MDD can present with psychotic symptoms, in which case an antipsychotic in addition to an antidepressant may be temporarily required.

not respond to first-line treatment, the next step may include adding lamotrigine (if started with lithium), bupropion, or SSRIs. In severe cases, consider ECT.

Schizophrenia

Lifetime prevalence is 1%. Peak onset is **18–25 years for men** and **25–35 years and perimenopausally for women.** Few patients have a complete recovery. There is a high incidence of substance abuse, and > 75% of patients smoke cigarettes. The suicide rate is 10%.

SYMPTOMS/EXAM

At least two of the following are required for one or more months, with **continuous signs for ≥ 6 months:**[*]

- **Delusions:** Fixed, false beliefs.
- **Hallucinations:** Usually auditory, but can be visual, olfactory (rare), or tactile.
- Disorganized speech.
- Grossly disorganized or catatonic behavior.
- **Negative symptoms:** Affective flattening, avolition, apathy, alogia.

DIFFERENTIAL

- **Brief psychotic disorder:** Symptoms are of **< 1 month's duration;** onset often follows a psychosocial stressor. Associated with a better prognosis.
- **Delusional disorder: Nonbizarre delusions for one or more months** in the absence of other psychotic symptoms; often chronic. (A *bizarre delusion* is defined as an absurd, totally implausible, strange false belief—e.g., the conviction that aliens from another planet have implanted electrodes into one's brain.)
- **Schizoaffective disorder:** Mood symptoms are present for a significant portion of the illness, but psychotic symptoms have been present **without a mood episode.**
- **Schizophreniform disorder:** Diagnosed by the same criteria as those for schizophrenia, but with a **duration of < 6 months.**
- **Other:** Mood disorder with psychotic features; substance-induced psychosis (e.g., amphetamines) or drug withdrawal (e.g., alcoholic hallucinosis); psychosis due to a general medical condition (e.g., brain tumor); delirium or dementia.

TREATMENT

Antipsychotic medications (neuroleptics). Hospitalize when the patient is a danger to himself or to others. Psychosocial treatments, individual supportive psychotherapy, and family therapy help prevent relapse.

---

[*]Only one of the above symptoms is required for diagnosis if delusions are bizarre, or if hallucinations include a running commentary or a conversation between two voices.

HIGH-YIELD FACTS

PSYCHIATRY

Delirium

Delirium is common in hospitalized medical or surgical patients (15–70%) and is a **medical, not psychiatric, disorder.** However, since delirium may mimic psychosis, psychiatrists are often consulted on this problem. Risk factors include elderly age, hospitalization, medications (benzodiazepines, anticholinergics and opioids), starting multiple new medications at once, preexisting cognitive deficits, electrolyte abnormalities, malnutrition, hypoxia, a windowless ICU environment, infections, vision or hearing deficits, and severe illness.

SYMPTOMS/EXAM

- Delirium includes:
    - **Disturbance of consciousness.**
    - **Altered cognition** (e.g., memory, orientation, language disturbance).
    - **Acute onset.**
    - **History** suggesting a probable medical cause of delirium.
- The above symptoms typically fluctuate during the day ("waxing and waning").

DIFFERENTIAL

In contrast to delirium, dementia usually has an insidious onset; it includes chronic memory and executive function deficits, and symptoms tend not to fluctuate during the day (see Table 2.16-1).

DIAGNOSIS

An evaluation may include CBC, electrolytes, BUN/creatinine, glucose, a liver panel, UA, urine toxicology, vitamin B_{12}/folate, TSH, RPR, HIV, blood culture, serum calcium/phosphorus/magnesium, pulse oximetry, arterial blood gas, CSF, or serum drug screening.

TREATMENT

- Treat the underlying medical condition.
- Minimize or discontinue delirium-inducing drugs (benzodiazepines, anticholinergics), and simplify medication regimens if possible.
- Recommend reorientation techniques (clocks, wall calendar); provide an environment that will facilitate healthy sleep/wake cycles.
- Pharmacotherapy may be beneficial and includes low-dose antipsychotics (haloperidol, risperidone, olanzapine, quetiapine), usually for short-term use.

Depression and Anxiety Due to a General Medical Condition

- Depression can be 2° to drug intoxication (alcohol or sedative-hypnotics; antihypertensives such as methyldopa, clonidine, and propranolol) or to stroke, hypothyroidism, MS, or SLE.
- Anxiety may be caused by drugs (**caffeine, sympathomimetics, steroids**), endocrinopathies (pheochromocytoma, **hypercortisolism, hyperthyroidism, hyperparathyroidism**), metabolic disorders (**hypoxemia, hypercalcemia, hypoglycemia**), or SLE.

HIGH-YIELD FACTS

PSYCHIATRY

TABLE 2.16-1. Dementia vs. Delirium

	DEMENTIA	DELIRIUM
Onset	Chronic; months to years.	Acute; hours to days.
Course	Progressive; usually irreversible.	Abrupt onset; usually reversible.
Consciousness	Alert.	Fluctuating ability to focus and shift attention.
Cognition	Disrupted memory, orientation, and language.	Similar to dementia, but may include perceptual disturbances (hallucinations) and paranoia.
History	No acute change.	Evidence of a general medical condition causing the problem.
Causes	Alzheimer's disease, Huntington's disease, vascular dementia, AIDS dementia, MDD in the elderly.	General medical condition (seizures, postictal state, infections, thyroid disorders, UTI, vitamin deficiencies); substances (e.g., cocaine, opioids, PCP); head trauma, kidney disease, sleep deprivation.

PERSONALITY DISORDERS

Defined as enduring patterns of inner experience and behavior that deviate from cultural standards; are pervasive and inflexible; begin in adolescence or early adulthood; are stable over time; and → distress or impairment (see Table 2.16-2).

SOMATOFORM DISORDERS

Somatization Disorder

Pain symptoms at four or more sites that are not intentionally produced and cannot be explained by a general medical condition. Onset is before the age of 30; much more prevalent in women.

Conversion Disorder

- Presents with **sensory symptoms, motor deficits, or "psychogenic seizures"** that are not intentionally produced and cannot be explained by an organic etiology.
- Relation to a **stressful event** suggests association with psychological factors.

Table 2.16-2. **Signs and Symptoms of Personality Disorders**

CLUSTER	DISORDERS	CHARACTERISTICS	CLINICAL DILEMMA/STRATEGY
Cluster A: "weird"	Paranoid	Distrustful, suspicious; interpret others' motives as malevolent.	Patients are suspicious and distrustful of doctors and rarely seek medical attention.
	Schizoid	Isolated, detached "loners." Restricted emotional expression.	Be clear, honest, noncontrolling, and nondefensive. Avoid humor. Maintain emotional distance.
	Schizotypal	Detached "loners" who also have cognitive or perceptual distortions (e.g., magical thinking).	
Cluster B: "wild"	Borderline	Unstable mood/relationships, feelings of emptiness. Impulsive.	Patients change the rules, demand attention, and feel they are special.
	Histrionic	Excessively emotional and attention seeking. Sexually provocative.	Will manipulate staff and doctor ("splitting").
	Narcissistic	Grandiose, need admiration, sense of entitlement. Lack empathy.	Be firm: Stick to treatment plan. Be fair: Do not be punitive or
	Antisocial	Violate rights of others, social norms, laws. Impulsive. Lack remorse.	derogatory. Be consistent: Do not change rules.
Cluster C: "worried and wimpy"	Obsessive-compulsive	Preoccupied with perfectionism, order, control. Inflexible morals, values.	Patients are controlling and may sabotage their treatment. Words may be inconsistent with actions.
	Avoidant	Socially inhibited, rejection sensitive. Fear being disliked or ridiculed.	Avoid power struggles. Give clear recommendations, but do not push
	Dependent	Submissive, clingy, need to be taken care of. Difficulty making decisions.	patients into decisions.

Hypochondriasis

Preoccupation over > 6 months with **fear of having a serious disease** based on misinterpretation of symptoms. Patients are not reassured by ⊖ medical evaluations, but symptoms are not delusions.

Pain Disorder

A pain syndrome that is exacerbated by or related to psychological factors.

Body Dysmorphic Disorder

Preoccupation with an **imagined defect** in appearance. Multiple visits to surgeons and dermatologists are common.

VOLITIONAL/INTENTIONAL DISORDERS

Factitious Disorder

- Symptoms are intentionally feigned for **2° gain** (e.g., assuming a sick role).
- More common in men and in health care workers.

HIGH-YIELD FACTS

PSYCHIATRY

Monoamine Oxidase Inhibitors (MAOIs)

- Includes **phenelzine, selegiline,** and **tranylcypromine.** MAOIs are also considered to be **second-line agents** due to their relatively poor side effect profile compared to the newer antidepressants.
- **Side effects:**
  - Common side effects include orthostatic hypotension, insomnia, weight gain, edema, and sexual dysfunction.
  - May → **tyramine-induced hypertensive crisis.** Dietary restrictions include aged cheeses, sour cream, yogurt, pickled herring, cured meats, and alcoholic beverages.
  - Potentially fatal **serotonin syndrome** can occur if MAOIs are combined with SSRIs, TCAs, meperidine, fentanyl, or indirect sympathomimetics (e.g., those found in **OTC cold remedies**).

Antipsychotics

First-Generation ("Typical") Antipsychotics

- **Mechanism of action:** Act through DA receptor blockade.
- **Applications:** Used for psychotic disorders and acute agitation. Cheap and effective. Include the following:
  - **High-potency agents** (haloperidol, fluphenazine): Associated with more extrapyramidal symptoms (EPS).
  - **Low-potency agents** (thioridazine, chlorpromazine): Associated with more sedation, anticholinergic effects, and hypotension.
- **Side effects:** Key side effects include the following:
  - EPS: See Table 2.16-4.
  - **Hyperprolactinemia:** Amenorrhea, gynecomastia, galactorrhea.
  - **Anticholinergic effects:** Dry mouth, blurry vision, urinary retention, constipation.

Aged cheeses and red wine can precipitate a hypertensive crisis in patients taking MAOIs.

> **Side effects of MAOIs—**
>
> **The 6 H's**
>
> **H**epatocellular jaundice/necrosis
> **H**ypotension (postural)
> **H**eadache
> **H**yperreflexia
> **H**allucinations
> **H**ypomania

TABLE 2.16-4. Extrapyramidal Symptoms and Treatment

Symptom	Description	Treatment
Acute dystonia	Involuntary muscle contraction or spasm (e.g., torticollis, oculogyric crisis).	Give an anticholinergic (benztropine) or diphenhydramine. To prevent, give prophylactic benztropine with an antipsychotic.
Akathisia	Subjective/objective restlessness.	↓ neuroleptic and try β-blockers (propranolol). Benzodiazepines or anticholinergics may help.
Dyskinesia	Pseudoparkinsonism (e.g., shuffling gait, cogwheel rigidity).	Give an anticholinergic (benztropine) or DA agonist (amantadine). ↓ dose of neuroleptic or discontinue (if tolerated).
Tardive dyskinesia	Stereotypic oral-facial movements. Likely from DA receptor sensitization. Often irreversible (50%).	Discontinue or ↓ dose of neuroleptic, attempt treatment with more appropriate drugs, and consider changing neuroleptic (e.g., to clozapine or risperidone). **Giving anticholinergics or ↓ neuroleptic may initially worsen tardive dyskinesia.**

- Neuroleptic malignant syndrome.
- **Other:** Cardiac arrhythmias, weight gain, sedation.

SECOND-GENERATION ("ATYPICAL") ANTIPSYCHOTICS

- **Mechanism of action:** Act through $5\text{-}HT_2$ and DA antagonism.
- **Applications:** Currently first-line therapy for schizophrenia. Benefits are **fewer EPS and anticholinergic effects** than first-generation agents.
    - **Risperidone, olanzapine, quetiapine, ziprasidone,** and **aripiprazole** are commonly used.
    - **Clozapine** is second-line therapy and is used for treatment-refractory patients.
- **Side effects:**
    - May cause **sedation, weight gain, type 2 DM, and QT prolongation.** Obtain baseline values, and monitor the patient's weight, lipid profile, and glucose levels
    - Common side effects of clozapine include sedation, constipation, weight gain, and sialorrhea (drooling). Clozapine may also cause **agranulocytosis** and seizures (requires weekly CBCs during the first six months and then biweekly).

Mood Stabilizers

Lithium toxicity treatment may include hemodialysis.

- **Lithium:**
    - **Applications:** Used for long-term maintenance or prophylaxis of bipolar disorder. Effective in mania and in augmenting antidepressants in depression and OCD. ↓ suicidal behavior/risk in bipolar disorder. Has a **narrow therapeutic index** and requires monitoring of serum levels.
    - **Side effects:**
        - Include thirst, polyuria, fine tremor, weight gain, diarrhea, nausea, acne, and hypothyroidism. **Monitor renal and thyroid function.**
        - Lithium toxicity presents with a **coarse tremor, ataxia,** vomiting, confusion, seizures, and arrhythmias.
- **Valproic acid:**
    - **Applications:** First-line agent for acute mania and bipolar disorder; effective in rapid cyclers (those with four or more episodes per year).
    - **Side effects:**
        - Sedation, weight gain, hair loss, tremor, ataxia, GI distress.
        - Pancreatitis, thrombocytopenia, and fatal hepatotoxicity are uncommon.
        - Monitor platelets, LFTs, and serum drug levels.
- **Carbamazepine:**
    - **Applications:** Second-line agent for acute mania and bipolar disorder.
    - **Side effects:**
        - Common side effects include nausea, sedation, rash, and ataxia.
        - Rare side effects include hepatic toxicity, hyponatremia, bone marrow suppression, and **Stevens-Johnson syndrome.**
        - Monitor blood counts, transaminases, and electrolytes. Drug interactions complicate its use.
- **Other anticonvulsants (lamotrigine, gabapentin, topiramate):**
    - Efficacy is not well documented.
    - Do not require blood level monitoring and do not cause weight gain.
    - **Lamotrigine or lithium** may be used as first-line agents for **bipolar depression.** Lamotrigine is associated with Stevens-Johnson syndrome.

The two measurements most often used in pulmonary function testing are FEV_1 (forced expiratory volume in one second) and FVC (forced vital capacity).

- An FEV_1/FVC ratio < 70% indicates **obstruction** (e.g., COPD, asthma, chronic bronchitis, bronchiectasis).
- The severity of FEV_1 is used to grade obstructive airway diseases.
- An FVC < 80% is suggestive of **restriction** (e.g., obesity, kyphosis, inflammatory/fibrosing lung disease, interstitial lung disease).
- Other points to keep in mind when looking at a set of PFTs (see Table 2.17-1) are as follows:
    - Total lung capacity (TLC) will be ↓ in **restrictive** processes and ↑ in **obstructive** processes.
    - DL_{CO}, defined as the diffusing capacity of carbon monoxide, measures the gas exchange capacity of the capillary-alveolar interface.

Defined as a room-air O_2 saturation < 88% or a PaO_2 < **55 mmHg** on ABG measurement or evidence of cor pulmonale. Think about the **cause of hypoxia** in order to determine the next step:

- **Ventilation-perfusion (V/Q) mismatch:**
    - Examples include asthma, COPD, nonmassive pulmonary embolus (PE), and pneumonia.
    - **Responds to O_2.**
    - Associated with an ↑ alveolar-arterial oxygen (A-a) gradient.
- **Hypoventilation:**
    - Commonly due to **oversedation** from medications.
    - **Responds to O_2.**
    - Characterized by a **normal A-a gradient.**
- **Decreased diffusion:**
    - Think about interstitial or parenchymal lung diseases.
    - Characterized by an ↑ **A-a gradient.**
    - **Responds to O_2.**
    - Associated with a **very low DL_{CO}.**
- **High altitude:**
    - Characterized by a **normal A-a gradient.**
    - **Responds to O_2.**

*Hypoxia due to shunt physiology will **not** correct with supplemental O_2*

Hypoxia can lead to apnea in infants, so be sure to use supplemental O_2 to maintain O_2 saturations.

TABLE 2.17-1. PFTs in Common Settings

	FEV₁/FVC	TLC	DL_{CO}
Asthma	Normal/↓	Normal	Normal/↑
COPD	↓	↑	Normal/↑
Fibrotic disease	Normal/↑	↓	↓
Extrathoracic restriction	Normal	↓	Normal

- **Shunt physiology:**
  - Think about acute respiratory distress syndrome (**ARDS**), massive PE, patent foramen ovale, or patent ductus arteriosus (**PDA**).
  - Typically **does not respond to O_2 (must use positive pressure).**
  - Characterized by an ↑ **A-a gradient.**

TREATMENT

Always treat hypoxic patients with adequate amounts of O_2 to maintain saturations of > 90% or a PaO_2 > 60 mmHg. Definitive treatment entails removing the underlying cause of the hypoxia.

BRONCHIOLITIS

Involves inflammation in smaller airways; occurs most often in infants from two months to one year of age. **RSV** accounts for the vast majority of cases. Other viral causes include adenovirus, influenza, and parainfluenza.

SYMPTOMS

Patients are typically **infants.** Symptoms begin as those of a **URI** (sore throat, runny nose) and **progress** over the next 3–7 days to lower respiratory symptoms (cough, wheezing).

EXAM

Patients may have cough, fever, **tachypnea,** and **intercostal retractions.** Look for cyanosis, expiratory wheezing, and crackles.

DIAGNOSIS

- Look for **hyperinflation** of the lungs on CXR with flattening of the diaphragms and mild interstitial infiltrates.
- RSV may be diagnosed with **ELISA** or fluorescent antibody test.

TREATMENT

- **Supplemental O_2** (oxygen tent).
- Aerosolized **albuterol.**
- In cases of RSV, use **ribavirin** in patients with severe disease or underlying cardiac or pulmonary problems.

CYSTIC FIBROSIS (CF)

An **autosomal-recessive** disorder with mutations located in the CFTR gene → abnormal transfer of sodium and chloride. Multiple exocrine glands and cilia in various organs become dysfunctional. The **most common** genetic disease in the United States and among **Caucasians, affecting 1 in 3200.**

SYMPTOMS

- Patients typically present in childhood or adolescence. Look for patients with **recurrent pulmonary infections,** sinusitis, **bronchiectasis, infertility,** or **pancreatic insufficiency** (diabetes, malabsorption, steatorrhea).
- Infants may present with **meconium ileus** or **intussusception.**

Think of methemoglobinemia in a patient with a low O_2 saturation on pulse oximetry but a normal PaO_2 on ABG. Treatment is with methylene blue.

Intubate infants with ↑ PCO_2 levels or ↑ O_2 requirements.

EXAM

Patients may have short stature. Lung exam often reveals **wheezing, crackles, or squeaks. Clubbing** may be present. Hyperinflation is seen early, followed by peribronchial cuffing, mucus plugging, and bronchiectasis.

DIAGNOSIS

- Diagnosis is made with a sweat chloride test of **> 60 mEq/L** (must be confirmed on two different days).
- Genetic testing can confirm the presence of many of the genetic mutations.

TREATMENT

- Manage the disease with attention to nutrition, **chest physiotherapy, bronchodilators, pancreatic enzymes, mucolytics** (DNase), and stool softeners (fiber).
- Patients need supplemental **fat-soluble vitamins (A, D, E, K)** to address fat malabsorption.
- **Chronic** and **chronic intermittent oral antibiotics (azithromycin)** or **inhaled antibiotics (tobramycin)** may also be beneficial. *Pseudomonas aeruginosa* is common, and therapies are tailored to treat the infecting organism.
- In severe end-stage pulmonary disease, bilateral **lung transplant** should be considered, since it is **the only definitive treatment.**

COMPLICATIONS

Associated with both **pseudomonal** and **staphylococcal** infections.

ASTHMA

Asthma is chronic inflammation of the airways. Patients may be atopic (the classic triad is eczema, wheezing, and seasonal rhinitis).

Think of GERD in a patient with chronic cough that worsens when the patient lies supine.

SYMPTOMS

- Look for **intermittent wheezing,** coughing, chest tightness, or shortness of breath.
- Symptoms may be seasonal or may occur after exposure to **triggers** (URIs, dust, pets, cold air) or with exercise.

EXAM

- Determine the severity of the attack by assessing **mental status, the ability to speak in full sentences,** the presence of cyanosis, use of accessory muscles, and, of course, vital signs. Oxygen saturation monitoring is not adequate, as ventilation is more important than oxygenation.
- Look for wheezing or rhonchi along with a prolonged expiratory phase. Patients with severe exacerbations may have ↓ wheezing. These patients will need prompt assessment of their gas exchange (with ABG analysis) along with aggressive treatment (see below).

DIFFERENTIAL

Not all that wheezes is asthma! Rule out foreign-body aspiration, laryngeal spasm or irritation, GERD, and CHF. In patients with chronic cough, think about allergic rhinitis. PFTs can help differentiate asthma from COPD and chronic bronchitis (see below), although there are overlapping findings.

DIAGNOSIS

- CXR may show **hyperinflation** (suggesting air trapping) but can also be normal.
- Definitive diagnosis is made by demonstration of **obstruction** on PFTs:
    - **Reversibility** with bronchodilators as defined by an ↑ in FEV_1 or FVC by 12% and 200 mL.
    - **Methacholine challenge** testing in a monitored setting can be used to confirm the diagnosis (not often used).

TREATMENT

- **Chronic asthma:** See Table 2.17-2.
- **Acute asthma exacerbation:** Recognizing the severity of the attack and instituting the correct therapy are the keys to treatment:
    - Initiate **short-acting β-agonist** (albuterol) therapy (nebulizer or MDI).
    - Administer a **systemic corticosteroid** such as methylprednisolone or prednisone.
    - Begin **inhaled corticosteroids** as well.
    - Follow patients closely with **peak flows** and tailor therapy to the response.
    - Chronic antibiotics (without evidence of infection), anticholinergics, cromolyn, and leukotriene antagonists are generally **not useful** in this setting.

A ⊖ methacholine challenge excludes asthma.

Inhaled corticosteroids are safe for use in pregnancy.

Be sure to check an ABG in any patient with an asthma exacerbation. A normal P_{CO_2} suggests that the patient is tiring out and about to crash..

TABLE 2.17-2. Medications for Chronic Treatment of Asthma

TYPE	SYMPTOMS (DAY/NIGHT)	FEV_1	MEDICATIONS
Severe persistent	Continual Frequent	≤ 60%	High-dose inhaled corticosteroids + long-acting inhaled β-agonists. Possible PO steroids. PRN short-acting bronchodilator.
Moderate persistent	Daily > 1 night/week	60–80%	Low- to medium-dose inhaled corticosteroids + long-acting inhaled β-agonists. PRN short-acting bronchodilator.
Mild persistent	> 2/week but < 1/day > 2 nights/month	≥ 80%	Low-dose inhaled corticosteroids. PRN short-acting bronchodilator.
Mild intermittent	≤ 2 days/week ≤ 2 nights/month	≥ 80%	No daily medications. PRN short-acting bronchodilator.

Reproduced, with permission, from Le T et al. *First Aid for the USMLE Step 2 CK,* 6th ed. New York: McGraw-Hill, 2007: 417.

Think α_1-antitrypsin deficiency in young patients with COPD and bullae.

A combination of emphysema and chronic bronchitis, COPD generally involves the destruction of lung parenchyma. This results in ↓ elastic recoil, which in turn → air trapping. **TLC** ↑ due to a **rise** in the **residual volume (RV)**. Chronic bronchitis is defined as chronic productive cough for three months in each of two successive years.

SYMPTOMS

Look for cough, dyspnea, wheezing, and a **history of smoking.** Dyspnea is usually progressive. In advanced disease, weight loss may be seen.

EXAM

- **Emphysema ("pink puffer"):** ↓ breath sounds, minimal cough, dyspnea, pursed lip breathing, hypercarbia/hypoxia late, barrel chest.
- **Chronic bronchitis ("blue bloater"):** Rhonchi; productive cough; cyanosis but with mild dyspnea; hypercarbia/hypoxia early. Patients are frequently overweight with peripheral edema.
- **Look for clubbing.**
- Patients may also have evidence of **cor pulmonale** (right heart failure from pulmonary hypertension).

DIAGNOSIS

- PFTs may suggest the diagnosis in patients who smoke.
- **FEV_1/FVC is < 80%.**
- The condition is **not reversible** with bronchodilators.
- ↓ DL_{CO} occurs in more advanced disease.
- TLC is ↑.
- CXR shows hyperlucent, **hyperinflated** lungs with **flat diaphragms** and a narrow cardiac silhouette (see Figure 2.17-1).

Only O_2 therapy and smoking cessation have been shown to improve survival in patients with COPD.

TREATMENT

- **Chronic COPD:**
    - The mainstays of treatment are inhaled β-agonists **(albuterol)** and **anticholinergics (ipratropium).**
    - **O_2 therapy** is indicated for patients with an O_2 saturation < 88% or a **PaO_2 < 55 mmHg** or PaO_2 55–60 and evidence of cor pulmonale. It is also indicated with desaturations < 88% during exercise or at night.
    - **Smoking cessation is key.**
    - Inhaled corticosteroids **do not** play a major role unless there is significant reversible airway disease on PFTs.
    - Remember to **vaccinate** COPD patients against **influenza** (yearly) and **pneumococcal pneumonia** (at least once).
- **Acute COPD exacerbations:**
    - Defined as **increasing dyspnea** or a **change in cough or sputum production.**
    - Check a **CXR** to look for causes of the exacerbation (pneumonia, CHF).
    - Administer **O_2** to maintain a saturation of 90–95% (no need to go higher!).
    - Initiate an inhaled **β-agonist (albuterol)** and **anticholinergics (ipratropium).**

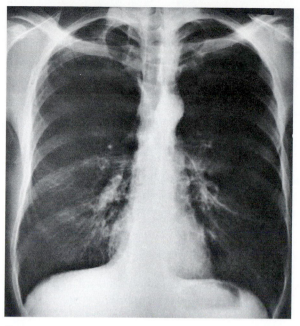
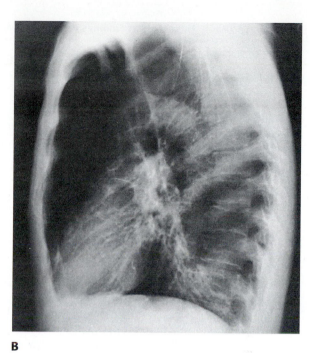

A   B

FIGURE 2.17-1.   COPD.

Note the hyperinflated and hyperlucent lungs, flat diaphragms, increased AP diameter, narrow mediastinum, and large upper lobe bullae on AP (A) and lateral (B) CXR. (Reproduced, with permission, from Stobo JD et al. *The Principles and Practice of Medicine*, 23rd ed. Stamford, CT: Appleton & Lange, 1996: 135.)

- **Systemic steroids** (prednisone) may ↓ the length of hospital stay but should be tapered over 3–14 days.
- **Empiric antibiotics** with coverage of *Streptococcus, H. influenzae,* and *Moraxella* (e.g., amoxicillin, TMP-SMX, doxycycline, azithromycin, clarithromycin) **are indicated** in an acute setting.
- Spirometry in an acute setting is **not helpful** in guiding therapy.

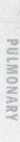

Always treat hypoxic patients with O_2. CO_2 retention won't kill the patient, but hypoxia will.

PLEURAL EFFUSION

Effusions are characterized as either transudative or exudative based on composition.

SYMPTOMS/EXAM

- Patients are usually short of breath and may complain of pleuritic chest pain. Some may be asymptomatic or have symptoms of an underlying process (e.g., CHF, pneumonia, cancer).
- Exam reveals ↓ **breath sounds, dullness** to percussion, and ↓ tactile fremitus on the side with the effusion.

DIAGNOSIS

- **Thoracentesis.**
- Obtain the following assays on the pleural fluid to aid in management: Gram stain and culture, acid-fast bacilli (AFB), total protein, serum LDH, glucose, triglycerides, cell count with differential, and pH. Serum total protein and LDH values will also be needed (see Table 2.17-3).

TABLE 2.17-3. Thoracentesis Findings in Transudative and Exudative Pleural Effusions

	PLEURAL/SERUM PROTEIN (RATIO)	PLEURAL/SERUM LDH (RATIO)	PLEURAL LDH
Transudative	< 0.5 *and*	< 0.6 *and*	< 200
Exudative	> 0.5 *or*	> 0.6 *or*	> 200

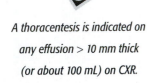

A thoracentesis is indicated on any effusion > 10 mm thick (or about 100 mL) on CXR.

- If the fluid is **transudative,** no further workup is needed; focus on treating the underlying cause (e.g., diuresing the patient).
- If the fluid is **exudative,** refer to Table 2.17-4 to help determine the cause.

TREATMENT

- If the CXR shows an effusion > 10 mm thick (or about 100 mL), always do a **thoracentesis.** This may be therapeutic (to relieve dyspnea) as well as diagnostic.
- **Indications for chest tube (any one of these)** are as follows:
    - A pleural WBC count > 100,000 or frank pus.
    - Glucose < 40.
    - pH < 7.0.

Always do a pleural biopsy if you suspect TB. Send the fluid for cytology if you suspect malignancy.

COMPLICATIONS

- An untreated pleural effusion may quickly become infected and turn into an empyema.
- Over time, effusions may become loculated and require video-assisted thoracoscopy (VATS) drainage or surgical decortication.
- The major complications of thoracentesis include pneumothorax and bleeding (remember, the neurovascular bundle runs along the inferior side of the rib).

TABLE 2.17-4. Assays for Exudative Fluid and Their Associated Differential Diagnosis

PLEURAL ASSAY	VALUE	DIFFERENTIAL
Glucose	< 60	Empyema or parapneumonia, TB, RA, malignancy.
WBC	> 10,000	Empyema or parapneumonia, RA, malignancy.
RBC	> 100,000	Gross blood—think of trauma, PE.
Cellular differential	Lymphocytes PMNs Eosinophils	TB, sarcoid, malignancy. Empyema, PE. Bleeding, pneumothorax.
pH	< 7.20	Complicated effusion or empyema.
Triglycerides	> 150	Diagnostic of chylothorax.

Defined as air that becomes trapped in the pleural space. This can be traumatic, spontaneous, or iatrogenic. Spontaneous pneumothorax can be due to underlying lung pathology such as COPD or CF.

SYMPTOMS/EXAM

Look for patients who develop acute shortness of breath and pleuritic chest pain. Look for **tachypnea,** ↓ tactile fremitus, ↓ breath sounds, **tympany** on percussion on the side involved, and tracheal deviation toward the affected side.

DIAGNOSIS

CXR will reveal the diagnosis. Look for a distinct lack of lung markings within the pneumothorax, along with collapse of the lung on that side (see Figure 2.17-2.). Tracheal deviation may be present (especially with tension).

TREATMENT

- Insertion of a chest tube is required in patients with a pneumothorax > 30%.
- Smaller pneumothoraces may be managed simply with supplemental O_2 and observation.
- Treat pain with morphine and NSAIDs.
- For patients with recurrent pneumothorax, consider pleurodesis.

Tension Pneumothorax

- In this emergent complication of pneumothorax, defects in the chest wall act as a one-way valve. This allows air to be drawn into the pleural space and become trapped. The result is **rapid decompensation,** hypotension, and circulatory collapse → **shock.**

Suspect pneumothorax with shortness of breath and chest pain plus underlying COPD, CF, chest procedures (e.g., central lines), or trauma.

The differential for shortness of breath/chest pain includes pneumothorax, MI, PE, and dissection.

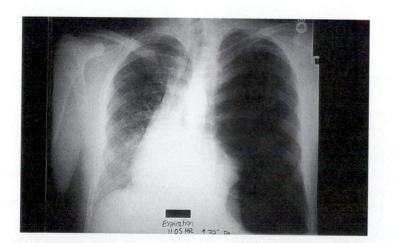

FIGURE 2.17-2.   Tension pneumothorax.

Note the hyperlucent lung field, hyperexpanded lower diaphragm, collapsed lung, tracheal deviation, mediastinal shift, and compression of the opposite lung on AP CXR. (Reproduced, with permission, from Le T et al. *First Aid for the USMLE Step 2 CK,* 6th ed. New York: McGraw-Hill, 2007: 426.)

HIGH-YIELD FACTS

PULMONARY

A tension pneumothorax is an emergency! If you suspect this, don't wait for imaging; insert a needle to decompress the chest.

Consider PE in any hospitalized patient who has dyspnea.

- Common scenarios in which to think of tension pneumothorax include **penetrating trauma**, positive-pressure ventilation, and COPD.
- **Dx:** Diagnostic clues include those of a **pneumothorax** along with **tachycardia, hypotension,** ↑ O_2 requirements, and ↑ JVP. The trachea deviates **away** from the side with tension.
- **Tx:** If you suspect that the patient has a tension pneumothorax, **don't wait for imaging!** Insert a needle to decompress the chest and then insert a chest tube.

PULMONARY EMBOLUS (PE)

Remember **Virchow's triad** when thinking of risk factors for venous thromboembolism (VTE):

- **Stasis:** Immobility, CHF, obesity, ↑ JVP.
- **Endothelial injury:** Trauma, surgery, recent fracture, prior DVT.
- **Hypercoagulable state:** Pregnancy, OCP use, coagulation disorder, malignancy, burns.

SYMPTOMS

Think about PE or DVT in **any patient with risk factors** and complaints of leg pain or swelling, acute-onset chest pain (especially pleuritic), shortness of breath, or syncope.

EXAM

Findings on exam include tachypnea, tachycardia, cyanosis, a loud P2 or S2, ↑ JVP, and signs of right heart failure. Patients may occasionally have hemoptysis or a low-grade fever.

DIFFERENTIAL

Most signs and symptoms of PE are nonspecific, so be sure to think about other entities that can present this way, including **acute MI, pneumonia, CHF,** and **aortic dissection.**

DIAGNOSIS

See Figure 2.17-3 for a diagnostic algorithm. Initial assessment should include the following:

- **ABG,** which may show a 1° respiratory alkalosis and an ↑ A-a gradient.
- **CXR** findings can include the following:
  - **Normal** (most common!).
  - A wedge-shaped infarct (Hampton's hump).
  - Oligemia in the affected lobe (Westermark's sign).
  - Pleural effusion.
- **ECG** may reveal an S wave in lead I, a Q wave in lead III, and T-wave inversion in lead III (not very sensitive or specific).
- The **pretest probability** of PE will help determine the diagnostic utility of the V/Q scan. If either the pretest probability or the V/Q scan results are intermediate, some type of confirmatory testing will be needed.
- In a nonhospitalized patient, a ⊖ D-dimer assay, when combined with some form of imaging, may help rule out DVT with good negative predictive value (NPV).
- **CT angiography,** if available, may also be useful as a confirmatory test when the V/Q scan is indeterminate (often used first line).
- **Pulmonary angiography** is still considered the **gold standard** for the diagnosis of PE and may be needed if other testing is intermediate.

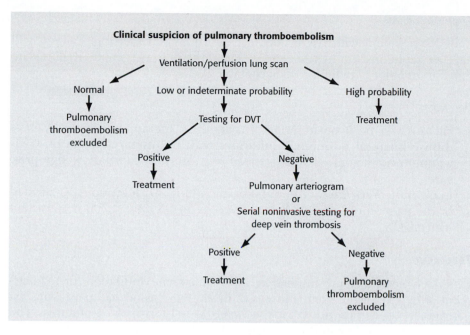

FIGURE 2.17-3. Diagnostic approach to pulmonary embolism.

(Reproduced, with permission, from Tierney LM et al. *Current Medical Diagnosis & Treatment: 2005.* New York: McGraw-Hill, 2005: 281.)

TREATMENT

- Treat VTE patients with anticoagulation.
    - Initially use **IV heparin or low-molecular-weight heparin.**
    - Patients who are not anticoagulated adequately within 24 hours have a high rate of recurrence.
    - Patients should then be transitioned to warfarin therapy, with a goal INR of 2.0–3.0.
- In patients with documented large **central PEs** (saddle PEs) and hypotension or shock, consider administering **tPA** along with heparin. The duration of therapy will vary with risk factors:
    - For patients with a **first event** and **reversible** or time-limited risk factors (e.g., surgery, pregnancy), treat for at least **3–6 months.**
    - Consider **lifelong anticoagulation** in patients with **chronic risk factors** (malignancy, paraplegia, recurrent DVTs, or PEs).
- In patients who cannot safely be anticoagulated, an IVC filter may be useful. Although these filters can ↓ the risk of PE, they are associated with a **higher risk** of recurrent DVT.

Don't forget to order DVT prophylaxis for all of your hospitalized patients!

ACUTE RESPIRATORY DISTRESS SYNDROME (ARDS)

ARDS is a common problem in the ICU and is a significant cause of mortality. It can be 2° to a range of underlying conditions, all with a similar end result of widespread inflammation in the lung parenchyma → (noncardiogenic) pulmonary edema and alveolar damage. Smokers and patients with cirrhosis are at higher risk for developing ARDS. Common etiologies are as follows:

- **Direct:** Pneumonia, aspiration.
- **Indirect:** Sepsis (most common), transfusions, pancreatitis, trauma.

Think of ARDS in a patient with a PaO_2/FiO_2 ratio < 200.

SYMPTOMS/EXAM

Look for a patient with risk factors, usually in an **ICU setting.** Patients will have an **acute** onset of hypoxia and will be difficult to oxygenate. Requires intubation in order to maintain an acceptable PaO_2.

DIAGNOSIS

- Patients will be hypoxic despite maximal O_2 therapy and typically have **diffuse bilateral pulmonary infiltrates with pulmonary edema** on CXR without evidence of volume overload (e.g., **normal capillary wedge pressure**).
- Look at the **PaO_2/FiO_2 ratio** (ratio of the arterial O_2 level on ABG divided by the fraction of inhaled O_2 the patient is on). A ratio < **200** is consistent with ARDS.

TREATMENT

Patients typically require intubation and mechanical ventilation for management of hypoxia. **Low tidal volumes** (6 mL/kg) and associated permissive hypercapnia (i.e., letting the PCO_2 rise) leads to a $\downarrow\downarrow$ risk of barotrauma. The use of **positive end-expiratory pressure (PEEP)** is used to improve oxygenation and thus $\downarrow$ FiO_2 requirement and associated O_2 toxicity. Look for the **underlying cause** and focus treatment on that, as you are stabilizing the patient and treating hypoxia.

SOLITARY PULMONARY NODULE (SPN)

Defined as a radiodense lesion seen on chest imaging that is **< 3 cm in diameter** and is not associated with infiltrates, adenopathy, or atelectasis. Most SPNs are detected on routine CXR in patients who are otherwise **asymptomatic.**

SYMPTOMS/EXAM

- **Benign** processes include histoplasmosis, coccidioidomycosis, TB, and hamartoma. Characteristics and risk factors include the following:
  - **Very fast** or **no growth** on serial imaging two years apart.
  - **Diffuse, central, or laminar** "popcorn" calcification pattern.
  - Patients who are **lifelong nonsmokers, are < 30 years of age,** and have **no history of malignancy.**
- **Malignant** lesions include lung cancer or metastases. Risk factors include the following:
  - Size > **2 cm.**
  - **Spiculation** (i.e., ragged edges).
  - Upper lobe location.
  - Occurring in patients who are **smokers, are > 30 years of age,** or have a **prior diagnosis of cancer.**

The appearance of laminar or "popcorn" calcification within an SPN likely represents a benign hamartoma.

DIAGNOSIS/TREATMENT

- Start by examining old radiographs to determine age and change in size. Lesions with > 1 malignant feature should be further evaluated with high-resolution CT imaging.
- If imaging points to a malignancy, biopsy tissue via bronchoscopy, needle aspiration, or VATS. If there is a low probability of malignancy, evaluate

with serial CXRs every three months for one year and then every six months for one year.

■ **Surgery** is the procedure of choice, particularly **thoracoscopy** or **thoracotomy** if the patient is a surgical candidate.

SARCOIDOSIS

An idiopathic illness characterized by the formation of **noncaseating granulomas** in various organs. Most patients have pulmonary involvement.

SYMPTOMS/EXAM

Typical features include **fever, cough, malaise, weight loss, dyspnea,** and **arthritis,** particularly of the knees and ankles.

DIFFERENTIAL

Sarcoidosis is a **diagnosis of exclusion,** so be sure to rule out other diseases that present similarly, such as **TB, lymphoma,** fungal infection, idiopathic pulmonary fibrosis, HIV, and berylliosis.

DIAGNOSIS

Look for **bilateral hilar lymphadenopathy** on CXR and/or infiltrates. PFTs will show a **restrictive** or **mixed restrictive-obstructive** pattern. Patients may also have **hypercalcemia.** Tissue biopsy will show **noncaseating granulomas without organisms.**

TREATMENT

Therapy includes systemic **corticosteroids** such as prednisone. Gear other medications toward the control of symptoms such as coughing or wheezing.

> **Features of sarcoidosis—**
>
> **GRUELING**
>
> **G**ranulomas
> **R**heumatoid arthritis
> **U**veitis
> **E**rythema nodosum
> **L**ymphadenitis
> **I**nterstitial fibrosis
> **N**egative PPD
> **G**ammaglobulinemia

OBSTRUCTIVE SLEEP APNEA (OSA)

Characterized by recurrent episodes of upper airway collapse during sleep → **intermittent hypoxia and recurrent arousals.**

SYMPTOMS

Patients and their bed partners may complain that they **snore.** Patients may also have **excessive daytime sleepiness,** neurocognitive impairment, morning headache, unrefreshing sleep, or impotence. They may report choking or gasping during sleep and may have witnessed apnea episodes at home.

EXAM

Patients are typically **obese** and **hypertensive.** They may also have a **large neck circumference.** Look for **retrognathia** and large tonsils. Patients with severe OSA may have peripheral edema.

DIFFERENTIAL

Rule out other causes of excessive daytime sleepiness, including **obesity hypoventilation syndrome,** narcolepsy, and restless leg syndrome.

DIAGNOSIS

Overnight polysomnography (sleep study) is the gold standard for diagnosis. Severity is measured by the apnea-hypopnea index (AHI), defined as the number of apneas and/or hypopneas per hour of sleep. An **AHI > 5** is diagnostic of OSA.

TREATMENT

Encourage weight loss. The most effective treatment is with **continuous positive airway pressure (CPAP)** to keep the airways open during sleep. Surgery such as uvulopalatopharyngoplasty (UPPP) is effective in 40–50% of cases.

COMPLICATIONS

Patients with OSA are at ↑ risk of **motor vehicle accidents** as well as for developing **hypertension, LV dysfunction, pulmonary hypertension,** and insulin resistance.

SECTION III

High-Yield CCS Cases

INITIAL MGMT	CONTINUING MGMT	F/U
Emergency room STAT • IV normal saline • Blood culture • CT—Head • Ceftriaxone and vancomycin • LP-CSF: ↑ WBCs, ↑ protein, ↓ CSF/blood glucose ratio, gram-⊕ cocci, ↑ opening pressure • IV dexamethasone **Emergency room W/U** • CBC: ↑ WBC count • Chem 8 • CT—head: ⊖ • CXR: ⊖ **Rx** • Acetaminophen	**Ward W/U** • CSF culture: ⊕ for S. pneumoniae • Blood culture: ⊖ **Rx** • Continue ceftriaxone + vancomycin + steroids	• Improved within 48 hours • Discharge home • Follow up in one month

Final Dx - Bacterial meningitis

INITIAL MGMT	CONTINUING MGMT	F/U
Emergency room STAT • O$_2$ • IV labetalol • BP in both arms • CT—head: White matter changes consistent with hypertension • ECG: LVH • CXR **Emergency room W/U** • Cardiac/BP monitoring • CPK-MB, troponin × 3: ⊖ • CBC • Chem 8 • UA	**ICU W/U** • Continuous cardiac monitoring • Lipid profile • Echocardiography: EF < 45% **Rx** • Labetalol or metoprolol if good control previously • ACEIs (low EF) • HCTZ	• Transfer to the floor • Counsel patient re medication compliance • Discharge home • Follow up in one week

Final Dx - Hypertensive emergency

Altered Mental Status/Loss of Consciousness

CASE 6

HX	PE	DDX
84 yo F brought in by her son complains of forgetfulness (e.g., forgets phone numbers, loses her way home) along with difficulty performing some of her daily activities (e.g., bathing, dressing, managing money, answering the phone). The problem has gradually progressed over the past few years.	VS: P 90, BP 120/60, RR 12 Gen: NAD Lungs: WNL CV: WNL Abd: WNL Ext: WNL Neuro: On mini-mental status exam, patient cannot recall objects, follow three-step commands, or spell "world" backward; cranial nerves intact; strength and sensation intact	• Alzheimer's disease • B_{12} deficiency • Chronic subdural hematoma • Depression • Hypothyroidism • Intracranial tumor • Neurosyphilis • Pressure hydrocephalus • Vascular dementia

CASE 7

HX	PE	DDX
79 yo M is brought in by his family complaining of a seven-week history of difficulty walking accompanied by memory loss and urinary incontinence. Since then he has had ↑ difficulty with memory and more frequent episodes of incontinence.	VS: P 92, BP 144/86, RR 14 Gen: NAD Lungs: WNL CV: WNL Abd: WNL Ext: WNL Neuro: Difficulty with both recent and immediate recall on mini-mental status exam; spasticity and hyperreflexia in upper and lower extremities; problem initiating gait (gait is shuffling, broad-based, and slow)	• Alzheimer's disease • B_{12} deficiency • Chronic subdural hematoma • Frontal lobe syndromes • Huntington's disease • Intracranial tumor • Meningitis • Normal pressure hydrocephalus • Parkinson's disease • Vascular dementia

CASE 8

HX	PE	DDX
The on-call physician is called to see a 46 yo M patient because of seizures. The patient was admitted to the surgical ward two days ago, after emergency trauma surgery. The nurse reports that the patient was anxious, agitated, irritable, and tachycardic last night. Later on, the nurse noted nausea, diarrhea, sweating, and insomnia. The patient had tremors, startle response, and hallucinations earlier tonight.	VS: T 37°C (99°F), P 133, BP 146/89, RR 22, O_2 sat 92% room air Gen: Sweating; cigarette burns on hands; multiple tattoos and rings Chest: WNL Abd: Hepatomegaly Ext: Evidence of recent surgery Neuro: Tremor, confusion, delirium, clouded sensorium, and evidence of peripheral neuropathy	• Alcohol withdrawal • Amphetamine psychosis • Delirium • Sedative withdrawal • SLE

INITIAL MGMT	CONTINUING MGMT	F/U
Office W/U • CBC • Chem 14 • TSH • Serum B_{12} • Serum folic acid • VDRL/RPR • CT—head **Rx** • Donepezil		• Patient counseling • Support group • Advance directives • Family counseling

Final Dx - Alzheimer's disease

INITIAL MGMT	CONTINUING MGMT	F/U
Emergency room W/U • CBC • Chem 8 • LFTs • TSH • CT—head: Enlarged lateral ventricles with no prominence of cortical sulci • LP • Serum B_{12} • Serum folic acid	**Ward W/U** • Neurosurgery consult • Neurology consult • Ventriculoperitoneal shunt	• Advance directives • Family counseling • Supportive care

Final Dx - Normal pressure hydrocephalus

INITIAL MGMT	CONTINUING MGMT	F/U
Ward W/U • CBC: MCV 110 fL • Chem 8: Hypokalemia, hypomagnesemia • Urine toxicology: WNL • LFTs: GGT 40 U/L • CT—head: Cerebral atrophy, no subdural hematoma **Rx** • Thiamine before IV D_5W NS • Pyridoxine • Folic acid • IV diazepam • Atenolol • Replete K and Mg	**Ward W/U** • Chem 8: Corrected hypokalemia, hypomagnesemia **Rx** • IV normal saline • IV diazepam • Atenolol • Naltrexone (for maintenance therapy if indicated)	• Follow up in four weeks • Patient counseling • Smoking cessation • Dietary supplements • Addiction unit consult • Social work consult

Final Dx - Alcohol withdrawal

CASE 9

HX	PE	DDX
24 yo M is brought to the ER in a drowsy state. His wife reports that he was working at home when he suddenly stiffened, fell backward, and lost consciousness. While he was lying on the ground, he was noted to have no respiration for about one minute, followed by jerking of all four limbs for about five minutes. He was unconscious for another five minutes.	VS: T 37°C (98.2°F), P 90, BP 120/80, RR 12 Gen: NAD Lungs: WNL CV: WNL Abd: WNL Ext: WNL Neuro: In a state of confusion and lethargy but oriented; no focal neurologic deficits	• Alcohol withdrawal • Cardioembolic stroke • Frontal lobe epilepsy • Migraine headache • Psychiatric conditions • Seizures • Syncope • Vascular conditions

CASE 10

HX	PE	DDX
72 yo M is brought to the ER complaining of syncope. He underwent a coronary artery bypass graft (CABG) three years ago. He reports fatigue and dizziness over the past five days. The patient's fall was broken by his wife, and as a result he has no head trauma. His wife reports loss of consciousness of about three minutes' duration. Prior to the syncopal episode, the patient recalls a prodrome of lightheadedness. His medications include propranolol, digoxin, and diltiazem.	VS: T 37°C (98.1°F), P 35, BP 114/54, RR 15 Gen: NAD Lungs: WNL CV: Irregular S1 and S2, bradycardia Abd: WNL Ext: WNL Neuro: Alert and oriented; CN II–XII intact; 5/5 motor strength in all extremities	• Aortic stenosis • Asystole • Dilated cardiomyopathy • Heart block • MI • Myocarditis • Myopathies • Restrictive cardiomyopathy • Vasodepressor/vasovagal response

INITIAL MGMT	CONTINUING MGMT	F/U
Emergency room W/U • CBC • Chem 8 • LFTs • ABG • Serum calcium, magnesium, phosphate • ECG • EEG • CT—head • MRI—brain • UA • Urine toxicology	**Ward W/U** • Continue IV • O_2 **Rx** • Neurology consult	• Follow up in 3–4 weeks • Patient counseling • Family counseling • Advise patient to use seat belts • Advise patient not to drive

Final Dx - Grand mal seizure (complex tonic-clonic seizure)

INITIAL MGMT	CONTINUING MGMT	F/U
Emergency room W/U • IV normal saline • CBC • Chem 8 • LFTs • ECG: Third-degree AV block • Cardiac enzymes • Serum troponin I • Serum calcium, magnesium, phosphate • CXR • UA • O_2 • Continuous cardiac monitoring **Rx** • Temporary transvenous cardiac pacemaker • Withhold AV nodal agents	**ICU W/U** • Continuous cardiac monitoring • ECG • Lipid profile • Echocardiography **Rx** • Lipid-lowering agents • Cardiology consult • Cardiac catheterization, angiocardiography • Permanent cardiac pacemaker	• Cardiac rehabilitation program • Smoking cessation • Counsel patient to limit alcohol intake • Counsel patient not to drive • Low-fat, low-sodium diet

Final Dx - Complete heart block

CASE 11

HX	PE	DDX
25 yo F with no significant past medical history is brought to the ER after having been found unresponsive with an empty bottle lying next to her.	VS: T 38°C (99.8°F), P 50, BP 110/50, RR 9, O_2 sat 92% room air Gen: Drowsy HEENT: Pinpoint pupils Lungs: WNL CV: Bradycardia Abd: WNL Ext: WNL Neuro: Opens eyes to painful stimuli Limited PE with ABCs	• Acetaminophen overdose • Narcotic overdose • TCA overdose

CASE 12

HX	PE	DDX
60 yo M was found unconscious by his wife, who called the paramedics. She left him in bed at 7 A.M. to go to her volunteer job. When she returned for lunch at 1 P.M., she found an empty bottle of amitriptyline next to him. When paramedics arrived, he was noted to be in respiratory distress and was transferred to the ER.	VS: T 38°C (101°F), P 110, BP 95/45, RR 35, O_2 sat 89% on 100% face mask Gen: Acute distress; shallow, rapid breathing HEENT: Dilated pupils Lungs: WNL CV: Tachycardia Abd: WNL Neuro: Opens eyes to painful stimuli **Limited PE**	• Anticholinergic toxicity • TCA intoxication

INITIAL MGMT	CONTINUING MGMT	F/U
Emergency room STAT • Suction airway • Fingerstick blood sugar • IV normal saline • IV naloxone: Patient responded • Dextrose 50% • IV thiamine • ABG **Emergency room W/U** • CBC • ECG • Urine pregnancy • Urine toxicology • UA • Serum acetaminophen, salicylate • INR • Serum lactate • CXR, PA	**ICU W/U** • Gastric lavage: Pill fragments • Continuous monitoring: Patient started to become drowsy again (monitor events) **Rx** • IV naloxone: Patient responded • Psychiatry consult • Suicide precautions	• Monitor for at least 24 hours

Final Dx - Narcotic overdose

INITIAL MGMT	CONTINUING MGMT	F/U
Emergency room STAT • Intubate **Emergency room W/U** • Cardiac/BP monitoring • Chem 14 • CBC • ABG • Serum lactate • Serum osmolality • Blood ketones • Urine toxicology: $\oplus$ for TCAs • ECG: Widened QRS • Serum magnesium • CXR, PA • Cardiac enzymes • CT—head **Rx** • IV D_5W 0.9 NS • Thiamine • Central line placement • NG tube gastric lavage • Activated charcoal • IV bicarbonate	**ICU W/U** • Continuous monitoring of urine output q 1 h • Continuous BP monitoring • Continuous cardiac monitoring • Neuro check **Rx** • Cardiology consult • Lidocaine for TCA-induced ventricular arrhythmias • IV magnesium sulfate, one time	• Psychiatry consult

Final Dx - Tricyclic antidepressant (TCA) intoxication

HIGH-YIELD CASES

Fatigue/Weakness

CASE 13

HX	PE	DDX
68 yo M presents following a 20-minute episode of slurred speech, right facial drooping and numbness, and weakness of the right hand. His symptoms had totally resolved by the time he got to the ER. He has a history of hypertension, diabetes mellitus, and heavy smoking.	VS: T 37°C (98°F), P 75, BP 150/90, RR 16, O_2 sat 100% room air Gen: NAD Neck: Right carotid bruit Lungs: WNL CV: WNL Abd: WNL Ext: WNL Neuro: WNL	• Intracranial tumor • Seizure • Stroke • Subdural or epidural hematoma • TIA

CASE 14

HX	PE	DDX
40 yo F presents with numbness, lower extremity weakness, and difficulty walking. She reports having had a URI approximately two weeks ago. She says that her weakness started from her lower limbs to her hip and then progressed to her upper limbs. She also complains of lightheadedness on standing and shortness of breath.	VS: Afebrile, P 115, BP 130/80 with orthostatic changes, RR 16 Gen: NAD Lungs: WNL CV: WNL Ext: WNL Neuro: Loss of motor strength in lower limbs; absent DTRs in patella and Achilles tendon; sensation intact	• Conversion disorder • Guillain-Barré syndrome • Myasthenia gravis • Paraneoplastic neuropathy • Poliomyelitis • Polymyositis

HIGH-YIELD CASES

INITIAL MGMT	CONTINUING MGMT	F/U
Emergency room STAT • Assess ABCs • O$_2$ • Blood glucose • IV normal saline • CT—head **Emergency room W/U** • Continuous cardiac monitoring • BP monitoring • ECG • CBC • Chem 8 • CXR • PT/PTT, INR • Neurology consult **Rx** • ASA	**Ward W/U** • Repeat neurologic exam • Continuous cardiac monitoring • BP monitoring • Telemetry • Lipid profile, Hb$_{Alc}$ • Echocardiography: EF 60% • Carotid duplex: > 75% stenosis in right carotid artery **Rx** • Vascular surgery consult • Patient is scheduled for elective carotid endarterectomy • ASA	• Counsel patient re smoking cessation, exercise • Treat hypertension • Treat diabetes • Diabetic diet • Diabetic teaching • Treat cholesterol • Low-fat, low-sodium diet

Final Dx - Transient ischemic attack (TIA)

INITIAL MGMT	CONTINUING MGMT	F/U
Emergency room W/U • CBC • Chem 8 • TSH • ESR • CRP • RF • VDRL • Serum B$_{12}$ • Serum folic acid • ECG • Serum CPK • CXR • LP: ↑ CSF protein • HIV testing, ELISA	**Ward Rx** • Immunoglobulins • Plasmapheresis • Rehabilitative medicine consult • Neurology consult • Immunology consult • Spirometry	• Follow up in 3–4 weeks • Patient counseling • Family counseling • Advise patient to use seat belts

Final Dx - Guillain-Barré syndrome

HIGH-YIELD CASES

CASE 15

HX	PE	DDX
40 yo F presents with fatigue, weight gain, sleepiness, cold intolerance, constipation, and dry skin.	VS: T 36°C (97°F), BP 100/60, HR 60 Gen: Obese Skin: Dry HEENT: Scar on neck from previous thyroidectomy Lungs: WNL CV: WNL Neuro: Delayed relaxation of DTRs	• Anemia • Depression • Diabetes • Hypothyroidism

CASE 16

HX	PE	DDX
16 yo M complains of myalgia, fatigue, and sore throat. He also reports loss of appetite and nausea but no vomiting. He reports that his girlfriend recently had similar symptoms that lasted a few weeks.	VS: T 38°C (101°F), P 85, BP 125/80, RR 18 Gen: Maculopapular rash HEENT: Posterior and auricular lymphadenopathy and pharyngitis with diffuse exudates and petechiae at junction of hard and soft palates Lungs: WNL CV: WNL Abd: Soft, nontender; mild hepatosplenomegaly Ext: WNL Neuro: WNL	• CMV • Hepatitis • Infectious mononucleosis • 1° HIV infection • Streptococcal pharyngitis • Toxoplasmosis

CASE 17

HX	PE	DDX
40 yo F complains of feeling tired, hopeless, and worthless. She also reports depressed mood, inability to sleep, and impaired concentration. She has been missing work. She denies any suicidal thoughts or attempts and denies having hallucinations. She has no history of alcohol or drug abuse and has not lost a loved one within the last 12 months. She is married and has one child and a supportive husband.	VS: P 70, BP 120/60, RR 12 Gen: NAD Lungs: WNL CV: WNL Abd: WNL Ext: WNL Neuro: WNL	• Adjustment disorder • Anemia • Anxiety • Cancer • Chronic fatigue syndrome • Dementia • Depression • Fibromyalgia • Hypothyroidism

INITIAL MGMT	CONTINUING MGMT	F/U
Office W/U • CBC • Chem 14 • TSH: ↑ • FT$_4$: ↓ • ECG • Lipid profile • Depression index **Rx** • Thyroxine		• Check TSH after one month

Final Dx - Hypothyroidism

INITIAL MGMT	CONTINUING MGMT	F/U
Office W/U • CBC: ↑ WBC count • Peripheral smear: Atypical lymphocytes • Chem 14: ↑ SGOT and SGPT • ESR • CRP • Mono test: ⊕ • Serum EBV titer: ↑, rapid strep **Rx** • Acetaminophen or NSAIDs • Hydrate; patient counseling		• Follow up in two weeks with CBC • Advise patient to rest at home • Avoid sports

Final Dx - Infectious mononucleosis

INITIAL MGMT	CONTINUING MGMT	F/U
Office W/U • CBC • Chem 14 • TSH • Urine/serum toxicology **Rx** • Suicide contract • SSRI (e.g., sertraline) or • SNRI (e.g., mirtazapine) • Psychiatry consult		• Follow up in one week • Supportive psychotherapy • Exercise program • Patient counseling

Final Dx - Major depression

HIGH-YIELD CASES

Cough/Shortness of Breath

CASE 18

HX	PE	DDX
2 yo M is brought in by his mother because of sudden-onset shortness of breath and cough. He had a URI four days ago. Earlier in the day he was playing with peanuts with his brother. His immunizations are up to date.	VS: T 37°C (98°F), P 110, BP 80/50, RR 38, O_2 sat 99% room air Gen: Respiratory distress; using accessory muscles HEENT: WNL Neck: WNL Lungs: Inspiratory stridor; ↓ breath sounds in right lower base CV: Tachycardia Abd: WNL	• Angioedema • Asthma • Croup • Epiglottis • Foreign-body aspiration • Laryngitis • Peritonsillar abscess • Pneumonia • Retropharyngeal abscess

CASE 19

HX	PE	DDX
75 yo F presents with chest pain and shortness of breath. She reports having fallen five days ago and has a long cast for her femoral fracture.	VS: Afebrile, BP 120/75, HR 100, RR 24 Gen: Respiratory distress HEENT: WNL Lungs: Rales, wheezing, ↓ breath sounds in left lower lung CV: Loud P2 and splitting of S2 Abd: WNL	• CHF • Lung cancer • MI • Pericarditis • Pneumothorax • Pulmonary embolism • Syncope

CASE 20

HX	PE	DDX
5 yo M is brought to the ER with a harsh barking cough. He has a history of URIs with coryza, nasal congestion, and sore throat. His symptoms have been present for about a week.	VS: T 38°C (101°F), BP 110/65, HR 100, RR 22 Gen: Pallor and mild respiratory distress with intercostal retraction and nasal flaring HEENT: WNL Lungs: Stridor, hoarseness, barking cough CV: WNL Abd: WNL	• Bacterial tracheitis • Croup • Diphtheria • Epiglottitis • Measles • Peritonsillar abscess • Retropharyngeal abscess

INITIAL MGMT	CONTINUING MGMT	F/U

Emergency room STAT
- CXR, PA and lateral
- XR—neck
- Bronchoscopy: Foreign body is removed and patient improves

Rx
- Consider IV methylprednisolone before removal of the foreign body

F/U:
- Follow up in two weeks

Final Dx - Foreign-body aspiration

INITIAL MGMT	CONTINUING MGMT	F/U

Emergency room W/U
- IV normal saline
- NPO
- CBC
- Chem 14
- ABG: Hypoxia and hypocapnia
- CXR: Left lower lobe atelectasis, Hampton's humps
- CT—chest: Pulmonary embolism
- ECG
- DVT U/S: Venous DVT
- Heparin IV and warfarin

Ward W/U
- Continuous cardiac and BP monitoring
- Pulmonary medicine consult
- PT/PTT, INR

Rx
- Discontinue heparin two days after INR is therapeutic
- Warfarin

F/U:
- Follow up in two weeks with PT/INR
- Chest physical therapy
- Warfarin
- Rehabilitative medicine consult

Final Dx - Pulmonary embolism

INITIAL MGMT	CONTINUING MGMT	F/U

Emergency room W/U
- O_2
- CBC
- Chem 8
- Throat culture
- XR—neck: Subglottic narrowing

Ward Rx
- Humidified air
- Epinephrine
- Dexamethasone

F/U:
- Follow up in one month
- Family counseling

Final Dx - Croup

CASE 21

HX	PE	DDX
75 yo M presents with shortness of breath on exertion along with cough and blood-streaked sputum. He reports progressive malaise and weight loss together with loss of appetite over the past six months. He smokes 40 packs of cigarettes per year.	VS: Afebrile, BP 130/85, HR 90, RR 15 Gen: WNL Chest: Barrel-shaped chest, gynecomastia Lungs: Rales, wheezing, ↓ breath sounds, dullness on percussion in left upper lung CV: WNL Abd: Mild tenderness in RUQ with mild hepatomegaly Ext: Finger clubbing; dark-colored, pruritic rash on both forearms	• Lung cancer • Lymphoma • Sarcoidosis • Tuberculosis

CASE 22

HX	PE	DDX
60 yo M presents with ↑ dyspnea, sputum production, and a change in the color of his sputum to yellow over the past three days. He is a smoker with a history of COPD.	VS: T 38°C (100.6°F), P 90, BP 130/70, RR 28, O_2 sat 92% on 2-L NC Gen: Moderate respiratory distress Lungs: Rhonchi at left lower base; diffuse wheezing CV: WNL Abd: WNL Ext: WNL	• Bronchitis • CHF • COPD exacerbation • Lung cancer • Pneumonia • URI

INITIAL MGMT	CONTINUING MGMT	F/U

Office W/U
- CBC: ↓ hemoglobin
- Chem 8
- LFTs: ↑ transaminase
- ABG
- ESR: ↑
- CXR: Infiltrate and nodules in upper left lobe
- Sputum cytology: Adenocarcinoma
- Sputum culture
- PPD: ⊖
- CT—chest: Left upper lobe mass

Office W/U
- PFTs
- Oncology consult
- Surgery consult
- Dietary consult
- Bronchoscopy with biopsy
- CT—abdomen and pelvis
- CT—head
- Antiemetic medication

- Smoking cessation
- Patient counseling
- Family counseling
- Follow up in 3–4 weeks with CXR and CBC
- Counsel patient to limit alcohol intake

Final Dx - Lung cancer

INITIAL MGMT	CONTINUING MGMT	F/U

Emergency room STAT
- O_2
- IV normal saline
- IV steroids
- Albuterol by nebulizer
- Ipratropium by nebulizer
- Sputum culture
- Blood culture

Emergency room W/U
- CBC: ↑ WBC count
- CXR: Left lower lobe infiltrate
- ECG
- ABG
- Peak flow: < 200 L/min
- Sputum Gram stain: Gram-⊕ cocci
- Chem 8

Rx
- Third-generation cephalosporin + azithromycin vs. levofloxacin or gatifloxacin IV

Ward W/U
- Peak flow: 300 L/min
- FEV_1: 2 L
- Sputum culture: ⊕ for S. pneumoniae sensitive to levofloxacin
- Blood culture: ⊖

Rx
- Change to levofloxacin
- Change IV prednisone

- Taper prednisone over the next two weeks
- Smoking cessation
- Consider pneumonia vaccine and flu shot

Final Dx - Chronic obstructive pulmonary disease (COPD) exacerbation/pneumonia

CASE 23

HX	PE	DDX
50 yo Mexican immigrant M presents with cough productive of bloody sputum accompanied by night sweats, weight loss, and fatigue of three months' duration.	VS: T 38°C (100°F), BP 130/85, HR 90, RR 22 Gen: Pallor Lungs: ↓ breath sounds in upper lobes of both lungs CV: WNL Abd: WNL	• Bronchiectasis • Fungal lung infection • Lung cancer • Lymphoma • Sarcoidosis • TB • Vasculitis

CASE 24

HX	PE	DDX
55 yo M presents with cough that is exacerbated when he lies down at night and improves when he props his head up on three pillows. He also reports worsening exertional dyspnea for the past two months (he now has dyspnea at rest). He has had a 25-pound weight gain since his symptoms began. His past medical history is significant for hypertension, an MI five years ago, hyperlipidemia, and smoking.	VS: P 70, BP 120/70, RR 28, O_2 sat 86% room air Gen: Moderate respiratory distress Neck: JVD Lungs: Bibasilar crackles CV: S1/S2/S3 RRR, 3/6 systolic murmur at apex Abd: WNL Ext: +2 bilateral pitting edema	• CHF • COPD exacerbation • MI • Pericardial tamponade • Pulmonary embolism • Pulmonary fibrosis • Renal failure

INITIAL MGMT	CONTINUING MGMT	F/U
Emergency room W/U • CXR: Infiltrate/nodules in upper lobes • AFB sputum/culture × 3 days: ⊕ stain • Sputum Gram stain and culture • PPD: 16 mm • CBC • Chem 14 • HIV testing • CT—chest: Infiltrates and cavity consistent with TB **Rx** • Respiratory isolation • Transfer to the ward	**Ward W/U** • Social worker consult **Rx** • INH + rifampin + pyrazin-amide + ethambutol • Vitamin B_6	• Sputum culture and smear at three months • LFTs • Ophthalmology consult • Family education • Family PPD placement • Report case to the local public health department

Final Dx - Tuberculosis (TB)

INITIAL MGMT	CONTINUING MGMT	F/U
Emergency room STAT • O_2 • IV • IV furosemide • CXR: Pulmonary edema • ECG: Old Q wave in anterior leads **Emergency room W/U** • Cardiac/BP monitoring • CPK-MB, troponin q 8 h • CBC • Chem 8: K 3.4 • Serum calcium, magnesium, phosphate **Rx** • IV KCl • Daily weight • Discontinue any β-blockers • SQ heparin • Low-fat, low-sodium diet	**Ward W/U** • TSH • Lipid profile • Echocardiography: Hypokinesia in anterior wall; EF 20% • Chem 8: K 3.7 **Rx** • Fluid restriction • Lisinopril • Atorvastatin • ASA • Digoxin • Spironolactone • Change IV furosemide • Restart β-blockers (when euvolemic)	• Cardiac rehabilitation • Counsel patient re smoking cessation, hypertension, exercise, relaxation, and lipids • Follow up in one week • Refer to cardiology; with ischemic cardiomyopathy and EF < 30%, patients may benefit from an automatic implantable cardiac defibrillator (AICD)

Final Dx - Congestive heart failure (CHF) exacerbation

CASE 25

HX	PE	DDX
5 yo F presents with shortness of breath. She has a history of recurrent pulmonary infection and fatty, foul-smelling stool. She has also shown failure to thrive and has a history of meconium ileus.	VS: T 38°C (101°F), BP 110/65, HR 110, RR 24 Gen: Pallor, mild respiratory distress, low weight and height for age, dry skin HEENT: Nasal polyps Lungs: Barrel-shaped chest, rales, dullness and ↓ breath sounds over lower lung fields CV: WNL Abd: Abdominal distention, hepatosplenomegaly	• Asthma • Cystic fibrosis • Failure to thrive • Malabsorption syndrome • Sinusitis

CASE 26

HX	PE	DDX
65 yo F with a history of hypertension and diabetes mellitus presents with LUQ pain accompanied by fever and a productive cough with purulent yellow sputum.	VS: T 38°C (101°F), P 105, BP 130/75, RR 22, O_2 sat 95% room air Gen: NAD Neck: WNL Lungs: ↓ breath sounds and rhonchi on left side CV: Tachycardia Abd: Tenderness in LUQ	• Bronchitis • Infectious mononucleosis • Lung abscess • Lung cancer • Pneumonia • Pyelonephritis • Spleen abscess

INITIAL MGMT	CONTINUING MGMT	F/U

Emergency room W/U
- CBC: ↓ hemoglobin
- Chem 8: ↑ sugar, ↓ albumin
- ABG: Hypoxia
- CXR: Hyperinflation
- Sputum Gram stain and culture
- O_2

Ward W/U
- PFTs
- Sweat chloride test: ⊕
- Pancreatic enzymes
- 24-hour fecal fat
- Dietary consult
- Genetics consult
- Cystic fibrosis specialist
- Pulmonary medicine, pediatrics consults

Rx
- IV normal saline
- O_2
- IV piperacillin
- Albuterol, inhalation

- Follow up in two months
- Chest physical therapy
- Regular multiple vitamins
- Influenza vaccine
- Pneumococcal vaccine
- Family counseling

Final Dx - Cystic fibrosis (CF)

INITIAL MGMT	CONTINUING MGMT	F/U

Office W/U
- CBC: ↑ WBC count
- Chem 8
- UA
- Sputum Gram stain: Gram-positive cocci
- Sputum culture: Pending
- CXR: Left lower lobe infiltrate
- U/S—abdomen

Ward W/U
- Sputum culture: ⊕ for *Streptococcus pneumoniae*

Rx
- IV normal saline
- PO levofloxacin
- Chest physiotherapy
- Acetaminophen
- SQ heparin

- Discharge home
- Continue PO levofloxacin × 14 days

Final Dx - Pneumonia

CASE 27

HX	PE	DDX
25 yo HIV-⊕ M presents with shortness of breath, malaise, dry cough, fatigue, and fever.	VS: T 38°C (101°F), BP 110/65, HR 110, RR 24 Gen: Pallor, mild respiratory distress, generalized lymphadenopathy HEENT: Oral thrush Lungs: Intercostal reaction; rales and ↓ breath sounds over both lung fields CV: WNL Abd: Soft, nontender; hepatosplenomegaly Ext: Reddish maculopapular rash	• CMV • Interstitial pneumonia • Kaposi's sarcoma • Legionellosis • *Mycobacterium avium-intracellulare* • *Pneumocystis carinii* pneumonia • TB

Chest Pain

CASE 28

HX	PE	DDX
40 yo F presents with sudden onset of 8/10 substernal chest pain that began at rest, has lasted for 20 minutes, and radiates to the jaw. The pain is accompanied by nausea. The patient has a prior history of hypertension, hyperlipidemia, and smoking.	VS: P 80, BP 130/60, RR 14, O_2 sat 99% room air Gen: Moderate distress Lungs: WNL CV: WNL Abd: WNL Ext: WNL	• Angina • Aortic dissection • Costochondritis • GERD • MI • Pericarditis • Pneumothorax • Pulmonary embolism

INITIAL MGMT	CONTINUING MGMT	F/U

Office W/U
- CBC
- CD4: 200
- Chem 8
- ABG: Hypoxia
- Sputum Gram stain and culture
- Sputum AFB smear
- Bronchial washings—*Pneumocystis* stain (bronchoscopy is a prerequisite along with thoracic surgery consult): $\oplus$
- CXR: Bilateral interstitial infiltrate
- PPD: $\ominus$

Office W/U
- LFTs
- VDRL
- Anti-HCV
- HBsAg
- Anti-HBc
- Serum *Toxoplasma* serology

Rx
- TMP-SMX or pentamidine (if patient cannot tolerate TMP-SMX)
- Prednisone
- Begin highly active antiretroviral therapy (HAART)

F/U
- Regular follow-up visits
- LFTs
- Influenza vaccine
- Pneumococcal vaccine
- Counsel patient re safe sex practices
- HIV support group
- Patient counseling
- Family counseling

Final Dx - *Pneumocystis jiroveci* pneumonia (PCP)

INITIAL MGMT	CONTINUING MGMT	F/U

Emergency room STAT
- O_2
- Chewable aspirin
- SL nitroglycerin
- IV normal saline
- IV morphine
- ECG: T-wave inversions

Emergency room W/U
- Cardiac/BP monitoring
- CPK-MB, troponin q 8 h: $\ominus$
- CBC
- Chem 14
- PT/PTT
- CXR
- Cardiac catheterization

ICU W/U
- ECG
- Lipid profile
- TSH
- Echocardiography: 60%
- Stress test: $\oplus$

Rx
- Enoxaparin
- ASA
- Clopidogrel
- β-blocker (atenolol)
- ACEI (enalapril)
- Atorvastatin
- Cardiology consult

F/U
- Cardiac rehabilitation
- Counsel patient re smoking cessation, hypertension, exercise, relaxation, and lipids
- Advise patient to rest at home
- Low-fat, low-sodium diet

Final Dx - Unstable angina

CASE 29

HX	PE	DDX
58 yo M was working in his office 30 minutes ago when he suddenly developed right-sided chest discomfort and shortness of breath. He has a prior history of asthma and emphysema.	VS: P 123, BP 101/64, RR 28, O_2 sat 91% room air Gen: Cyanosis, severe respiratory distress Trachea: Deviated to left Lungs: No breath sounds on right side with hyperresonance on percussion CV: Tachycardia; apical impulse displaced to the left Abd: WNL	• Angina • Aortic dissection • Asthma exacerbation • Pneumothorax • Pulmonary embolism • Tension pneumothorax

CASE 30

HX	PE	DDX
34 yo F presents with stabbing retrosternal chest pain that radiates to the back. The pain improves when she leans forward and worsens with deep inspiration. She had a URI one week ago.	VS: T 37°C (99.2°F), P 80, BP 130/70, RR 16, O_2 sat 98% room air Gen: NAD Neck: WNL Lungs: WNL CV: S1/S2, pericardial friction rub Abd: WNL Ext: WNL	• Angina/MI • Aortic dissection • Costochondritis • Esophageal rupture • GERD • Pericarditis • Pneumothorax • Pulmonary embolism

CASE 31

HX	PE	DDX
48 yo F presents with palpitation and anxiety. She reports that she feels hot and has to run the air conditioner all the time. She also reports hand tremors. She has lost 10 pounds over the past few months despite her good appetite.	VS: P 113, BP 145/85, RR 20 Gen: Mild respiratory distress, dehydration, sweaty palms and face, warm skin, hand tremor HEENT: Exophthalmos with lid lag, generalized thyromegaly, thyroid bruit Lungs: WNL CV: Tachycardia Abd: WNL Ext: Edema over the tibia bilaterally	• Anxiety • Atrial fibrillation • Early menopause • Hyperthyroidism • Mitral valve prolapse • Panic attack • Withdrawal syndrome

INITIAL MGMT	CONTINUING MGMT	F/U

Emergency room STAT
- IV normal saline
- O_2
- Needle thoracostomy
- Chest tube
- CXR: Collapsed right lung, mediastinal shift to left
- IV morphine

Emergency room W/U
- Cardiac/BP monitoring
- ECG: Sinus tachycardia
- CBC
- Chem 14
- PT/PTT

Ward W/U
- Thoracic surgery consult
- CXR: Inflated right lung

Rx
- Morphine
- Chest tube to water seal and vacuum device

Ward
- Pleurodesis if indicated

Final Dx - Tension pneumothorax

INITIAL MGMT	CONTINUING MGMT	F/U

Emergency room W/U
- Continuous cardiac and BP monitoring
- Stat ECG: Diffuse ST elevation, PR depression
- CPK-MB, troponin × 3
- CBC
- Chem 8
- CXR: No cardiomegaly
- ESR

Rx
- ASA or NSAIDs
- Start IV
- O_2

Ward W/U
- Discontinue continuous monitoring
- Echocardiography: Minimal pericardial effusion

Rx
- Reassure patient
- ASA

- Discharge home
- Follow up in two weeks

Final Dx - Pericarditis

INITIAL MGMT	CONTINUING MGMT	F/U

Office W/U
- CBC
- BMP
- Thyroid studies (T_4, T_3RU, T_3, TSH): ↑ T_3/T_4, ↓ TSH
- Serum thyroid autoantibodies: ⊕
- ECG
- CXR
- Nuclear scan—thyroid: ↑ uptake

Rx
- Propranolol
- Methimazole
- PTU

Office W/U
- Endocrinology consult

- Check thyroid studies in one month
- Patient counseling

Final Dx - Hyperthyroidism

HIGH-YIELD CASES

CASE 32

HX	PE	DDX
65 yo M presents with sudden onset of severe tearing anterior chest pain that radiates to the back. He is anxious and diaphoretic. He has a history of long-standing hypertension.	VS: T 36°C (97°F), BP 195/110 right arm, 160/80 left arm, HR 100, RR 30, O_2 sat 98% room air Gen: Acute distress Lungs: WNL CV: Tachycardia, S4, diastolic decrescendo heard best at left sternal border Abd: WNL Ext: Unequal pulse in both arms **Limited PE**	• Aortic dissection • MI • Pericarditis • Pulmonary embolism

CASE 33

HX	PE	DDX
34 yo F is brought to the ER after a car accident. She is gasping for air and complains of weakness, chest pain, and dizziness.	VS: Afebrile, BP 100/50, HR 115, RR 22, pulsus paradoxus Gen: Confusion, cyanosis, respiratory distress Neck: ↑ JVP, engorged neck veins, Kussmaul's sign Lungs: WNL CV: Muffled heart sounds, ↓ PMI Abd: WNL Ext: WNL	• Aortic dissection • Cardiogenic shock • MI • Pericardial tamponade • Pericarditis • Pneumothorax • Pulmonary embolism

INITIAL MGMT	CONTINUING MGMT	F/U
Emergency room STAT	**ICU W/U**	• Diet and lifestyle modifications
• ASA	• Continuous cardiac and BP monitoring	• Lipid/BP management
• O_2	• Blood type and cross-match	
• IV normal saline	• PT/PTT, INR	
• SL nitroglycerin	**Rx**	
• CXR: Widened mediastinum	• Continuing IV β-blockers	
• IV β-blockers	• Emergent surgery	
• ECG: LVH		
• IV morphine		
Emergency room W/U		
• Cardiac/BP monitoring		
• CPK-MB, troponin × 3: ⊖		
• CBC		
• Chem 8		
• TEE: Aortic dissection type A or		
• CT—chest with IV contrast: Aortic dissection		
Rx		
• Thoracic surgery consult		

Final Dx - Aortic dissection

INITIAL MGMT	CONTINUING MGMT	F/U
Emergency room W/U	**ICU W/U**	• CXR
• O_2	• Continuous cardiac and BP monitoring	• Echocardiography
• IV normal saline	• ECG	• Patient counseling
• NPO	• Echocardiography	
• Pulse oximetry	• CXR	
• ECG: Tachycardia, low voltage, nonspecific ST- and T-wave changes	• Cardiac surgery consult	
• CPK-MB	• ABG	
• CBC	**Rx**	
• Chem 8	• NPO to liquid	
• ABG	• O_2	
• Coagulation profile	• Follow up in two weeks	
• Blood type and cross-match		
• CXR: Cardiomegaly		
• Echocardiography: Tamponade		
• Pericardiocentesis		

Final Dx - Pericardial tamponade

CASE 34

HX	PE	DDX
28 yo F presents with palpitation, chest pain, nausea, and dizziness that last for almost 5–6 minutes. She has had several attacks over the past few weeks. During these episodes, she becomes diaphoretic and occasionally has diarrhea. In the course of some of her attacks, she describes feeling as if she might die.	VS: P 90, BP 125/75, RR 20 Gen: Mild respiratory distress, dehydration, sweating, cold hands HEENT: WNL Lungs: WNL CV: WNL Abd: WNL Ext: WNL	• Anxiety • Asthma attack • Atrial fibrillation • Early menopause • Hyperthyroidism • Hyperventilation • Hypoglycemia • Mitral valve prolapse • Panic attack • Pheochromocytoma • Pulmonary embolus • Substance abuse

CASE 35

HX	PE	DDX
32 yo F presents with occasional palpitation, chest pain, and dizziness. She also reports shortness of breath and chest tightness during her attacks.	VS: P 90–200 (variable), BP 125/75, RR 20 Gen: Mild cyanosis HEENT: WNL Lungs: Bibasilar crackles CV: Irregularly irregular, tachycardia Abd: WNL Ext: WNL	• Anxiety • Atrial fibrillation • Hyperthyroidism • Hyperventilation • Mitral valve prolapse • Panic attack

INITIAL MGMT	CONTINUING MGMT	F/U

Office W/U
- CBC
- Chem 8
- UA
- Urine toxicology: ⊖
- TFTs
- ECG
- CXR

Rx
- Reassure patient
- Benzodiazepines (e.g., alprazolam, lorazepam, clonazepam) or
- SSRIs

F/U
- Outpatient follow-up in four weeks
- Psychiatry consult
- Patient counseling
- Behavioral modification program
- Relaxation exercises

Final Dx - Panic attack

INITIAL MGMT	CONTINUING MGMT	F/U

Emergency room W/U
- IV normal saline
- O_2
- CBC
- Chem 8
- TFTs
- ECG: Atrial fibrillation
- CXR: Pulmonary vascular congestion
- Echocardiography: Enlarged left atrium

Rx
- Synchronous cardioversion
- Amiodarone (give prior to DC cardioversion if possible)
- Propranolol
- Heparin

ICU W/U
- ECG
- Continuous cardiac monitoring
- Continuous BP monitoring
- Warfarin
- ASA

F/U
- Follow up in two weeks
- Patient counseling

Final Dx - Atrial fibrillation

Abdominal Pain

CASE 36

HX	PE	DDX
38 yo M presents with RUQ abdominal pain of 48 hours' duration. The pain radiates to his right groin and scrotal area and comes in waves of severe intensity that prevent him from finding a comfortable resting position.	VS: T 36°C (96°F), BP 130/85, HR 110, RR 22 Gen: In pain Lungs: WNL CV: Tachycardia Abd: Soft, nontender, no distention, tenderness in right flank, no peritoneal signs, normal BS Rectal exam: WNL, guaiac ⊖	• Gastroenteritis • Nephrolithiasis • Pancreatitis • Perforated duodenal ulcer • Retrocecal appendicitis

CASE 37

HX	PE	DDX
60 yo M presents with generalized weakness, left flank discomfort, nausea, and constipation of two weeks' duration. He has lost 20 pounds over the past four months.	VS: T 37°C (99.2°F), P 90, BP 120/60, RR 18 Gen: NAD Lungs: WNL CV: WNL Abd: ↓ BS, left flank tenderness with deep palpation Rectal exam: WNL Ext: WNL Neuro: WNL	• Colorectal cancer • Renal abscess • Renal cell carcinoma

CASE 38

HX	PE	DDX
32 yo F presents with two days of progressive flank pain, urinary frequency, and a burning sensation during urination. She also reports associated fever and shaking chills.	VS: T 39.1°C (102°F), BP 130/85, HR 86, RR 18 Gen: Mild discomfort with exam Lungs: WNL CV: Tachycardia Abd: ⊕ BS, mild suprapubic tenderness, no peritoneal signs Back: Mild CVA tenderness on the left Pelvic: WNL Rectal exam: WNL, guaiac ⊖	• Acute cervicitis • Acute cystitis • Acute PID • Acute pyelonephritis • Acute urethritis • Ectopic pregnancy • Nephrolithiasis

INITIAL MGMT	CONTINUING MGMT	F/U
Emergency room W/U • CBC: Normal WBC count • Chem 8 • Serum amylase, lipase • UA: Microscopic hematuria • Urine culture • KUB: Radiopaque 3-mm stone • CT—kidney: Stone visualized in distal ureter **Rx** • Analgesia: Narcotics and NSAIDs • Counsel patient re oral hydration	• Serum calcium, magnesium, phosphate • Serum uric acid • Urine strain • Stone analysis: Calcium oxalate	• ↑ fluid intake • Follow up in four weeks • Patient counseling • Counsel patient to limit alcohol intake • Counsel patient to limit caffeine intake • Smoking cessation

Final Dx - Nephrolithiasis

INITIAL MGMT	CONTINUING MGMT	F/U
Office W/U • CBC: Hemoglobin 9.0 • Chem 14: Ca 15, BUN 40, creatinine 2.0 • UA: ⊕ for RBCs • CXR • U/S—complete abdominal: Left renal mass • Admit to ward **Rx** • IV normal saline • Bisphosphonate (pamidronate)	**Ward W/U** • Intact PTH: ↓ • Chem 7: Ca 10, BUN 20, creatinine 1.5 • CT—abdomen and chest: Left renal mass • Renal mass biopsy • Bone scan • CT—head • Ferritin, TIBC, serum iron **Rx** • Oncology consult • Surgery consult	

Final Dx - Renal cell carcinoma

INITIAL MGMT	CONTINUING MGMT	F/U
Office W/U • CBC: ↑ WBC count • Chem 8 • UA: WBC, bacteria, nitrite ⊕ • Urine culture: Pending • Urinary β-hCG: ⊖ • U/S—renal **Rx** • Ciprofloxacin (fluoroquinolone)	**Office W/U** • Urine culture: ⊕ for *E. coli*	• Follow up in 3–5 days • Patient counseling • Counsel patient re medication compliance • Counsel patient to limit alcohol intake

Final Dx - Pyelonephritis

CASE 39

HX	PE	DDX
10 yo African-American M presents with sudden onset of jaundice, dark-colored urine, back pain, and fatigue. He was started on TMP-SMX for an ear infection a few days ago. He has a family history of blood disorders.	VS: T 38°C (99.8°F), P 90, BP 110/50, RR 14 Gen: NAD Skin: Jaundice HEENT: Icterus, pallor Lungs: WNL CV: WNL Abd: WNL Ext: WNL	• Autoimmune hemolytic anemia • DIC • G6PD deficiency • Sickle cell anemia • Spherocytosis • Thalassemias • TTP

CASE 40

HX	PE	DDX
58 yo alcoholic M presents with a one-day history of sharp epigastric pain that radiates to his back. He is nauseated and has vomited several times. He also complains of anorexia. The patient reports heavy alcohol use over the past 2–3 days. He has no previous history of peptic ulcer disease.	VS: T 38.2°C (101°F), BP 138/68, HR 110, RR 22 Gen: WD/WN but agitated, lying on bed with knees drawn up Lungs: ↓ breath sounds over left lower lung CV: Tachycardia Abd: Tender and distended with ↓ BS	• Acute cholecystitis • Acute gastritis • Acute pancreatitis • Aortic dissection • Cholelithiasis • Intestinal perforation • MI • Perforated duodenal ulcers • Pneumonia

INITIAL MGMT	CONTINUING MGMT	F/U

Office W/U
- CBC stat and q 12 h: ↓↓ hemoglobin, ↓↓ hematocrit
- Peripheral smear: Bite cells, fragment cells
- Chem 14: ↑ indirect bilirubin
- PT/PTT, INR

Rx
- Discontinue TMP-SMX

Ward W/U
- Reticulocyte count: Elevated
- LDH: ↑
- Haptoglobin: ↓
- UA: Hemoglobinuria
- G6PD assay: Consistent with G6PD deficiency
- Type and cross two units of packed RBCs

Rx
- Start IV
- IV normal saline
- Transfuse two units of packed RBCs

- Discharge home
- Follow up in two months
- Educate patient/family

Final Dx - G6PD deficiency

INITIAL MGMT	CONTINUING MGMT	F/U

Emergency room W/U
- IV normal saline
- NPO
- Monitor, continue BP cuff
- NG tube suction
- ECG: No evidence of ischemia
- CBC
- Chem 14
- Serum amylase, lipase: ↑
- ABG
- O₂
- Pulse oximetry
- LFTs
- Serum calcium
- AXR, upright
- CXR

Rx
- NG tube
- IV meperidine

Ward W/U
- Monitor, continue BP cuff
- Continue NPO
- U/S—liver, gallbladder and bile duct, pancreas
- PT/PTT
- CT—abdomen
- Surgery consult
- GI consult
- Advance diet as tolerated

- Follow up in seven days
- Patient counseling
- Counsel patient to cease alcohol intake
- Smoking cessation

Final Dx - Acute pancreatitis

HIGH-YIELD CASES

CASE 41

HX	PE	DDX
1-day-old M born at home is brought to the ER because of bilious vomiting, irritability, poor feeding, lethargy, and an acute episode of rectal bleeding.	VS: T 38°C (100°F), P 170, BP 69/44, RR 43, O$_2$ sat 89% room air Skin: Evidence of poor perfusion Chest: WNL CV: WNL Abd: Distention; evidence of intestinal obstruction **Limited PE**	• Duodenal web • Intestinal atresia • Malrotation with volvulus • Meconium plug/ileus • Necrotizing enterocolitis

CASE 42

HX	PE	DDX
21-month-old M is brought to the ER because of intermittent abdominal pain that causes him to become still while drawing up his legs. He also presents with irritability and vomiting that initially was clear but then became bilious. The child seemed lethargic between the pain episodes. In the ER, the child passes some dark red stool.	VS: T 38.5°C (101°F), P 157, BP 81/59, RR 35, O$_2$ sat 93% room air Skin: No evidence of purpura Chest: WNL CV: WNL Abd: Soft and mildly tender; examination of RUQ fails to identify presence of bowel; ill-defined mass in the RUQ **Limited PE**	• Intoxication • Intussusception • Metabolic disease • Neurologic disease • Small bowel obstruction • Volvulus

INITIAL MGMT	CONTINUING MGMT	F/U

Emergency room STAT
- IV normal saline
- O$_2$
- ABG: Metabolic acidosis

Emergency room W/U
- CBC: ↑ WBC count, mildly ↓ hemoglobin
- Chem 8
- AXR: Airless rectum; large gastric bubble
- CXR: No evidence of diaphragmatic hernia

Rx
- NG tube suction
- IV bicarbonate (to correct acidosis if pH < 7.0)
- Pediatric surgery consult

Ward W/U
- Upper GI series: Bird's-beak, corkscrew appearance of proximal jejunum
- Barium enema: Cecum in RUQ

Rx
- NG tube suction
- IV normal saline

- Follow up in 48 hours
- Family counseling

Final Dx - Malrotation with volvulus

INITIAL MGMT	CONTINUING MGMT	F/U

Emergency room STAT
- IV normal saline
- O$_2$

Emergency room W/U
- CBC: ↑ WBC count
- Chem 14
- ABG: Metabolic acidosis
- AXR: Distended bowel with air-fluid levels; mass in right abdomen
- U/S—abdomen: Compatible with intussusception

Rx
- NG tube suction
- Barium enema: Coiled-spring appearance; disorder is relieved by air insufflation
- Pediatric surgery consult

Ward W/U
- AXR: Gastric bubble; no air-fluid levels
- ABG: Derangements being resolved

Rx
- D/C NG tube suction
- IV normal saline
- Advance diet

- Follow up in 48 hours
- Family counseling

Final Dx - Intussusception

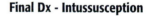

CASE 43

HX	PE	DDX
27-month-old M presents to the ER with seizures, irritability, anorexia, altered sleep patterns, emotional lability, and vomiting. His mother states that the family has been living for about a year in an old, poorly maintained building that has only recently begun to undergo renovation. Since she was laid off at the battery plant, the family has been considering moving out of town.	VS: T 37°C (99°F), P 129, BP 89/61, RR 20, O_2 sat 92% room air Neuro: Lethargy, ataxia, seizures Remainder of physical examination is noncontributory (except for some conjunctival pallor)	• Lead toxicity • Metabolic disease • Neurologic disease • Nonmetal intoxication • Other heavy metal toxicity

CASE 44

HX	PE	DDX
7-day-old alert M presents to a clinic with jaundice that started two days ago. The baby was born at term via an uneventful vaginal delivery and started breast-feeding after some delay. The mother states that she took the baby to the doctor's office at that time and that the baby's bilirubin was 14 mg/dL. The mother does not take any drugs. She is very concerned that the baby's jaundice is not improving and asks if the baby has kernicterus.	VS: T 37°C (99°F), P 129, BP 80/51, RR 29, O_2 sat 94% room air PE: WNL except for jaundice Neuro: WNL	• Breast-feeding jaundice • Hereditary spherocytosis • Physiologic hyperbiliru-binemia • Unconjugated hyper-bilirubinemia (Gilbert's/Crigler-Najjar)

CASE 45

HX	PE	DDX
31 yo M comes to the office complaining of midepigastric pain that usually begins 1–2 hours after eating and sometimes awakens him at night. He also has occasional indigestion. He is taking an antacid for his problem. He denies melena or hematemesis.	VS: T 37.1°C (99°F), BP 130/75, HR 100, RR 16 Gen: Pallor, no distress Lungs: WNL CV: WNL Abd: Epigastric tenderness Rectal exam: WNL	• Acute gastritis • Diverticulitis • GERD • Pancreatic disease • Peptic ulcer disease • Mesenteric ischemia

INITIAL MGMT	CONTINUING MGMT	F/U
Emergency room W/U • CBC: Hemoglobin 9 g/dL, MCV 75, blood smear reveals coarse basophilic stippling in RBCs • Chem 8 • Serum lead: 80 µg/dL • UA: Glycosuria • Free erythrocyte protoporphyrin: ↑ • Serum toxicology: ↑ lead levels **Rx** • IV normal saline • IM EDTA	**Ward Rx** • IV normal saline • Serum lead • IM EDTA (if necessary) • Family counseling	• Follow up in seven days • Family counseling • Lead paint assay in home

Final Dx - Lead intoxication with encephalopathy

INITIAL MGMT	CONTINUING MGMT	F/U
Office W/U • CBC: WNL, smear WNL • Direct Coombs' test: Noncontributory • Serum bilirubin: ↑ indirect bilirubin • TSH: WNL	**Office W/U** • Breast-feeding suppression test: Bilirubin levels ↓ on cessation of breast-feeding; levels ↑ again when breast-feeding restarted **Rx** • Continue breast feedings • Consider phototherapy (if bilirubin levels do not ↓)	• Follow up in seven days • Family counseling

Final Dx - Breast-feeding neonatal jaundice

INITIAL MGMT	CONTINUING MGMT	F/U
Office W/U • CBC • Chem 8 • Serum amylase, lipase • Serum *H. pylori* antibody • Stool *H. pylori* antibody **Rx** • Proton pump inhibitor • Clarithromycin (Biaxin) • Metronidazole		• Follow up in four weeks; patient reports that he is feeling better (if symptoms persist or if *H. pylori* is still present, may proceed to endoscopy) • Patient counseling • Counsel patient to limit alcohol intake • Smoking cessation

Final Dx - Gastritis (*H. pylori* infection)

CASE 46

HX	PE	DDX
45 yo M presents with a six-week history of jaundice, pale stools, tea-colored urine, and epigastric pain that radiates to the back. He also reports that he has bilateral lower extremity swelling.	VS: T 37°C (98°F), BP 130/70, HR 90, RR 16 Gen: Jaundice Lungs: WNL CV: WNL Abd: Palpable epigastric mass Ext: Lower extremity swelling with pain on dorsiflexion of ankle	• Cholangiocarcinoma • Colon/stomach cancer with metastases in the porta hepatis region causing biliary obstruction • Pancreatic cancer

CASE 47

HX	PE	DDX
60 yo F G0 presents with a two-month history of ↑ abdominal girth, ↓ appetite, and early satiety. She also has mild shortness of breath.	VS: T 36°C (97°F), BP 140/60, HR 90, RR 23 Gen: Pallor Breast: WNL Lungs: WNL CV: WNL Abd: Distended, nontender, normal BS, no palpable hepatosplenomegaly Pelvic: Solid right adnexal mass Rectal exam: Solid right adnexal mass; no involvement of recto-vaginal septum	• CHF • Liver cirrhosis • Ovarian cancer

CASE 48

HX	PE	DDX
32 yo F presents with sudden onset of left lower abdominal pain that radiates to the scapula and back and is associated with vaginal bleeding. Her last menstrual period was five weeks ago. She has a history of pelvic inflammatory disease and unprotected intercourse.	VS: T 37°C (99°F), P 90, BP 120/50, RR 14 Gen: Moderate distress 2° to pain Lungs: WNL CV: WNL Abd: RLQ tenderness, rebound, and guarding Pelvic: Slightly enlarged uterus with small amount of dark bloody discharge from cervix; right adnexal tenderness	• Ectopic pregnancy • Ovarian torsion • PID • Ruptured ovarian cyst

INITIAL MGMT	CONTINUING MGMT	F/U

Office W/U
- CBC
- Chem 14
- Bilirubin, ALT, AST, alkaline phosphatase
- CT—abdomen: Large necrotic pancreatic mass in head
- ERCP/EUS:Biopsy to obtain histology

Ward Rx
- Medical oncology consult; palliative care
- Surgery is not an option owing to advanced disease

Final Dx - Pancreatic cancer

INITIAL MGMT	CONTINUING MGMT	F/U

Office W/U
- CBC
- Chem 14
- CA-125: 900
- CT—abdomen and pelvis: 10- × 12-cm right complex ovarian cyst; large amounts of ascites
- CXR: Right moderate pleural effusion
- ECG
- Pap smear
- Mammogram
- Colonoscopy
- Gynecology consult

Ward Rx
- Blood type and cross-match
- PT/PTT, INR
- Exploratory laparotomy
- TAH-BSO, laparotomy
- Staging, laparotomy

- Carboplatin
- CA-125
- CBC
- Chem 14

Final Dx - Ovarian cancer

INITIAL MGMT	CONTINUING MGMT	F/U

Emergency room W/U
- Urinary β-hCG: ⊕
- Quantitative serum β-hCG: 2500
- CBC
- Chem 8
- Cervical Gram stain and G&C culture
- U/S—transvaginal: 2-cm right adnexal mass, no intrauterine pregnancy, free fluid in cul-de-sac

Rx
- IV normal saline

- Blood type and cross-match
- PT/PTT, INR
- Gynecology consult
- Laparoscopy
- Rh IgG (RhoGAM) if Rh-⊖

- Counsel patient on contraception
- Counsel patient re safe sex practices

Final Dx - Ectopic pregnancy

HIGH-YIELD CASES

CASE 49

HX	PE	DDX
74 yo M presents with LLQ abdominal pain, fever, and chills for the past three days. He also reports recent-onset episodes of alternating diarrhea and constipation. He consumes a low-fiber, high-fat diet.	VS: T 38°C (101°F), BP 130/85, HR 100, RR 22 Gen: Pallor, diaphoresis Lungs: WNL CV: Tachycardia Abd: LLQ tenderness, no peritoneal signs, sluggish BS Rectal exam: Guaiac ⊖	• Crohn's disease • Diverticular abscess • Diverticulitis • Gastroenteritis • Ulcerative colitis

CASE 50

HX	PE	DDX
41 yo F presents with sudden-onset RUQ abdominal pain of six hours' duration. She also reports nausea and emesis. The pain started after lunch and has become more severe and constant. She reports that the pain is exacerbated by deep breathing and that it radiates to her shoulder. She had a similar attack almost one year ago. She is taking OCPs and has three children.	VS: T 39.0°C (102°F), BP 130/82, HR 80, RR 16 Gen: WD, slightly obese, moderate distress Lungs: WNL CV: WNL Abd: Obesity, tenderness and guarding to palpation on RUQ, ⊕ Murphy's sign, ↓ BS Rectal exam: WNL, guaiac ⊖	• Acute appendicitis • Acute cholangitis • Acute cholecystitis • Acute hepatitis • Acute pancreatitis • Acute peptic ulcer disease with or without perforation • Biliary atresia • Cardiac ischemia • Cholelithiasis • Fitz-Hugh–Curtis syndrome (gonococcal perihepatitis) • Gastritis • Renal colic • Right-sided pneumonia • Small bowel obstruction

INITIAL MGMT	CONTINUING MGMT	F/U
Emergency room W/U • CBC: ↑ WBC count • Chem 14 • Serum amylase, lipase • UA • Urine culture: Pending • Blood culture: Pending • Stool culture and sensitivity • Stool for ova and parasites • CXR • KUB • CT—abdomen: Diverticulitis **Rx** • NPO • IV normal saline • IV metronidazole + ciprofloxacin	**Ward W/U** • Urine culture: Pending • Blood culture: Pending **Rx** • NPO or clear liquid diet • Surgery consult • Metronidazole + ciprofloxacin × 7–10 days • Discharge home in 3–4 days	• High-fiber diet • Colonoscopy four weeks after recovery

Final Dx - Diverticulitis

INITIAL MGMT	CONTINUING MGMT	F/U
Emergency room W/U • IV normal saline • NPO • Monitor, continue BP cuff • ECG • CBC • Chem 14 • Serum amylase, lipase • LFTs • Blood/urine cultures • AXR/CXR • Pregnancy test—urine • U/S—abdomen: Gallstones with gallbladder edema **Rx** • IM prochlorperazine • IV morphine • IV cefuroxime	**Ward W/U** • Blood type and cross-match • PT/PTT, INR • Surgery consult for cholecystectomy • Vitals q 4 h • CBC next day • Chem 8 next day **Rx** • NPO → advance diet as tolerated • Continue antibiotic therapy	• Follow up in two weeks • Patient counseling • Counsel patient to limit alcohol intake

Final Dx - Acute cholecystitis

CASE 51

HX	PE	DDX
24 yo F presents with bilateral lower abdominal pain that started with the first day of her menstrual period. The pain is associated with fever and a thick, greenish-yellow vaginal discharge. She has had unprotected sex with multiple sexual partners.	VS: T 38°C (100.4°F), P 90, BP 110/50, RR 14 Gen: Moderate distress 2° to pain Lungs: WNL CV: WNL Abd: Diffuse tenderness (greatest in the lower quadrants), no rebound, no distention, ↓ BS Pelvic: Purulent, bloody discharge from cervix; cervical motion and bilateral adnexal tenderness Rectal exam: WNL Ext: WNL	• Dysmenorrhea • Endometriosis • PID • Pyelonephritis • Vaginitis

CASE 52

HX	PE	DDX
25 yo M is brought to the ER because of abdominal pain and ↓ appetite for four days. This episode was preceded by ↑ urinary frequency, nausea, and vomiting.	VS: T 37°C (98°F), P 120, BP 100/60, RR 25 Gen: Moderate distress Skin: Poor skin turgor HEENT: Dry mucous membranes, "fruity breath" Lungs: WNL CV: Tachycardia Abd: Generalized tenderness Ext: WNL Neuro: WNL **Limited PE**	• Acute intestinal obstruction • Alcoholic ketoacidosis • Appendicitis • DKA • Drug intoxication • Gastroenteritis • Pancreatitis • Pyelonephritis

INITIAL MGMT	CONTINUING MGMT	F/U
Emergency room W/U	**Ward W/U**	• Counsel patient re safe sex practices
• Urinary β-hCG: $\ominus$	• Cervical culture: *N. gonorrhoeae*	• Treat partners
• CBC: ↑ WBC count	**Rx**	
• Chem 14	• Discontinue IV ceftriaxone when symptoms improve (usually in 24–48 hours)	
• Cervical Gram stain and G&C culture		
• U/S—pelvis		
• UA and urine culture	• Switch to doxycycline or clindamycin	
Rx		
• IV normal saline		
• IV ceftriaxone + PO doxycycline or PO azithromycin		
• Acetaminophen		

Final Dx - Pelvic inflammatory disease (PID)

INITIAL MGMT	CONTINUING MGMT	F/U
Emergency room STAT	**ICU W/U**	• Diabetic diet
• Glucometer: 480 mg/dL	• Continuous monitoring	• Diabetic teaching
• IV normal saline	• Random glucose q 1 h	• Hb_{A1c} q 3 months
Emergency room W/U	• Chem 8 q 4 h: ↓ K, glucose < 250	• Follow up in two weeks in the office
• Continuous monitoring	**Rx**	• Diabetic foot care
• Chem 14: Normal K, normal Na, ↑ anion gap	• Switch IV fluid to D_5W	• Ophthalmology consult
• CBC: ↑ WBC count	• IV potassium	• Lipid profile
• Serum amylase, lipase	• SQ insulin NPH	• Instruct patient in home sugar monitoring
• UA and urine culture: $\oplus$ glucose, $\oplus$ ketone	• SQ insulin regular	• Home sugar monitoring, glucometer
• Urine/serum toxicology	• Discontinue IV insulin two hours after starting long-acting insulin (NPH or Lantus)	
• Phosphate: ↓		
• ECG		
• ABG: Metabolic acidosis (pH = 7.1)		
• Quantitative serum ketones: ↑		
• Serum osmolality: Normal		
• CXR/AXR		
Rx		
• IV regular insulin, continue		
• Phosphate therapy		

Final Dx - Diabetic ketoacidosis (DKA)

HIGH-YIELD CASES

Constipation/Diarrhea

CASE 53

HX	PE	DDX
67 yo M presents with constipation, ↓ stool caliber, and blood in his stool for the past eight months. He also reports unintentional weight loss. He is on a low-fiber diet and has a family history of colon cancer.	VS: P 85, BP 140/85, RR 14, O_2 sat 98% room air Gen: NAD HEENT: Pale conjunctiva Lungs: WNL CV: WNL Abd: WNL Pelvic: WNL Rectal exam: Hemoccult ⊕	• Angiodysplasia • Colorectal cancer • Diverticulosis • GI parasitic infection (ascariasis, giardiasis) • Hemorrhoids • Hypothyroidism • Inflammatory bowel disease • Irritable bowel syndrome

CASE 54

HX	PE	DDX
28 yo M presents with diffuse abdominal pain, loose stools, perianal pain, mild fever, and weight loss over the past four weeks. He denies any history of travel or recent use of antibiotics.	VS: T 37°C (99°F), BP 130/65, HR 70, RR 14 Gen: NAD Lungs: WNL CV: WNL Abd: WNL Rectal exam: Perianal skin tags, hemoccult ⊕	• Crohn's disease • Diverticulitis • Gastroenteritis • Infectious colitis • Irritable bowel syndrome • Ischemic colitis • Lactose intolerance • Pseudomembranous colitis • Small bowel lymphoma • Ulcerative colitis

CASE 55

HX	PE	DDX
30 yo F presents with periumbilical crampy pain of six months' duration. The pain never awakens her from sleep. It is relieved by defecation and worsens when she is upset. She has alternating constipation and diarrhea but no nausea, vomiting, weight loss, or anorexia.	VS: Afebrile, P 85, BP 130/65, RR 14 Gen: NAD Lungs: WNL CV: WNL Abd: WNL Pelvic: WNL Rectal exam: Guaiac ⊖	• Celiac disease • Chronic pancreatitis • Colorectal cancer • Crohn's disease • Diverticulosis • Endometriosis • GI parasitic infection (ascariasis, giardiasis) • Hypothyroidism • Inflammatory bowel disease • Irritable bowel syndrome

INITIAL MGMT	CONTINUING MGMT	F/U

Office W/U
- CBC: ↓ hematocrit, ↓ MCV
- Chem 8: Normal
- Ferritin: ↓
- Serum iron: ↓
- TIBC: ↑
- TSH: Normal
- Stool for ova and parasites
- ESR: Normal
- Stool guaiac: ⊕

Office W/U
- GI consult
- Colonoscopy: Polyp with adenocarcinoma
- CT—abdomen and pelvis with contrast
- CEA

Rx
- Iron sulfate
- General surgery consult
- Plan partial colectomy

Final Dx - Colorectal cancer

INITIAL MGMT	CONTINUING MGMT	F/U

Office W/U
- CBC
- Chem 14
- Serum amylase, lipase
- Stool for ova and parasites
- Stool C. *difficile*
- AXR
- Colonoscopy: Crohn's disease

Rx
- 5-ASA
- Metronidazole (for perianal abscess or fistula)

- Follow up in two weeks
- Counsel patient re medication compliance and adherence

Final Dx - Crohn's disease

INITIAL MGMT	CONTINUING MGMT	F/U

Office W/U
- CBC
- Chem 14
- TSH
- Stool for ova and parasites
- Stool for WBCs
- Stool culture and sensitivity
- Transglutaminase antibody

Rx
- Educate patient
- Reassurance
- High-fiber diet
- Lactose-free diet

- Follow up in four weeks
- Call with questions

Final Dx - Irritable bowel syndrome

HIGH-YIELD CASES

CASE 56

HX	PE	DDX
8 yo M is brought to the clinic by his mother for intermittent diarrhea alternating with constipation together with vomiting and cramping abdominal pain. His mother also reports that he has had progressive anorexia.	VS: T 37°C (98°F), BP 110/65, HR 90, RR 16 Gen: Pale and dry mucosal membranes; lack of growth Lungs: WNL CV: WNL Abd: WNL Ext: Muscle wasting, especially in gluteal area	• Bacterial gastroenteritis • Celiac disease • Food allergy • Giardiasis • Protein intolerance • Viral gastroenteritis

CASE 57

HX	PE	DDX
28 yo M reports intermittent episodes of vomiting and diarrhea along with cramping abdominal pain for the past two days. He describes his stool as watery. He returned from Mexico three days ago.	VS: T 39°C (101.9°F), BP 135/85, HR 100, RR 22 Gen: Mild dehydration Lungs: WNL CV: WNL Abd: Mild tenderness, no peritoneal signs, hyperactive BS Rectal exam: WNL, guaiac ⊖	• *Campylobacter* infection • Cholera • *C. difficile* colitis • Crohn's disease • Giardiasis • Salmonellosis • Shigellosis • Traveler's diarrhea, *E. coli*

CASE 58

HX	PE	DDX
40 yo F presents with fever, anorexia, nausea, profuse and watery diarrhea, and diffuse abdominal pain. Last week she was on antibiotics for a UTI.	VS: T 38°C (100.4°F), BP 100/50, HR 100, RR 22, orthostatic hypotension Gen: WNL Lungs: WNL CV: Tachycardia Abd: Diffuse tenderness, no peritoneal signs, ⊕ BS Rectal exam: Guaiac ⊕	• Amebiasis • Food poisoning • Gastroenteritis • Giardiasis • Hepatitis A • Infectious diarrhea (bacterial, viral, parasitic, protozoal) • Inflammatory bowel disease • Pseudomembranous (*C. difficile*) colitis • Traveler's diarrhea

INITIAL MGMT	CONTINUING MGMT	F/U
Office W/U • CBC • Chem 14 • UA • Stool for ova and parasites • Stool occult blood • Stool Gram stain • Stool fat stain • Barium enema • CT—abdomen • Ferritin • Serum folate • Serum B$_{12}$ • Serum endomysial antibody: ⊕ titers • Serum transglutaminase antibody: ⊕ titers	**Ward W/U** • CXR: Normal • KUB: Normal • CT—abdomen: Normal • D-xylose tolerance test: Carbohydrate malabsorption • Peroral duodenal biopsy: Villi are atrophic or absent • Dietary consult **Rx** • Gluten-free diet • Prednisone • Vitamin D • Calcium	• Follow up in one week • Patient counseling • Pneumococcal vaccine

Final Dx - Celiac disease

INITIAL MGMT	CONTINUING MGMT	F/U
Emergency room W/U • CBC • Chem 14 • Stool culture • Fecal leukocyte stain • Stool for *C. difficile* • Stool Gram stain • Stool for ova and parasites • Stool occult blood • Stool fat stain • UA and urine culture	**Emergency room W/U** • Stool culture: ⊕ for *E. coli* • Stool Gram stain: ⊕ for gram-⊖ rods and ↑ leukocytes **Rx** • Oral hydration • Ciprofloxacin	• Follow up in one week • Patient counseling • Counsel patient to limit alcohol intake • Smoking cessation

Final Dx - Gastroenteritis

INITIAL MGMT	CONTINUING MGMT	F/U
Emergency room W/U • Stool culture • Stool *Giardia* antigen • Stool for ova and parasites • Stool WBCs: ⊕ • Stool for *C. difficile*: ⊕ • CBC: ↑ WBC count • Chem 14 **Rx** • IV normal saline • Metronidazole	**Ward W/U** • No orthostatic hypotension **Rx** • Send home on metronidazole (when diarrhea improves); no Lomotil/Imodium	• Counsel patient re oral hydration

Final Dx - Pseudomembranous (*C. difficile*) colitis

CASE 59

HX	PE	DDX
33 yo M presents with foul-smelling, watery diarrhea together with diffuse abdominal cramps and bloating that began yesterday. He also vomited once. He was recently in Mexico.	VS: T 37°C (98°F), BP 110/50, HR 85, RR 22, no orthostatic hypotension Gen: WNL Lungs: WNL CV: WNL Abd: No tenderness, no peritoneal signs, active BS Rectal exam: Guaiac ⊖	• Amebiasis • Food poisoning • Gastroenteritis • Giardiasis • Hepatitis A • Infectious diarrhea (bacterial, viral, parasitic, protozoal) • Inflammatory bowel disease • Pseudomembranous (*C. difficile*) colitis • Traveler's diarrhea

GI Bleeding

CASE 60

HX	PE	DDX
38 yo M presents with intermittent hematemesis of two weeks' duration. He has a history of epigastric pain for almost two years that occasionally worsens when he eats food or drinks milk. He also reports melena of three weeks' duration. His social history is significant for alcohol and tobacco use.	VS: T 37°C (98.9°F), BP 90/65, HR 110, RR 24 Gen: Pallor Lungs: WNL CV: WNL Abd: No tenderness, no peritoneal signs, normal BS Rectal exam: WNL, guaiac ⊕ **Limited PE**	• Duodenal ulcers • Esophageal tear • Gastric carcinoma • Gastric ulcer • Portal hypertension

INITIAL MGMT	CONTINUING MGMT	F/U

Office W/U
- Stool culture
- Stool *Giardia* antigen: $\oplus$
- Stool for ova and parasites
- Stool WBCs
- Stool for *C. difficile*
- CBC
- Chem 8

Rx
- Metronidazole

- Counsel patient re oral hydration

Final Dx - Giardiasis

INITIAL MGMT	CONTINUING MGMT	F/U

Emergency room STAT
- IV normal saline
- O_2
- Orthostatic vitals: Drop on standing
- Type and cross-match

Emergency room W/U
- CBC: Hematocrit 24
- Chem 14
- Upper GI series: Gastric antral lesion with adherent clot
- PT/PTT, INR
- CXR
- ECG

Rx
- NPO
- NG tube, iced saline lavage: Clears with 1 L of normal saline
- IV pantoprazole
- IV cimetidine

ICU W/U
- CBC q 4 h until hematocrit is stable; then frequency can be ↓

Rx
- GI consult
- Combination therapy with epinephrine injection followed by thermal coagulation
- Octreotide for varices
- Advance diet
- Ranitidine
- Pantoprazole
- Transfer to wards if patient remains stable
- *H. pylori* serology and eradication if $\oplus$

- Follow up in one week
- Patient counseling
- Counsel patient to cease alcohol intake
- Smoking cessation
- Dietary consult

Final Dx - Bleeding gastric ulcer

CASE 61

HX	PE	DDX
67 yo F presents with acute crampy abdominal pain, weakness, and black stool. She reports diffuse abdominal pain of three months' duration. Eating worsens the pain. She has had a five-pound weight loss over the last three months.	VS: T 37°C (98.9°F), BP 90/65, HR 100, RR 24 Gen: Mild dehydration Lungs: WNL CV: WNL Abd: Tender and mildly distended; no rigidity or rebound tenderness Rectal exam: WNL, guaiac ⊕ **Limited PE**	• Adenocarcinoma of the colon • Crohn's disease • Diverticular bleed • Infectious colitis • Ischemic colitis • Peptic ulcer disease • Ulcerative colitis

CASE 62

HX	PE	DDX
30 yo M presents with loose, watery stools that are streaked with blood and mucus. He has also had colicky abdominal pain and weight loss over the past three weeks. He denies any history of travel, radiation, or recent medication use (antibiotics, NSAIDs).	VS: T 37°C (99°F), BP 130/65, HR 70, RR 14 Gen: NAD Lungs: WNL CV: WNL Abd: WNL Rectal exam: Blood-stained stool	• Crohn's disease • Diverticulitis • Gastroenteritis • Infectious colitis • Internal hemorrhoid • Ischemic colitis • Pseudomembranous colitis • Radiation colitis • Ulcerative colitis

INITIAL MGMT	CONTINUING MGMT	F/U
Emergency room STAT • IV normal saline • O_2 **Emergency room W/U** • CBC • Chem 14 • Serum amylase: Normal • LDH: ↑ • PT/PTT • CXR • ECG • AXR • CT—abdomen: Pneumatosis coli • Blood type and cross-match **Rx** • NPO • Surgery consult (for bowel resection) • Broad-spectrum antibiotics • NG tube suction	**Ward W/U** • Hemoglobin and hema- tocrit q 4 h **Rx** • Advance diet • Monitor carefully for per- sistent fever, leukocytosis, peritoneal irritation, diar- rhea, and/or bleeding	• Follow up in four weeks • Patient counseling • Counsel patient to cease alcohol intake • Smoking cessation • Dietary consult

Final Dx - Ischemic colitis

INITIAL MGMT	CONTINUING MGMT	F/U
Office W/U • CBC: Mild anemia • Chem 14 • Serum amylase, lipase • Stool culture and sensitivity • Stool for ova and parasites • Stool WBCs • PT/PTT • Flexible sigmoidoscopy and rectal biopsy: Consistent with ulcerative colitis involving rectum and distal sigmoid colon **Rx** • IV steroids (for attack) or • 5-ASA enema/suppositories • Sulfasalazine		• Follow up in two weeks • Counsel patient re med- ication compliance and adherence

Final Dx - Ulcerative colitis

INITIAL MGMT	CONTINUING MGMT	F/U

Office W/U
- Urine pregnancy test
- Prolactin
- TSH
- FSH: ↑
- Wet mount
- Pap smear
- Mammogram
- DEXA scan

Rx
- Calcium
- Vitamin D
- SSRI (venlafaxine) for hot flashes
- Premarin (vaginal estrogen)
- Vaginal jelly for lubrication

- Follow up in 12 months
- Counsel patient re HRT—not recommended unless only short-term treatment is planned and if the patient has no CAD, breast cancer, or thromboembolic risk factors

Final Dx - Menopause

INITIAL MGMT	CONTINUING MGMT	F/U

Office W/U
- TSH
- FSH: ↑
- LH: ↑
- Karyotyping: Consistent with Turner's syndrome
- Lipid panel
- Fasting glucose

Rx
- Growth hormone therapy
- Estrogen + progestin
- Psychiatry consult for IQ estimation
- Vitamin D
- Calcium

Office W/U
- 2D echocardiography
- U/S—renal
- U/S—pelvis: Streaked ovaries
- Skeletal survey: Short fourth metacarpal
- Chem 13
- CBC
- UA
- Lipid profile
- Hearing test

Rx
- Continue growth hormone therapy until epiphysis is closed
- Combination estrogen and progestin
- Encourage weight-bearing exercises

- Stop growth hormone when bone age > 15 years
- Audiogram every 3–5 years
- Check yearly for hypertension
- Monitor aortic root diameter every 3–5 years

Final Dx - Turner's syndrome

HIGH-YIELD CASES

Vaginal Bleeding

CASE 74

HX	PE	DDX
21 yo F complains of prolonged and excessive menstrual bleeding and menstrual frequency for the past six months.	VS: T 36°C (97°F), P 65, BP 120/60, RR 14 Gen: NAD HEENT: WNL Lungs: WNL CV: WNL Abd: WNL GU: WNL	• Bleeding disorder • Dysfunctional uterine bleeding • Fibroids • Hyperthyroidism • Hypothyroidism • Pregnancy

CASE 75

HX	PE	DDX
27 yo F whose last menstrual period was seven weeks ago presents with lower abdominal cramping and heavy vaginal bleeding.	VS: T 36°C (97°F), BP 120/60, HR 80, RR 12 Gen: NAD Lungs: WNL CV: WNL Abd: Suprapubic tenderness with no rebound or guarding Pelvic: Active bleeding from cervix, cervical os open, seven-week-size uterus, mildly tender, no cervical motion tenderness, no adnexal masses or tenderness	• Cervical or vaginal pathology (polyp, infection, neoplasia) • Cervical polyp • Ectopic pregnancy • Menstrual period with dysmenorrhea • Spontaneous abortion

CASE 76

HX	PE	DDX
60 yo F G0 who had her last menstrual period 10 years ago presents with mild vaginal bleeding for the last two days. Her medical history is significant for type 2 diabetes, hypertension, and infertility.	VS: T 36°C (97°F), BP 120/60, HR 80, RR 14 Gen: NAD HEENT: WNL Lungs: WNL CV: WNL Abd: WNL Pelvic: WNL	• Atrophic endometritis • Cervical cancer • Endometrial cancer • Endometrial polyp

INITIAL MGMT	CONTINUING MGMT	F/U

Office W/U
- Qualitative urine pregnancy test
- TSH
- CBC: Hypochromic microcytic anemia
- Bleeding time
- PT/aPTT, INR
- U/S—pelvis
- Pap smear

Rx
- Iron sulfate
- NSAIDs
- OCPs

F/U
- Follow up in six months
- Counsel patient re safe sex practices

Final Dx - Dysfunctional uterine bleeding

INITIAL MGMT	CONTINUING MGMT	F/U

Emergency room W/U
- Qualitative urine pregnancy test: $\oplus$
- Quantitative serum β-hCG: 3000
- CBC: Hemoglobin 9
- Blood type and cross-match
- Rh factor
- U/S—pelvis: Intrauterine pregnancy sac, fetal pole, no fetal heart tones
- Gynecology consult

Rx
- Fluids, IV normal saline
- D&C

Ward W/U
- CBC

Rx
- Methylergonovine
- Doxycycline
- Counsel patient re birth control
- Grief counseling
- Pelvic rest for two weeks

F/U
- Follow up in three weeks

Final Dx - Spontaneous abortion

INITIAL MGMT	CONTINUING MGMT	F/U

Office W/U
- CBC
- Chem 14
- PT/PTT, INR
- Bleeding time
- Pap smear
- Endometrial biopsy: Poorly differentiated endometrioid adenocarcinoma
- U/S—pelvis: 10-mm endometrial stripe
- Gynecology consult

Ward W/U
- CXR
- ECG
- CA-125

Rx
- Exploratory laparotomy
- TAH-BSO
- Depending on staging, patient may benefit from adjuvant therapy (radiation vs. chemo vs. hormonal therapy)

Final Dx - Endometrial cancer

CASE 77

HX	PE	DDX
32 yo F G2P1011 presents with vaginal bleeding after intercourse for the last month. She has no history of abnormal Pap smears or STDs and has had the same partner for the last eight years. She uses OCPs.	VS: WNL Gen: NAD Abd: WNL Pelvic: Visible cervical lesion Rectal exam: $\ominus$, guaiac $\ominus$	• Cervical cancer • Cervical polyp • Cervicitis • Ectropion • Vaginal cancer • Vaginitis

Musculoskeletal Pain

CASE 78

HX	PE	DDX
28 yo F complains of multiple facial and bodily injuries. She claims that she fell on the stairs. She was hospitalized for some physical injuries seven months ago. She denies any abuse.	VS: P 90, BP 120/64, RR 22, O_2 sat 95% room air Gen: Moderate distress with shallow breathing HEENT: 2.5-cm bruise on forehead; 2-cm bruise on left cheek Chest/lungs: Severe tenderness on left fifth and sixth ribs; CTA bilaterally CV: WNL Abd: WNL Ext: WNL Neuro: WNL	• Accident proneness • Domestic violence • Substance abuse

CASE 79

HX	PE	DDX
28 yo F presents with joint pain and swelling along with a butterfly-like rash over her nasal bridge and cheeks that worsens after exposure to the sun. She also reports pleuritic chest pain, shortness of breath, myalgia, and fatigue over the past few months. She says that her joint pain tends to move from joint to joint and primarily involves her hands, wrists, knees, and ankles. She also has weight loss, loss of appetite, and night sweats.	VS: T 38°C (101°F), BP 140/95, HR 80, RR 18 Gen: Pallor, fatigue HEENT: Oral ulcers, malar rash Lungs: CTA, pleural friction rub CV: WNL Abd: WNL Ext: Maculopapular rash over arms and chest; effusion in knees, wrists, and ankles	• Dermatomyositis • Drug reaction • Photosensitivity • Polymyositis • SLE

INITIAL MGMT	CONTINUING MGMT	F/U
Office W/U • UA • Pap smear: HGSIL • Pelvic: Visible cervical lesion • G&C culture or PCR • Wet mount • Gynecology consult	**Office W/U** • Colposcopy • Cervical biopsy: Invasive squamous cell carcinoma of the cervix	• Radical hysterectomy versus radiation therapy • +/− adjuvant chemoradiotherapy • Console patient

Final Dx - Cervical cancer

INITIAL MGMT	CONTINUING MGMT	F/U
Emergency room W/U • XR—ribs: Fracture of left fifth and sixth ribs • Urine toxicology • CT—head • Skeletal survey: Old fracture in forearm **Rx** • Ibuprofen • Oxycodone PRN • Splint • Counsel patient re domestic abuse • Counsel patient re safety plan		• Support group referral • Social work referral

Final Dx - Domestic abuse

INITIAL MGMT	CONTINUING MGMT	F/U
Office W/U • CBC: ↓ hemoglobin • BMP • PT/PTT • ESR: ↑ • Serum ANA: ⊕ • UA: Proteinuria • CXR • Total complement: ↓ C3 and C4 **Rx** • NSAIDs	**Office W/U** • Anti-dsDNA or SLE prep: ⊕ • Bone densitometry **Rx** • Prednisone • NSAIDs • Rheumatology consult • Nephrology consult	• Follow up in four weeks with UA • Patient counseling • Counsel patient to cease alcohol intake • Smoking cessation • Sunblock

Final Dx - Systemic lupus erythematosus (SLE)

HIGH-YIELD CASES

CASE 80

HX	PE	DDX
35 yo M with a history of hypertension presents with pain and swelling in his left knee for the last three days. He was recently started on HCTZ for his hypertension. He is sexually active only with his wife and denies any history of trauma or IV drug abuse.	VS: T 38°C (100.7°F), P 80, BP 130/60, RR 12 Gen: In pain Skin: WNL HEENT: WNL Lungs: WNL CV: WNL Abd: WNL Ext: Left knee is swollen, erythematous, and tender with limited range of motion and effusion	• Bacterial arthritis • Gout • Infective endocarditis • Lyme disease • Pseudogout • Psoriatic arthritis • Reiter's arthritis

CASE 81

HX	PE	DDX
40 yo M with a history of diabetes mellitus presents with pain, swelling, and discoloration of his right leg for the last week. He denies any trauma.	VS: T 38°C (100.5°F), P 70, BP 120/60, RR 12 Gen: NAD Lungs: WNL CV: WNL Abd: WNL Ext: +2 edema in right lower extremity; warmth, erythematous discoloration of skin, 20-cm ulcer	• Calf tear or pull • Cellulitis • Deep venous thrombosis • Lymphedema • Osteomyelitis • Popliteal (Baker's) cyst • Venous insufficiency

CASE 82

HX	PE	DDX
50 yo M complains of a single episode of steady, diffuse, aching pain that affected his skeletal muscles and made it difficult for him to climb stairs. He states that he has never experienced anything like this before and that no one in his family has had a disease similar to his. Because of his ↑ LDL cholesterol, ↓ HDL cholesterol, and ↑ triglycerides, he was started on simvastatin and gemfibrozil about one year ago.	VS: T 37°C (99°F), P 85, BP 127/85, RR 20, O_2 sat 94% room air HEENT and neck: No dysarthria, dysphagia, diplopia, or ptosis; exam WNL Chest: WNL CV: WNL Abd: WNL Ext: Proximal muscle weakness that is more obvious in lower limbs; no evidence of myotonia	• Cocaine abuse • Inclusion body myositis • Myopathy due to drugs/toxins • Myotonic dystrophy • Polymyositis

INITIAL MGMT	CONTINUING MGMT	F/U

Office W/U
- CBC: ↑ WBC count
- Chem 14
- ESR: ↑
- PT/PTT, INR
- XR—left knee
- Joint aspiration fluid analysis: Gram stain ⊖, culture ⊖, ⊖ birefringent and needle-shaped crystals, WBC 8000
- Urethral Gram stain: ⊖

Rx
- NSAIDs or corticosteroids
- Discontinue HCTZ and start losartan

Ward W/U
- Blood culture: ⊖
- Urethral culture: ⊖
- Lyme serology: ⊖
- CBC: WBC is trending down

Rx
- Continue NSAIDs and corticosteroids until patient improves
- Low-purine diet

- Follow up in two weeks in the clinic
- Uric acid ↑
- Low-purine diet
- Start allopurinol or colchicine (to prevent an attack if serum uric acid > 12 or if the patient has tophaceous gout)

Final Dx - Gout

INITIAL MGMT	CONTINUING MGMT	F/U

Emergency room W/U
- CBC: ↑ WBC count
- Chem 14
- PT/PTT
- U/S—left lower extremity: ⊖ for deep venous thrombosis
- ESR
- X-ray
- Blood culture: Pending

Rx
- IV ampicillin-sulbactam
- Surgical consult: Debridement of ulcers

Ward W/U
- Blood culture: ⊖
- Blood glucose: Controlled on insulin regimen
- CBC: WBC is trending down

Rx
- Elevate the leg
- Switch to amoxicillin when patient is afebrile and symptoms improve (usually in 3–5 days)
- Discharge home

- Two weeks later his leg is back to normal
- Amoxicillin is discontinued after a course of 14 days

Final Dx - Cellulitis

INITIAL MGMT	CONTINUING MGMT	F/U

Emergency room W/U
- IV normal saline
- CBC
- BMP
- Serum CPK: ↑
- LDH: ↑
- EMG: Muscle injury
- UA: Myoglobinuria

Rx
- Counsel patient re medication side effects
- NSAIDs

Ward W/U
- CPK, LDH: ↑
- UA: ⊕ for myoglobin

Rx
- Stop the offending simvastatin and gemfibrozil

- Follow up in four weeks
- Patient counseling
- Rest at home
- Counsel patient re medication side effects

Final Dx - Myopathy due to simvastatin and gemfibrozil

CASE 83

HX	PE	DDX
21 yo F stripper complains of hot, swollen, painful knee joints following an asymptomatic dermatitis that progressed from macules to vesicles and pustules. She admits using IV drugs, binge drinking, and having sex with multiple partners. She states that about three weeks ago, during a trip to Mexico, she had dysuria, frequency, and urgency during her menses, followed a few days later by bilateral conjunctivitis.	VS: T 39°C (102°F), P 122, BP 138/82, RR 28, O$_2$ sat 96% room air HEENT and neck: WNL Chest: Four vesicles on thoracic skin CV: WNL Abd: Three vesicles and one pustule on abdominal skin Ext: Knee joints are hot, swollen, and tender; ↓ ROM due to severe pain	• *Chlamydia trachomatis* infection • *Neisseria gonorrhoeae* infection • Reactive arthritis • *S. aureus* infection • *Streptococcus* infection

CASE 84

HX	PE	DDX
25-month-old M is brought to the ER because of sudden respiratory distress. His mother does not remember the boy's immunization, developmental, or nutritional history. She calmly states that her son fell from a sofa a few days ago, and that this accident explains the boy's reluctance to walk. She adds that her son has been exposed to sick children lately and that she has used coin rubbing and cupping as folk medicine practices.	VS: T 37°C (99°F), P 129, BP 82/59, RR 40, O$_2$ sat 89% room air Gen: Undernourished HEENT: Circumferential cord marks around neck Lungs: Clear; pain with exam CV: Tachycardia; I/VI systolic murmur Abd: Bruising over nipples Ext: Circumferential burns of both feet and ankles with a smooth, clear-cut border; light brown bruises; pain on palpation of right lower limb Neuro/psych: Withdrawn, apprehensive	• Accidental trauma • Child abuse • Deliberate criminal violence (home invasion)

INITIAL MGMT	CONTINUING MGMT	F/U
Emergency room W/U • CBC: ↑ WBC count • GC culture assay: ⊕ • Blood culture: ⊖ • Arthrocentesis • Joint fluid analysis • Joint fluid culture: Pending • Throat culture: Pending • Anorectal culture: Pending • Urine β-hCG: ⊖ **Rx** • NSAIDs • Antibiotics: Azithromycin (for *C. trachomatis*), penicillin (if susceptible), ceftriaxone (if not resistant), or fluoroquinolones (if not resistant)	**Ward W/U** • Joint fluid analysis and culture: 60,000 leukocytes/mL, ⊕ for *N. gonorrhoeae* • Throat culture • Anorectal culture **Rx** • Azithromycin (for *C. trachomatis*), penicillin (if susceptible), ceftriaxone (if not resistant), or fluoroquinolones (if not resistant) • Joint drainage and irrigation (if indicated) • Arthroscopy (if indicated)	• Follow up in one week • Patient counseling • Counsel patient re safe sex practices • Treat sexual partner • Counsel patient to cease illegal drug use • Counsel patient to cease alcohol intake • Smoking cessation • Rest at home

Final Dx - Septic arthritis due to *N. gonorrhoeae* infection

INITIAL MGMT	CONTINUING MGMT	F/U
Emergency room W/U • CBC • PT/aPTT • Electrolyte panel, BUN, creatinine • CXR: Posterior rib fractures • Skeletal survey: Posterior rib fractures; obliquely oriented callus formation in right femur • CT—head: Short-length skull fractures; small subdural hemorrhages • Ophthalmologic exam: Bilateral retinal hemorrhages **Rx** • Admission to hospital • IV fluids • Neurosurgery consult • Ventilator (if necessary)	**Ward W/U** • Child abuse report • Social work/Child Protective Services evaluation in hospital • Ventilator (if necessary) • IV fluids	• Child Protective Services

Final Dx - Nonaccidental trauma (child abuse)

CASE 85

HX	PE	DDX
36 yo F complains of malaise, anorexia, unintended weight loss, and morning stiffness together with swollen and painful wrist, knee, and ankle joints of two years' duration. Initially, she disregarded her symptoms, as they were insidious. However, over time they persisted and ↑ in severity. An acute disabling episode prompted her to visit the office.	VS: T 38°C (100°F), P 95, BP 132/86, RR 20, O₂ sat 95% room air HEENT and neck: Cervical lymphadenopathy Chest: WNL CV: WNL Ext: Symmetric wrist, knee, and ankle joint swelling with tenderness and warmth; subcutaneous nodules over both olecranon prominences; no ulnar deviation of fingers, boutonnière deformity, or swan-neck deformity; no evidence of carpal tunnel syndrome; knee valgus is observed	• Gout • Lyme disease • Osteoarthritis • Paraneoplastic syndrome • Rheumatoid arthritis • Sarcoidosis

CASE 86

HX	PE	DDX
45 yo F bus driver comes to the clinic complaining of pain radiating down the leg that followed back pain. The pain is aggravated by coughing, sneezing, straining, or prolonged sitting.	VS: T 37°C (99°F), P 86, BP 128/86, RR 20, O₂ sat 93% room air Trunk: Lumbar spine mobility ↓ due to pain Ext: ⊕ straight leg raising (Lasègue) sign; ⊕ crossed straight leg sign Neuro: Weak plantar flexion of foot; loss of Achilles tendon reflex	• Cauda equina syndrome • Compression fracture • Facet joint degenerative disease • Lumbar disk herniation • Spinal stenosis • Tumor involving the spine causing radiculopathy

INITIAL MGMT	CONTINUING MGMT	F/U
Office W/U • CBC: Hypochromic normocytic anemia, thrombocytosis • ESR: ↑ • XR—joints: Soft tissue swelling, juxta-articular demineralization, joint space narrowing, erosions in juxta-articular margin • RF: High titer **Rx** • Ibuprofen or celecoxib • Intra-articular triamcinolone (for acute disabling episodes)	**Office W/U** • RF: High titer • Joint fluid analysis: Abnormalities suggesting inflammation **Rx** • Methotrexate (if unresponsive to NSAIDs) • Etanercept (if unresponsive to methotrexate); place PPD • Hydroxychloroquine for mild disease	• Follow up in four weeks • Patient counseling • Physical therapy • Occupational therapy • Rest at home • Exercise program • Splint extremity • Ophthalmologic consult if using hydrochloroquine

Final Dx - Rheumatoid arthritis

INITIAL MGMT	CONTINUING MGMT	F/U
Office W/U • None initially **Rx** • Conservative treatment • Pain control (NSAIDs)	**Office W/U** • MRI—lumbar spine: Disk herniation at L5–S1 level (MRI is not routinely ordered for a disk herniation; it is ordered if conservative treatment fails) **Rx** • Conservative treatment • Orthopedic surgery consult (if conservative treatment fails)	• Follow up in two weeks • Patient counseling • Rest at home

Final Dx - Lumbar disk herniation

Child with Fever

CASE 87

HX	PE	DDX
40-day-old M is brought to the ER because of irritability and lethargy, vomiting, and ↓ oral intake of three days' duration. Today his parents noted that he had a fever of 101.5°F, and he subsequently had a seizure. The baby's weight at delivery was 2500 grams, and he has been well.	VS: T 39°C (102°F), P 160, BP 77/50, RR 40, O_2 sat 92% room air Gen: Irritable infant Lungs: Clear CV: Tachycardia; I/VI systolic murmur Abd: WNL Neuro/psych: Bulging fontanelle, ↓ responsiveness	• CNS fungal infection (in immunocompromised patients) • HIV infection (in immunocompromised patients) • Meningitis (viral or bacterial) • Osteomyelitis • Pneumonia • Sepsis • UTI

CASE 88

HX	PE	DDX
4-month-old M is brought to the ER because of apneic episodes following a runny nose, cough, labored breathing, wheezing, and fever of two days' duration. His asthmatic mother was diagnosed with rubella infection during her pregnancy. The baby was delivered prematurely at 28 weeks. The boy has a history of respiratory difficulty and tachycardia, and he has missed several of his health maintenance appointments.	VS: T 39°C (102°F), P 160, BP 77/50, RR 40, O_2 sat 88% room air Gen: Irritable infant Lungs: Tachypnea, intercostal retractions, nasal flaring, expiratory wheezing, bilateral crackles CV: Tachycardia; continuous II/VI murmur Abd: WNL Neuro/psych: Fontanelle is soft and flat; infant is irritable	• Asthma • CHF • Cystic fibrosis • Pneumonia • RSV bronchiolitis

INITIAL MGMT	CONTINUING MGMT	F/U

Emergency room W/U
- CBC
- Blood cultures
- Electrolyte panel, BUN, creatinine, glucose
- CXR
- UA and urine culture
- LP: Cell count, differential, bacterial culture, viral PCR pending
- ABG: Metabolic acidosis, hyponatremia

Rx
- Empiric IV antibiotics (ampicillin and cefotaxime)
- Admission to the hospital
- IV fluid bolus
- IV fluids with dextrose

Ward W/U
- Serum glucose: 75 mg/dL
- Urine culture: $\ominus$
- Blood culture: $\oplus$ for S. *pneumoniae*
- Ventilator (if necessary)

Rx
- IV fluids, (D5½ NS)
- IV antibiotics × 10–14 days.

- Follow up in 48 hours of discharge from hospital
- Family counseling

Final Dx - Meningitis

INITIAL MGMT	CONTINUING MGMT	F/U

Emergency room W/U
- CBC: WBC 14,000
- Blood culture
- Electrolyte panel, BUN, creatinine, glucose
- CXR: Hyperinflation, bilateral patchy interstitial infiltrates, ↑ pulmonary blood flow, prominent left atrium and ventricle
- UA and urine culture
- ABG: Hypoxemia
- RSV PCR: Pending

Rx
- Empiric IV antibiotics
- Admission to the ICU
- IV fluid bolus
- Supplemental O_2
- Nebulized albuterol trial

ICU W/U
- Serum glucose: 70 mg/dL
- Urine culture: $\ominus$
- CXR: No change
- Blood culture: $\ominus$
- RSV PCR $\oplus$
- Ventilator (if necessary)
- Echocardiogram: Patent ductus arteriosus

Rx
- IV fluids (D51/2 NS)
- Supplemental O_2
- Nebulized albuterol (if effective)
- Cardiology consult

- Follow up in 48 hours of discharge from hospital
- Family counseling

Final Dx - Bronchiolitis with patent ductus arteriosus (PDA)

HIGH-YIELD CASES

CASE 89

HX	PE	DDX
8-month-old F is brought to the urgent care clinic because of abrupt onset of fever that lasted a couple of days with one seizure episode (the girl and her parents were camping in a remote area). The fever resolved after a rash appeared on the girl's chest and abdomen. Her parents did not notice any lethargy, poor feeding, or vomiting. She has no history of seizures.	VS: T 37°C (100°F); other vital signs WNL HEENT and neck: Bilateral cervical lymphadenopathy, ears WNL, ophthalmologic exam WNL Trunk: Macular rash Neuro: Alert and active; no abnormalities	• Fifth disease • Measles • Meningitis • Roseola infantum • Rubella

CASE 90

HX	PE	DDX
3-day-old M presents to the ER with ↑ temperature, lethargy, respiratory distress, and poor feeding for the past 24 hours. His Apgar scores at birth were 6 and 8. His mother had a prolonged rupture of membranes (30 hours).	VS: T 39°C (102°F), P 170, BP 74/51, RR 70, O$_2$ sat 90% room air Lungs: Grunting respiration, chest indrawing with breathing, ↓ air entry CV: No murmurs or rubs Abd: Distended; ⊖ BS Neuro: Lethargy	• *Bordetella* lung infection • *Chlamydia* lung infection • Complicated congenital lung abnormalities (e.g., sequestration) • Foreign body causing obstruction • Group B streptococcus bacterial pneumonia

Fever

CASE 91

HX	PE	DDX
49 yo F presents to the ER with fever of three days' duration. Since she turned 49 (about seven months ago), she has had recurrent infections that have been treated with antibiotics. She has also been treated with anthracyclines and alkylating agents for another disease for the past 18 months. However, she has not seen a doctor lately. She works in a manufacturing plant that produces cosmetics.	VS: T 39°C (102°F), P 132, BP 108/77, RR 29, O$_2$ sat 88% room air Lungs: No evidence of consolidation CV: WNL Abd: WNL Ext: WNL Neuro: WNL	• Deep abscess (unknown location) • Pneumonia • Pyelonephritis • Sepsis • Severe infection (unknown location)

INITIAL MGMT	CONTINUING MGMT	F/U
Office W/U • CBC: WNL **Rx** • Hydrate • Acetaminophen		• Follow up in seven days or as needed • Family counseling

Final Dx - Roseola infantum (exanthem subitum)

INITIAL MGMT	CONTINUING MGMT	F/U
Emergency room W/U • CBC: ↑ WBC count • Random serum glucose: 60 mg/dL • CXR: Patchy infiltrates, pleural effusion, gastric dilation • Blood cultures: Pending • Viral culture • ABG: P_{O_2} 50 mmHg, P_{CO_2} 55 mmHg **Rx** • O_2 • Fluids, D_5 ¼ NSS • Empiric IV antibiotics • Respiratory and hemodynamic support (if necessary)	**Ward W/U** • Random serum glucose: 65 mg/dL • Blood cultures: Group B streptococcus • ABG: P_{O_2} 60 mmHg, P_{CO_2} 50 mmHg **Rx** • Antibiotics • Ventilatory and hemodynamic support (if necessary) • Antiviral drugs (if appropriate) • Bronchoscopy (if indicated)	• Follow up in 48 hours • Family counseling

Final Dx - Pneumonia

INITIAL MGMT	CONTINUING MGMT	F/U
Emergency room W/U • CT—abdomen: WNL • CBC: Neutropenia • CXR: Bilateral infiltrates in both lungs • Sputum cultures: ⊕ for several bacterial species, including *Klebsiella* • Blood cultures: ⊕ for *Klebsiella* • UA: WNL • Urine cultures: ⊖ **Rx** • IV antibiotics (empiric cefepime or quinolone) • Acetaminophen • IV normal saline	**Ward W/U** • Bone marrow biopsy, needle: Low myelogenous progenitor cell lines • CT—chest, spiral: Widespread bilateral infiltrates in both lungs **Rx** • IV antibiotics (appropriate for *Klebsiella*); tailor antibiotics to sensitivities • IV normal saline • G-CSF (for neutropenia)	• Follow up in four weeks • Patient counseling • Counsel patient to cease alcohol intake • Smoking cessation • Chest physical therapy

Final Dx - Lung infection (bilateral pneumonia) in a neutropenic patient

HIGH-YIELD CASES

CASE 92

HX	PE	DDX
43 yo F presents to the ER with fever, fatigue, malaise, and diffuse musculoskeletal pain of two days' duration. She complains of difficulty moving her right eye. The patient has a history of diabetes mellitus and mitral valve prolapse with regurgitation.	VS: T 40°C (104°F), P 134, BP 113/83, RR 31, O_2 sat 93% room air Ophthalmology: Visual field defects, conjunctival hemorrhage Funduscopy: Abnormal spots Lungs: WNL CV: Regurgitant murmur Abd: WNL Ext: Petechiae on feet Neuro: CN III palsy	• Complicated pyelonephritis • Infective endocarditis • Infective process (undetermined location) • Intracranial infection • Sepsis

CASE 93

HX	PE	DDX
60 yo M presents with fever and altered mental status eight hours after undergoing a diverticular abscess drainage.	VS: T 39°C (102°F), P 110, BP 60/35, RR 22, O_2 sat 92% on 2-L NC Gen: Acute distress HEENT: WNL Lungs: WNL CV: Tachycardia Abd: Lower abdominal tenderness Neuro: WNL	• Cardiogenic shock • Hypovolemic shock • Septic shock

INITIAL MGMT	CONTINUING MGMT	F/U

Emergency room W/U
- ESR: 59 mm/hr
- CBC: ↑ WBC
- CXR: Some areas of patchy consolidation
- Blood cultures: Pending
- Echocardiography: Mobile mass attached to a valve
- ECG: RBBB
- UA: Microscopic hematuria

Rx
- IV normal saline
- O_2
- Empiric IV antibiotics (oxacillin and gentamicin)
- Acetaminophen

Ward W/U
- Blood cultures: ⊕ for *S. viridans*

Rx
- IV antibiotics
- Acetaminophen
- IV normal saline

- Follow up in four weeks
- Patient counseling
- Counsel patient to cease alcohol intake
- Smoking cessation

Final Dx - Infective endocarditis

INITIAL MGMT	CONTINUING MGMT	F/U

Emergency room STAT
- O_2
- IV normal saline/central line
- Blood culture: Pending
- Wound culture
- UA and urine culture

Emergency room W/U
- CBC: ↑ WBC count
- Chem 14
- ABG: Metabolic acidosis
- ECG
- Serum amylase, lipase
- Serum lactate: 6
- Cardiac enzymes
- CXR
- CT—abdomen: Persistent diverticular abscess

Rx
- Ampicillin-gentamicin-metronidazole or piperacillin-tazobactam or ticarcillin-clavulanate

ICU W/U
- Urine output q 1 h
- 2D echocardiography
- Blood culture: ⊕ for *E. coli* sensitive to gentamicin and ceftriaxone
- Wound culture: ⊕ for *E. coli* sensitive to gentamicin and ceftriaxone

Rx
- Tailor antibiotics to sensitivities
- Surgery consult

Final Dx - Septic shock

CASE 94

HX	PE	DDX
17 yo F G0 whose last menstrual period was two days ago presents with fever, vomiting, myalgia, and a generalized skin rash.	VS: T 39°C (102°F), BP 75/30, HR 120 Gen: NAD Skin: Diffuse macular erythema; hyperemic mucous membranes Lungs: WNL CV: WNL Pelvic: Menstrual flow; foul-smelling tampon **Limited PE**	• Meningococcemia • Rocky Mountain spotted fever • Streptococcal toxic shock syndrome • Toxic shock syndrome • Typhoid fever

Outpatient Potpourri

CASE 95

HX	PE	DDX
50 yo F presents with a painless lump in her right breast. She first noted this mass one month ago. There is no nipple discharge.	VS: Afebrile, P 70, BP 110/50, RR 12 Gen: NAD Skin: WNL HEENT: WNL Lymph nodes: ⊖ Breast: 3-cm, hard, immobile, non-tender mass with irregular borders; no nipple discharge Lungs: WNL CV: WNL Abd: WNL	• Breast cancer • Fibroadenoma • Fibrocystic disease • Mastitis • Papillomas

CASE 96

HX	PE	DDX
62 yo F complains of vaginal itching, painful intercourse, and a clear discharge.	VS: WNL Gen: NAD Lungs: WNL CV: WNL Pelvic: Vulvar erythema, thin and pale mucosa with areas of erythema, clear discharge, mucosa bleeds easily during exam	• Atrophic vaginitis • Bacterial vaginosis • Candidal vaginitis • Cervicitis (chlamydia, gonorrhea) • Trichomonal vaginitis

INITIAL MGMT	CONTINUING MGMT	F/U

Emergency room STAT
- O_2 inhalation
- IV normal saline
- Tampon removal

Emergency room W/U
- CBC with differential
- Chem 14
- UA
- Blood culture: Pending
- Urine culture: Pending

Rx
- IV clindamycin + vancomycin
- Methylprednisone

ICU W/U
- Blood culture: ⊖
- Urine culture: ⊖

Rx
- Continue IV clindamycin and vancomycin
- Wound care

Final Dx - Toxic shock syndrome

INITIAL MGMT	CONTINUING MGMT	F/U

Office W/U
- Mammography: Suspicious of tumor
- FNA biopsy: Malignancy

Rx
- Surgery consult

Final Dx - Breast cancer

INITIAL MGMT	CONTINUING MGMT	F/U

Office W/U
- Vaginal pH: 6
- Chlamydia PCR
- Gonorrhea PCR
- Wet mount
- Pap smear

Rx
- Vaginal jelly for lubrication
- Counsel patient re local HRT
- Premarin (vaginal estrogen)

- Follow up as needed

Final Dx - Atrophic vaginitis

CASE 97

HX	PE	DDX
33 yo Rh-negative F who currently lives in a battered-women's shelter calls the on-call physician because she noticed ↓ fetal movements. She is a G1P0 pregnant F at 36 weeks' gestational age. She states that fetal growth has been normal and that her obstetric ultrasound at 18 weeks showed a single normal fetus. The patient has no known preexisting diseases and does not smoke, drink alcohol, or take medications or illicit drugs. She received a dose of anti-D at 28 weeks.	VS: T 37°C (99°F), P 96, BP 141/91, RR 26, O_2 sat 93% room air Gen: No jaundice Eyes: Normal vision Lungs: No rales CV: No gallops or murmurs Pelvic: Fundal height in centimeters is appropriate for gestational age; cephalic presentation; speculum exam reveals unripe cervix, no ferning, nitrazine ⊖ Ext: Slight pedal edema	• Preeclampsia • Pregnancy-induced hypertension

CASE 98

HX	PE	DDX
30 yo F presents for her regular checkup. She denies any complaints but is concerned about her BP, as it has been high on both of her previous visits over the past two months.	VS: P 75, BP 160/90 (no difference in BP between both arms), RR 12 Gen: WNL HEENT: WNL Breast: WNL Lungs: WNL CV: WNL Abd: WNL Pelvic: WNL Ext: WNL Neuro: WNL	• Cushing's disease • Essential hypertension • Hyperaldosteronism • Hyperthyroidism • Pheochromocytoma • Renal artery stenosis • White coat hypertension/anxiety

CASE 99

HX	PE	DDX
6 yo M is brought by his mother with continuous oozing of blood from the site of a tooth extraction he underwent two days ago. The bleeding initially stopped but restarted spontaneously a few hours later. His mother denies any history of epistaxis, easy bruising, petechiae, or bleeding per rectum. The patient's mother has a brother with hemophilia.	VS: Afebrile, P 80, BP 80/50, RR 14 Gen: NAD Skin: WNL HEENT: Blood oozing from site of extracted tooth Lungs: WNL CV: WNL Abd: WNL Ext: WNL	• DIC • Hemophilia • ITP • Liver disease • TTP • Vitamin K deficiency • von Willebrand's disease

INITIAL MGMT	CONTINUING MGMT	F/U
Office W/U • BUN, Creatinine, ALT, AST • CBC • Chem 8 • UA: ⊕ protein • Random serum glucose • Serum uric acid **Rx** • Complete bed rest • Monitor, continue BP cuff • Fetal monitoring	**Ward W/U** • UA: Protein 0.3 g/L/24 hrs; normal sediment • LFTs: WNL **Rx** • Complete bed rest • Monitor, continue BP cuff • Fetal monitoring	• Patient counseling • Counsel patient to cease alcohol intake • Smoking cessation • Admit to labor and delivery for induction of labor • Obstetric consult

Final Dx - Antenatal disorder: Pregnancy-induced hypertension

INITIAL MGMT	CONTINUING MGMT	F/U
Office W/U • Lipid profile • Chem 14 • CBC • UA: +1 protein • ECG: LVH • Echocardiography: LVH • TSH **Rx** • Lisinopril • Exercise program • Low-sodium diet	**Office W/U** • Consider workup for 2° hypertension given the patient's young age (MRI/MRA renal arteries, urine catecholamines, urine cortisol)	• Follow up in one month

Final Dx - Essential hypertension

INITIAL MGMT	CONTINUING MGMT	F/U
Office W/U • CBC • Peripheral smear • Bleeding time • PTT: Prolonged • PT, INR • Plasma factor VIII: 3% • Plasma factor IX **Rx** • Factor VIII therapy • Genetics consult • Consel parents		• Console and reassure patient • Patient counseling • Family counseling

Final Dx - Hemophilia

HIGH-YIELD CASES

CASE 100

HX	PE	DDX
27 yo F complains of pain during intercourse. She has a long history of painful periods.	VS: WNL Gen: NAD Lungs: WNL CV: WNL Pelvic: Normal vaginal walls, normal cervix, mild cervical motion tenderness; uterus tender, retroverted, and fixed; right adnexa slightly enlarged and tender	• Endometriosis • PID • Vaginismus • Vaginitis

INITIAL MGMT	CONTINUING MGMT	F/U

Office W/U
- Wet mount
- Chlamydia DNA probe
- Gonorrhea DNA probe
- U/S—pelvis: Retroverted uterus of normal size; 2- × 3-cm cyst on the right adnexa that may represent a hemorrhagic corpus luteum or endometrioma

Rx
- NSAIDs
- OCPs

- If initial treatment with OCPs and NSAIDs does not relieve pain, refer to a gynecologist for a trial of GnRH analogs, progestins, or danazol.
- Follow up as needed

Final Dx - Endometriosis

APPENDIX

Acronyms and Abbreviations

Abbreviation	Meaning
A-a	alveolar-arterial (oxygen gradient)
ABC	airway, breathing, circulation
ABG	arterial blood gas
AC	alternating current
ACEI	angiotensin-converting enzyme inhibitor
ACh	acetylcholine
ACL	anterior cruciate ligament
ACLS	advanced cardiac life support (protocol)
ACTH	adrenocorticotropic hormone
ADA	American Diabetes Association
ADH	antidiuretic hormone
ADHD	attention-deficit hyperactivity disorder
AED	antiepileptic drug
AF	atrial fibrillation
AFB	acid-fast bacillus
AFI	amniotic fluid index
AFP	α-fetoprotein
AHI	apnea-hypopnea index
AICD	automatic implantable cardiac defibrillator
AIDS	acquired immunodeficiency syndrome
ALL	acute lymphocytic leukemia
ALS	amyotrophic lateral sclerosis
ALT	alanine aminotransferase
AMA	antimitochondrial antibody
AML	acute myelogenous leukemia
ANA	antinuclear antibody
ANC	absolute neutrophil count
AP	anteroposterior
APC	activated protein C
aPTT	activated partial thromboplastin time
ARB	angiotensin receptor blocker
ARDS	acute respiratory distress syndrome
ARF	acute renal failure
ARR	absolute risk reduction
5-ASA	5-aminosalicylic acid
ASA	acetylsalicylic acid
ASD	atrial septal defect

Abbreviation	Meaning
ASMA	anti–smooth muscle antibody
ASO	antistreptolysin O
AST	aspartate aminotransferase
ATN	acute tubular necrosis
AV	arteriovenous, atrioventricular
AVM	arteriovenous malformation
AVN	avascular necrosis
AXR	abdominal x-ray
AZT	azidodeoxythymidine (zidovudine)
BAL	British anti-Lewisite
BID	twice daily
BMP	basic metabolic panel
BMT	bone marrow transplant
BP	blood pressure
BPH	benign prostatic hyperplasia
BPP	biophysical profile
BPPV	benign paroxysmal positional vertigo
BS	bowel sounds
BSA	body surface area
BUN	blood urea nitrogen
CABG	coronary artery bypass graft
CAD	coronary artery disease
CALLA	common ALL antigen
CBC	complete blood count
CBT	cognitive-behavioral therapy
CCB	calcium channel blocker
CD	cluster of differentiation
CEA	carcinoembryonic antigen
CF	cystic fibrosis
CGD	chronic granulomatous disease
cGMP	cyclic guanosine monophosphate
CH_{50}	total hemolytic complement
CHF	congestive heart failure
CI	confidence interval
CIN	cervical intraepithelial neoplasia
CIS	carcinoma in situ
CK	creatine kinase
CK-MB	creatine kinase, MB fraction
CLL	chronic lymphocytic leukemia
CML	chronic myelogenous leukemia
CMV	cytomegalovirus
CN	cranial nerve

Abbreviation	Meaning
CNS	central nervous system
COPD	chronic obstructive pulmonary disease
CPAP	continuous positive airway pressure
CPR	cardiopulmonary resuscitation
CrCl	creatinine clearance
CREST	calcinosis, Raynaud's phenomenon, esophageal dysmotility, sclerodactyly, telangiectasia (syndrome)
CRF	chronic renal failure
CRP	C-reactive protein
CSF	cerebrospinal fluid
CST	contraction stress test
CT	computed tomography
CTA	clear to auscultation
CVA	costovertebral angle
CVID	common variable immunodeficiency
CVS	chorionic villus sampling
CXR	chest x-ray
D&C	dilation and curettage
D4T	didehydrodeoxythymidine (stavudine)
D_5NS	5% dextrose in normal saline solution
D_5W	5% dextrose in water
DA	dopamine
DBP	diastolic blood pressure
DC	direct current
DCIS	ductal carcinoma in situ
DDAVP	1-deamino (8-D-arginine) vasopressin
ddC	dideoxycytidine (zalcitabine)
ddI	dideoxyinosine
DES	diethylstilbestrol
DEXA	dual-energy x-ray absorptiometry
DHEA	dehydroepiandrosterone
DHEAS	dehydroepiandrosterone sulfate
DIC	disseminated intravascular coagulation
DIP	distal interphalangeal (joint)
DKA	diabetic ketoacidosis
DL_{CO}	diffusing capacity of carbon monoxide
DM	diabetes mellitus
DNR	do not resuscitate
DPoA	durable power of attorney
DRE	digital rectal exam
dsDNA	double-stranded DNA
DTaP	diphtheria, tetanus, acellular pertussis (vaccine)
DTRs	deep tendon reflexes
DTs	delirium tremens
DUB	dysfunctional uterine bleeding
DVT	deep venous thrombosis
DWI	diffusion-weighted imaging
EBV	Epstein-Barr virus
ECG	electrocardiography
ECT	electroconvulsive therapy

Abbreviation	Meaning
ED	erectile dysfunction
EDTA	calcium disodium edetate
EEG	electroencephalography
EF	ejection fraction
EGD	esophagogastroduodenoscopy
ELISA	enzyme-linked immunosorbent assay
EM	erythema multiforme
EMG	electromyography
EPS	extrapyramidal symptoms
ER	emergency room, estrogen receptor
ERCP	endoscopic retrograde cholangiopancreatography
ESR	erythrocyte sedimentation rate
ESWL	extracorporeal shock-wave lithotripsy
ETEC	enterotoxigenic *E. coli*
EtOH	ethanol
FAP	familial adenomatous polyposis
Fe_{Na}	fractional excretion of sodium
FEV_1	forced expiratory volume in one second
FFP	fresh frozen plasma
FiO_2	fraction of inspired oxygen
FISH	fluorescent in situ hybridization
FNA	fine-needle aspiration
FOBT	fecal occult blood test
FSH	follicle-stimulating hormone
FTA-ABS	fluorescent treponemal antibody absorption (test)
FTT	failure to thrive
5-FU	5-fluorouracil
FUO	fever of unknown origin
FVC	forced vital capacity
G&C	gonorrhea and chlamydia (culture)
G6PD	glucose-6-phosphate dehydrogenase
GA	gestational age
GAD	generalized anxiety disorder
GBM	glomerular basement membrane
GBS	group B streptococcus, Guillain-Barré syndrome
GCS	Glasgow Coma Scale
G-CSF	granulocyte colony-stimulating factor
GERD	gastroesophageal reflux disease
GFR	glomerular filtration rate
GGT	gamma-glutamyltransferase
GI	gastrointestinal
GM-CSF	granulocyte-macrophage colony-stimulating factor
GnRH	gonadotropin-releasing hormone
GTCS	generalized tonic-clonic seizure
GTD	gestational trophoblastic disease
GU	genitourinary
H&P	history and physical
HAART	highly active antiretroviral therapy
HACEK	*Haemophilus, Actinobacillus, Cardiobacterium, Eikenella, Kingella*

Abbreviation	Meaning
HAV	hepatitis A virus
Hb	hemoglobin
HbA$_{1c}$	hemoglobin A$_{1c}$
HBeAg	hepatitis B early antigen
HBsAg	hepatitis B surface antigen
HBV	hepatitis B virus
hCG	human chorionic gonadotropin
HCO$_3$	bicarbonate
HCTZ	hydrochlorothiazide
HCV	hepatitis C virus
HDCV	human diploid cell vaccine
HDL	high-density lipoprotein
HDV	hepatitis D virus
HEENT	head, eyes, ears, nose, and throat
HEV	hepatitis E virus
HHNK	hyperglycemic hyperosmolar nonketotic state
5-HIAA	5-hydroxyindole acetic acid
Hib	*Haemophilus influenzae* type b
HIDA	hepato-iminodiacetic acid (scan)
HIPAA	Health Insurance Portability and Accountability Act
HIV	human immunodeficiency virus
HLA	human leukocyte antigen
HMG-CoA	hydroxymethylglutaryl coenzyme A
HNPCC	hereditary nonpolyposis colorectal cancer
HPV	human papillomavirus
HR	heart rate
HRIG	human rabies immunoglobulin
HRT	hormone replacement therapy
HSV	herpes simplex virus
5-HT	5-hydroxytryptamine
HTLV	human T-cell leukemia virus
HUS	hemolytic-uremic syndrome
HVA	homovanillic acid
IBD	inflammatory bowel disease
IBS	irritable bowel syndrome
ICP	intracranial pressure
ICU	intensive care unit
Ig	immunoglobulin
IM	intramuscular
INH	isoniazid
INR	International Normalized Ratio
IPV	inactivated poliovirus vaccine
ITP	idiopathic thrombocytopenic purpura
IUD	intrauterine device
IUGR	intrauterine growth restriction
IV	intravenous
IVC	inferior vena cava
IVIG	intravenous immunoglobulin
IVP	intravenous pyelography
JVD	jugular venous distention
JVP	jugular venous pressure
KOH	potassium hydroxide
KUB	kidney, ureter, bladder

Abbreviation	Meaning
LA	left atrial
LAP	leukocyte alkaline phosphatase
LBP	low back pain
LCL	lateral cruciate ligament
LDH	lactate dehydrogenase
LDL	low-density lipoprotein
LEEP	loop electrosurgical excision procedure
LFT	liver function test
LGSIL	low-grade squamous intraepithelial lesion
LH	luteinizing hormone
LKMA	liver/kidney microsomal antibody
LLQ	left lower quadrant
LMN	lower motor neuron
LP	lumbar puncture
LTB	latent tuberculosis
LUQ	left upper quadrant
LV	left ventricular
LVEF	left ventricular ejection fraction
LVH	left ventricular hypertrophy
MAI	*Mycobacterium avium-intracellulare*
MAOI	monoamine oxidase inhibitor
MCA	middle cerebral artery
MCHC	mean corpuscular hemoglobin concentration
MCL	medial collateral ligament
MCP	metacarpophalangeal (joint)
MCV	mean corpuscular volume
MDD	major depressive disorder
MDI	metered-dose inhaler
MEN	multiple endocrine neoplasia
MgSO$_4$	magnesium sulfate
MGUS	monoclonal gammopathy of undetermined significance
MHA-TP	microhemagglutination assay—*Treponema pallidum*
MI	myocardial infarction
MMR	measles, mumps, rubella (vaccine)
6-MP	6-mercaptopurine
MRA	magnetic resonance angiography
MRCP	magnetic resonance cholangiopancreatography
MRI	magnetic resonance imaging
MRSA	methicillin-resistant *S. aureus*
MS	multiple sclerosis
MSAFP	maternal serum α-fetoprotein
MTP	metatarsophalangeal (joint)
NAD	no acute distress
NBTE	nonbacterial thrombotic endocarditis
NCS	nerve conduction study
NE	norepinephrine
NG	nasogastric
NHL	non-Hodgkin's lymphoma
NK	natural killer (cells)
NNRTI	non-nucleoside reverse transcriptase inhibitor

Abbreviation	Meaning
NNT	number needed to treat
NPO	nil per os (nothing by mouth)
NPV	negative predictive value
NRTI	nucleoside reverse transcriptase inhibitor
NS	normal saline
NSAID	nonsteroidal anti-inflammatory drug
NSCLC	non–small cell lung cancer
NST	nonstress test
NTD	neural tube defect
O&P	ova and parasites
OA	osteoarthritis
OCD	obsessive-compulsive disorder
OCP	oral contraceptive pill
OR	odds ratio, operating room
ORIF	open reduction with internal fixation
OTC	over the counter
PA	posteroanterior
$PaCO_2$	partial pressure of carbon dioxide in arterial blood
p-ANCA	perinuclear antineutrophil cytoplasmic antibody
PaO_2	partial pressure of oxygen in arterial blood
PCL	posterior cruciate ligament
PCO_2	partial pressure of carbon dioxide
PCOS	polycystic ovarian syndrome
PCP	phencyclidine hydrochloride, *Pneumocystis carinii* (now *P. jiroveci*) pneumonia
P_{Cr}	plasma creatinine
PCR	polymerase chain reaction
PCT	porphyria cutanea tarda
PCV	polycythemia vera
PDA	patent ductus arteriosus
PDE-5	phosphodiesterase type 5
PE	physical exam, pulmonary embolus
PEA	pulseless electrical activity
PEEP	positive end-expiratory pressure
PFT	pulmonary function test
PG	prostaglandin
PI	protease inhibitor
PID	pelvic inflammatory disease
PIP	proximal interphalangeal (joint)
PIV	parainfluenza virus
PMI	point of maximal impulse
PMN	polymorphonuclear (leukocyte)
P_{Na}	plasma sodium
PNH	paroxysmal nocturnal hemoglobinuria
PNS	peripheral nervous system
PO	per os (by mouth)
PO_4	phosphate
POC	product(s) of conception
P_{osm}	plasma osmolarity
PPD	purified protein derivative

Abbreviation	Meaning
PPH	postpartum hemorrhage
PPI	proton pump inhibitor
PPROM	preterm premature rupture of membranes
PPV	positive predictive value
PR	progesterone receptor
PRN	as needed
PROM	premature rupture of membranes
PSA	prostate-specific antigen
PSGN	poststreptococcal glomerulonephritis
PT	prothrombin time
PTH	parathyroid hormone
PTHrP	parathyroid hormone–related peptide
PTSD	post-traumatic stress disorder
PTT	partial thromboplastin time
PTU	propylthiouracil
PUD	peptic ulcer disease
PUVA	psoralen and ultraviolet A
PVS	persistent vegetative state
PWI	perfusion-weighted imaging
RA	rheumatoid arthritis
RAST	radioallergosorbent testing
RBBB	right bundle branch block
RBC	red blood cell
RCT	randomized controlled trial
RDW	red cell distribution width
REM	rapid eye movement
RF	rheumatoid factor
RIBA	recombinant immunoblot assay
RLQ	right lower quadrant
RNA	ribonucleic acid
RPR	rapid plasma reagin
RR	relative risk, respiratory rate
RRR	relative risk reduction, regular rate and rhythm
RSV	respiratory syncytial virus
RT	reptilase time
RTA	renal tubular acidosis
RUQ	right upper quadrant
RV	residual volume, right ventricular
SAAG	serum-ascites albumin gradient
SAB	spontaneous abortion
SAD	seasonal affective disorder
SAH	subarachnoid hemorrhage
SBP	spontaneous bacterial peritonitis, systolic blood pressure
SCID	severe combined immunodeficiency
SCLC	small cell lung cancer
SERM	selective estrogen receptor modulator
SIADH	syndrome of inappropriate secretion of antidiuretic hormone
SIRS	systemic inflammatory response syndrome
SLE	systemic lupus erythematosus
SMA	superior mesenteric artery

Abbreviation	Meaning
SNRI	selective norepinephrine reuptake inhibitor
SPEP	serum protein electrophoresis
SPN	solitary pulmonary nodule
SQ	subcutaneous
SRS	somatostatin receptor scintigraphy
SSRI	selective serotonin reuptake inhibitor
STD	sexually transmitted disease
SVT	supraventricular tachycardia
T_3	triiodothyronine
T_3RU	T_3 resin uptake
T_4	thyroxine
TAH-BSO	total abdominal hysterectomy and bilateral salpingo-oophorectomy
TB	tuberculosis
3TC	dideoxythiacytidine (lamivudine)
TCA	tricyclic antidepressant
Td	diphtheria toxoid
TD	traveler's diarrhea
TdT	terminal deoxynucleotidyl transferase
TEE	transesophageal echocardiography
TENS	transcutaneous electrical nerve stimulation
TFT	thyroid function test
TIA	transient ischemic attack
TIBC	total iron-binding capacity
TID	three times daily
TIG	tetanus immunoglobulin
TIPS	transjugular intrahepatic portosystemic shunt
TLC	total lung capacity
TMP-SMX	trimethoprim-sulfamethoxazole
TNF	tumor necrosis factor
TNM	tumor, node, metastasis (staging)
tPA	tissue plasminogen activator
TPN	total parenteral nutrition
TPO	thyroid peroxidase
TRALI	transfusion-related acute lung injury

Abbreviation	Meaning
TSH	thyroid-stimulating hormone
TT	thrombin time
TTG	tissue transglutaminase
TTP	thrombotic thrombocytopenic purpura
TURP	transurethral resection of the prostate
UA	urinalysis
U_{Cr}	urine creatinine
UMN	upper motor neuron
U_{Na}	urinary sodium
U_{osm}	urine osmolarity
UPEP	urinary protein electrophoresis
UPPP	uvulopalatopharyngoplasty
URI	upper respiratory infection
UTI	urinary tract infection
UVA	ultraviolet A
UVB	ultraviolet B
VATS	video-assisted thoracoscopy
VCUG	voiding cystourethrography
VDRL	Venereal Disease Research Laboratory
VF	ventricular fibrillation
VMA	vanillylmandelic acid
V/Q	ventilation-perfusion (ratio)
VRE	vancomycin-resistant enterococcus
VS	vital signs
VSD	ventricular septal defect
VT	ventricular tachycardia
vWF	von Willebrand's factor
VZV	varicella-zoster virus
WAGR	Wilms' tumor, aniridia, GU abnormalities, mental retardation (syndrome)
WBC	white blood cell
WD/WN	well developed, well nourished
WNL	within normal limits
W/U	workup
XR	x-ray

Index

Pregnancy (*Continued*)
  obstetric complications of, 221–226
    gestational trophoblastic disease (GTD), 224–226
    intrauterine growth restriction (IUGR), 221, 223
    oligohydramnios and polyhydramnios, 223, 224
    Rhesus (Rh) isoimunization, 223–224
    third-trimester bleeding, 224, 225
  teratogens in, 221, 222
Prenatal care and nutrition, 214
Prenatal diagnostic testing, 215
  amniocentesis, 215
  chorionic villus sampling (CVS), 215
  triple marker screen/quadruple test quad screen, 215
Presbycusis, 18
Preterm labor, 226–227
Preterm premature rupture of membranes (PPROM), 226
Prolactinoma, 74
Propionibacterium acnes, 27
Prostate cancer, 134–135, 362–363
  recommended screening guidelines, 30
Prostatic nodules and abnormal PSA, workup of, 29
Prostatitis, 154, 364–365
Proteinuria, 191–192
Pseudohematuria, 191
Pseudohyponatremia, 181
Pseudomembranous colitis, 356–357
Pseudomonas, 144, 145, 150, 151, 160
Pseudomonas aeruginosa, 294
Psoriasis, 22–23
Psychiatric emergencies, 286–287
  neuroleptic malignant syndrome, 286
  serotonin syndrome, 286–287
  suicide risk assessment, 286
Psychotic disorders, 278
  schizophrenia, 278
Puerperium, 219–221
  intrapartum and postpartum fevers, 219, 220

mastitis, 219, 221
postpartum hemorrhage (PPH), 219
  common causes of, 220
Pulmonary edema, 46
Pulmonary embolus (PE), 300–301, 324–325
  diagnostic approach to, 301
Pulmonary function tests (PFTs), 292
Pulseless electrical activity (PEA), 52
Pyelonephritis, 154, 340–341
Pyloric stenosis, 259–260
Pyoderma gangrenosum, 91

R

Raccoon eyes, 51, 204
Radioallergosorbent testing (RAST), 19
Radionuclide tracer (thallium or technetium), 38
Raynaud's phenomenon, 88, 166
Reed-Sternberg cells, 127
Renal amyloidosis, 193
Renal artery stenosis, 39, 41
Renal cell carcinoma, 340–341
Renal failure, 128, 166
  acute (ARF), 187–188
    causes of, 187
  chronic (CRF), 39, 189–190
Renal tubular acidosis (RTA), 196
Respiratory distress syndrome/hyaline membrane disease, 250
Respiratory syncytial virus (RSV), 265–266
Retinopathy, 68
Rett's disorder, 285
Rheumatic fever, 33
Rhesus (Rh) isoimunization, 223–224
Rhinophyma, 24
Rheumatoid arthritis (RA), 167–168, 378–379
Rinne test, 19
Rome III criteria, 93
Rosacea, 24
Roseola infantum (exanthem subitum), 382–383

Rotavirus, 95, 158
  vaccine, 246
Roth's spots, 43
Rubella, 251
Ruptured globe, 61

S

Salmonella, 95, 115, 158
Salter-Harris fracture, 174
Sarcoidosis, 185, 303
Schilling test, 112
Schistosomiasis, 134
Schizophrenia, 278
Schwannoma, 207
Scleroderma, 88, 176–177
  limited vs. diffuse, 177
Seizures, 200–201, 223
  febrile, 266
Selective serotonin reuptake inhibitors (SSRIs), 287
Sepsis, 160–161
  severity of, 161
Septic shock, 384–385
Severe combined immunodeficiency (SCID), 254
Sexual assault, 49–50
Sexually transmitted diseases (STDs), 155–156
  cervicitis/urethritis, 156
  genital herpes, 155
  pelvic inflammatory disease (PID), 156
  syphilis, 155
Sheehan's syndrome (postpartum hypopituitarism), 219, 221
Shigella, 95, 158
Shoulder dislocation, 173
Shoulder dystocia, 227–228
Sickle cell anemia, 113, 114–115
Sinusitis, 148–149
  acute, 148–149
  chronic, 149
Sipple's syndrome, 75
Skin tumors, 136–138
  basal cell carcinoma, 137
  melanoma, 136–137
  squamous cell carcinoma, 137–138
Sodium (Fe_{Na}), fractional excretion of, 181